Current Topics in Comparative Pathobiology

Volume 1

Current Topics in Comparative Pathobiology

Edited by THOMAS C. CHENG

INSTITUTE FOR PATHOBIOLOGY AND
DEPARTMENT OF BIOLOGY
LEHIGH UNIVERSITY
BETHLEHEM, PENNSYLVANIA

Volume 1

ACADEMIC PRESS New York and London 1971

ACADEMIC PRESS, INC.
111 Fifth Avenue, New York, New York 10003

United Kingdom Edition published by
ACADEMIC PRESS, INC. (LONDON) LTD.
24/28 Oval Road, London NW1 7DD

LIBRARY OF CONGRESS CATALOG CARD NUMBER:

PRINTED IN THE UNITED STATES OF AMERICA

Contents

List of Contributors

Numbers in parentheses indicate the pages on which the authors' contributions begin.

SHIH L. CHANG (201), Environmental Control Administration, Public Health Service, U.S. Department of Health, Education, and Welfare, Cincinnati, Ohio

LIONEL E. MAWDESLEY-THOMAS (87), Huntingdon Research Centre, Huntingdon, England

SAMMY M. RAY, Marine Laboratory (171), Texas A&M University, Galveston, Texas

EDWARD A. STEINHAUS † (1), Center for Pathobiology, University of California, Irvine, California and Division of Entomology, Berkeley, California

Y. TANADA (1), Center for Pathobiology, University of California, Irvine, California and Division of Entomology, Berkeley, California

† Deceased, October 20, 1969.

Editor's Note

I would like to take advantage of the occasion of the genesis of this series to call attention to two commemorable events—one regretfully sad, and the other joyous. The first is the passing of a giant and a leader among comparative pathobiologists, Edward A. Steinhaus, on October 20, 1969. The second is the official establishment of the Institute for Pathobiology at Lehigh University for which your Editor has the privilege of serving as the first Director.

Ed Steinhaus was a most unusual person. Not only was he an outstanding scientist, administrator, and teacher, he was a friend and confidant of all who knew him. His brilliant career was launched in 1939 upon receiving his doctorate from Ohio State University. His initial interest was insect bacteriology but, true to his fashion, his pursuits broadened with time. He developed interests in immunology, virology, teratology, and parasitology, and is generally recognized as one of the pioneers in biological control. After a brief association with the Rocky Mountain Laboratory of the United States Public Health Service, he joined the faculty of the University of California and rose through the ranks until he was appointed the first Dean of Biological Sciences at the Irvine campus. Dean Steinhaus envisioned the type of comparative pathobiology this series, hopefully, will advance.

Dr. Steinhaus was a strong advocate of the application of science for the welfare of man and his environment. He envisioned and practised the utilization of scientific knowledge to lighten the burdens of man and to preserve his habitat. Pathobiology, as I envision it, serves this function.

Dr. Steinhaus encouraged the development of "Centers of Pathobiology" (1968. *J. Invertebr. Pathol.* **11**, i–iv). As the result of the farsightedness of the Lehigh University administration, a new institute dedicated to this purpose now exists at Lehigh. This is not to say that no other laboratories exist with similar goals. A number of academic and governmental institutions have been established throughout the world devoted to similar goals although the Lehigh venture appears to be the only functional one at this time with the type of broad basis advocated by Steinhaus.

Hopefully, in Lehigh's time-honored tradition of scientific excellence and the application of science for the welfare of man and the maintenance of his environment, the new Institute will become a landmark.

THOMAS C. CHENG

Preface

This is the first volume of a new annual series entitled *Current Topics in Comparative Pathobiology.* The idea for initiating this series had its origin some time ago during conversations with a number of microbiologists, parasitologists, comparative pathologists, and immunologists. A unanimous opinion was expressed at that time that there is much to be gained from the evaluation of pathobiological phenomena from a truly comparative viewpoint. By "comparative" is meant an analytical and critical evaluation of comparable processes as they apply to all categories of animals, invertebrates as well as poikilothermic and homeothermic vertebrates. Furthermore, the idea was fostered that the study of infectious diseases and their consequences, among other pathologic phenomena, should be viewed from a broader spectrum than is customarily the case. In other words, an animal parasitologist interested in the invasion processes of a nematode, for example, should be acutely aware of parallel processes involving viruses and bacteria, and a virologist interested in cellular alterations should be aware of similar phenomena resulting from intracellular parasitism by protozoa. With this ecumenical approach in mind, arrangements were made with Academic Press to launch this series.

Since "pathobiology" is a relatively new term in biological circles, it appears appropriate to devote some space to its explanation. Pathobiology may be defined as the basic discipline concerned with resolving the fundamental nature of disease and the causative agents and processes of such, in addition to the reactions provoked. The term "disease" is employed in its broadest sense and includes degenerative and infectious processes as well as other types of alterations resulting from injury or insult, irrespective of duration. Consequently, pathobiology is not purely a descriptive and/or diagnostic science, but one concerned with all of the factors contributing to and resulting from the disease state.

The intent of this continuing series is not to publish the usual type of report found in most scientific journals. Rather, we intend to present a series of definitive and critical reviews by recognized authorities. The hope is that the interdisciplinary approach will serve to broaden the reader's viewpoint and excite new ideas for continued research in the broad area of pathobiology.

Because the majority of scientists are most familiar with one specific area, each of the reviews comprising this and subsequent volumes need not be comprehensively comparative in themselves; however, as the reader scans the entire continuing spectrum, the comparative nature of the subject will become evident.

Because of the intentional ecumenical nature of this series, articles traditionally considered to fall within the realms of virology, microbiology, protozoan and metazoan parasitology, entomology, biological control, epidemiology and epizootiology, environmental biology, nutrition and food science, toxicology, oncology, immunology, geratology, comparative physiology and biochemistry, developmental biology (teratology), and cytology (including ultrastructure) will receive the major emphasis. It is noted, however, that in contributions dealing with parasitism, the emphasis should be on the interaction of the host and parasite rather than on the parasite alone. Similarly, articles dealing with toxins and other insulting molecules should not be concerned solely with these agents but with their effects as well.

The policy is to include one or more comprehensive reviews of specific topics in each volume. Such contributions should include not only a synthesis of known information but also point out research trends, advance concepts and theories, and suggest new approaches. In general, each contribution will be by invitation although individuals wishing to submit appropriate articles for consideration may do so by negotiating with the editor.

Although most of the topics to be included will deal with the pathobiology of animals, invertebrate and vertebrate, occasionally the editor may see fit to include a section primarily concerned with plant pathobiology, but the subject material must be of fundamental and general interest.

As stated, *Current Topics in Comparative Pathobiology* is intended to reflect an interdisciplinary approach. Such is the trend in modern biology and science in general. It is our hope that this series will aid in dissolving the artificial boundaries that sometimes separate investigators working on one group of organisms from those interested in another.

It is our good fortune and honor to be able to include in this inaugural volume the last piece of scientific writing by Dr. Edward A. Steinhaus, co-authored with his former student Dr. Y. Tanada of the University of California, Berkeley, who has risen to a position of authority in his own right.

We are also most pleased to incorporate in this volume the contribution by Dr. L. E. Mawdesley-Thomas. As this distinguished English investigator has pointed out, the study of neoplasms in fish can serve as a useful model for understanding the nature of such abnormal growths. His scholarly treatment of the subject, especially his classification, should stimulate increased emphasis in this area of research.

Also we are delighted to be able to incorporate the contribution by Dr. Sammy M. Ray. This author is widely known for his pioneering work on the biology and chemistry of marine toxins, especially the paralytic shellfish toxin, and his succinct review of this timely topic will without doubt be greatly appreciated.

The final section in this volume represents a timely review and discussion by Dr. S. L. Chang of the species of small, free-living amebas which in relatively recent years have been shown to be pathogenic to man and animals if accidentally introduced. These amebas, at least certain strains, are excellent examples of pathogenic, facultative parasites and serve not only to remind those interested in parasitism that the phenomenon of facultative parasitism is an important and interesting one, perhaps occurring more frequently than is generally suspected, but also to once again call attention to the fact that a more thorough understanding of facultative parasitism will undoubtedly contribute to our understanding of the ontogeny of obligatory parasitism.

THOMAS C. CHENG

Current Topics in Comparative Pathobiology

Volume 1

Diseases of the Insect Integument

Edward A. Steinhaus† and Y. Tanada

CENTER FOR PATHOBIOLOGY,
UNIVERSITY OF CALIFORNIA,
IRVINE, CALIFORNIA

AND

DIVISION OF ENTOMOLOGY,
BERKELEY, CALIFORNIA

† Deceased October 20, 1969.

I. Introduction

The body wall or integument constitutes the principal barrier between the insect on one hand, and infectious microorganisms and injury on the other; it is the insect's first line of defense. Nevertheless, the integument itself is subject to diseases and pathological changes. These changes are manifested in both the cuticle and the epidermis, or in either one of them.

David (1967) has presented an excellent review and discussion on the insect integument in relation to the invasion of pathogens. Our report also touches upon invasion, which is one aspect of disease manifestation, but the reader is encouraged to refer to David's publication for a much more thorough discussion of this aspect.

When reference is made to "the diseases of the integument," it is not meant to imply that the maladies concerned always attack only the integument and none of the other organs or tissues of the insect. As we shall see, some afflictions may be centered almost entirely in the integument, but in many instances, especially when the epidermis (often called the "hypodermis") is involved, the disease is known to occur among other tissues of the body as well. In the present case, however, we are concerned with diseases as they are manifested in the body wall and its parts.

When one examines and observes the exterior of an insect's body, what the eye perceives depends upon the interests of the observer, and upon his training and experience. If he is familiar with the insect and its appearance, the slightest departure from normal may be noted, but it is surprising how frequently a person thoroughly familiar with the normal may overlook indications of physical abnormalities and signs of disease. Or, the integument may be suffering from a disease of such a nature that only the most meticulous scrutiny will reveal external signs of the malady. However, a pathologist may have a tendency to see abnormality or disease where none exists, so he must guard against interpreting extremes of normal variations as disease. Even when an aberration or sign is obviously apparent, to characterize, define, and delimit it accurately a comparison with a normal healthy specimen is a safeguard and highly recommended for precision.

The procedures and methodology for making a physical examination or a general inspection of a diseased insect have been described elsewhere (Steinhaus and Marsh, 1962; Steinhaus, 1963), and the reader is asked to consult these and other sources to obtain a full understanding of certain aspects of the subject treated in this chapter. In general, the observational methods used to discern diseases of the integument of insects are similar to those used to study the external signs of general diseases, except that in the case of the former histological and ultramicroscopic methods are used to study the changes that take place in the integument itself, including the epidermis.

Before considering the diseased (including abnormal) integument, it is proper that we briefly review the principal features of the healthy integument, or the integument of the healthy insect.

II. The Integument of the Healthy Insect

The integument is the basic structure of the insect's exoskeleton, which is essentially an elongate, hollow, continuous ellipsoid with complex evaginations and invaginations. It is, in itself, one of the principal organ systems of the insect. Although other structures derived from the embryonic ectoderm, such as the epithelial tissue lining, the foregut, and the hindgut, are widely considered to be part of this system, in this chapter we are primarily concerned with the external body wall. It consists essentially of an epidermis that deposits, on its outer surface, an acellular durable cuticle usually containing a polysaccharide called chitin and, on its inner surface, the thin basement membrane.

In addition to the earlier treatise by Richards (1951) on the integument of arthropods, the readers, for detailed information on insect integument, should refer to two recent reviews, one by Locke (1964) on the formation and structure of the insect integument, and the other by Noble-Nesbitt (1967) on the insect cuticle.

A. The Epidermis

The epidermis is by far the most important of the three layers since it secretes the other two and plays the main role in molting. It is comprised of cubical or columnar cells in the form of a simple epithelium; occasionally, specialized cells are present. The size of individual epidermal cells, subject to the influence of temperature and nutrition, varies according to species and in different areas of the insect's body. They are usually larger in larvae than in adults. In some species no mitosis occurs, and larval growth may be accounted for by an increase in the size of epidermal cells, rather than an increase in number.

Pigment granules, mitochondria, and vacuoles appear to be commonly present in the cytoplasm of epidermal cells, frequently at the distal ends. Golgi bodies may also be present. Some authorities believe the granules to be related to nutritional reserves of the insect. In some insects integument color may depend on various factors, such as hormone, diet, light, and genetic differences. In the cabbageworm, *Pieris rapae crucivora*, the pupal color is apparently controlled by a hormone associated with the brain and prothoracic ganglion (Ohtaki, 1960; Hidaka and Ohtaki, 1963). Exposure of the cabbageworm larva to light of different colors and intensities, however, may also affect pupal color. When a mature larva is exposed to yellow or orange light just prior to pupation, a green pupa is formed, but a larva placed in darkness forms a brown pupa. The larva of *Cerura vinula* changes color from green to dark red when it stops feeding and prepares a cocoon. The red color is caused by an accumulation of ommochrome pigments, first in the epidermal cells and later in the fat body. According to Bückmann (1959), the color change is brought about by a hormone, ecdysone, of the thoracic gland which is activated by the brain.

The concentration of the insectoverdin pigments in the larval cuticle of the tobacco hornworm, *Manduca sexta*, varies with the diet and genetic differences (Dahlman, 1969). There are definitely more bile pigment proteins per gram of dried cuticle from larvae reared on plant food than from that of larvae fed an artificial diet. In *Locusta migratoria cinerascens*, there are several distinct zones in the pars intercerebralis, and the destruction of one of the zones causes a general depigmentation of gregarian grasshoppers (Girardie, 1967). Implantation of the pars intercerebralis has an opposite effect and produces almost entirely black individuals. Thus certain cells in the pars intercerebralis secrete a melanotropic hormone.

Granules in the integument have been variously identified as urates, glycogen, fat, ascorbic acid, and melanin precursors. Granules called "chromatin droplets" are sometimes found extracellularly among the epidermal cells; they give a positive Feulgen reaction and, according to some investigators, may represent a stage in the dissolution of nuclei from dermal glands and oenocytes. The nuclei of epidermal cells are generally spherical or oval in shape and are commonly located toward the basal end of the cells. Nucleoli or plasmasomes have been demonstrated in some cases.

Lower (1964), in a study on the arthropod integument, has stated that the three general groups of insects (Endopterygota, Apterygota, and Exopterygota) each have their own characteristic epidermal type. The first, found in the highly evolved winged insects (Endopterygota), is a single layer of cuboidal cells of uniform thickness and well-defined cell membranes. The nuclei of these cells are relatively large and located near the basal cell membrane. The cytoplasm is transparent, has few granules, and is usually colorless.

The second type of epidermis is found in primitive wingless insects (Apterygota). It shows no uniformity in thickness of the cell layer, nor are the cell membranes distinct; in many places the epidermis is a syncytium. The cells themselves tend to be ovate, and the nuclei, which are highly variable in size, are found in different positions throughout the cells.

The last type of epidermis is found in the Exopterygota, winged insects linking the primitive and the highly evolved. The more primitive members of this group have retained the primitive type of epidermis, while higher members tend to possess the advanced type with some modifications. Since adult winged insects do not molt, the epidermis no longer functions, and frequently the cells degenerate into a thin protoplasmic layer in which the cell membranes become indistinct and the cell areas are indicated primarily by nuclei.

In addition to general epithelial cells, there are several kinds of specialized cells in the epidermis (e.g., secretory or gland cells). These cells, known as dermal glands, are connected to the exterior by a duct running through the cuticle. Secretions of different types are produced by these glands, including wax, many types of ill-smelling scent compounds, and irritating skin poisons. Certain dermal glands are believed to secrete the outer waxy covering of the epicuticle.

Some epidermal cells become specialized to form the flexible hairs or bristles of insects. The epidermal cell forming the hair itself is called a trichogen cell, while the cell forming the socket for the hair is called a tormogen cell. A hair or bristle originating from the epidermis is called a seta. Specialized setae (scales, poison hairs, and sensory setae) also originate in this manner.

Oenocytes, important in intermediary metabolism, have been shown to originate in the epidermis (Wigglesworth, 1933). They are large cells, commonly more than 100 μ in diameter, having a homogeneous eosinophilic cytoplasm and a round nucleus. The cells may develop pseudopodia, the nuclei may become branched, and the cytoplasm vacuolated. Fat droplets, pigment, and glycogen granules may appear in the cytoplasm. The cells themselves are usually amber in color, but may be yellow, brown, red, green, or colorless (Richards, 1951).

Although oenocytes originate in the epidermis and may remain there, situated between the bases of the epidermal cells and the basement membrane, this is not always true. They may break through the basement membrane and form clusters of cells separated from the epidermis; they may project into the body cavity but remain attached to the epidermis; or they may become dispersed and embedded in the fat body. Some investigators believe that oenocytes may play a role in molting and cuticle production. Delachambre (1966) studied the epidermal oenocytes of *Tenebrio molitor* nymphs histochemically and observes that they synthesize lipoproteins that contain sterols. He believes that oenocytes secrete the sterols required for building the different layers of the adult cuticle. Wigglesworth (1933, 1948) also suggests a secretory role for the oenocytes. In the house cricket, *Acheta domesticus*, Philogène and McFarlane (1967) believe that the oenocytes secrete substances necessary for the wax layer of the epicuticle, contribute to the polysaccharide material involved in chitin synthesis, and function in phenolic metabolism before sclerotization.

B. The Basement Membrane

The basement membrane is a very thin layer of neutral mucopolysaccharide secreted by a type of hemocyte (Wigglesworth, 1956), or by the epidermis, and coating the entire inner surface of the epidermis. It is rarely thicker than 1 μ. Little is known about the chemical composition of the membrane, but it is believed to resemble that of the innermost part of the cuticle. The basement membrane serves to bind the inner surfaces of the epidermal cells, forming a boundary between them and the body cavity. It may also play a part in absorption of the materials needed by the cells for their nutrition, respiration, and growth (Lower, 1964). No other definite functions have been assigned to it.

C. *The Cuticle*

The cuticle is generally considered to be the nonliving portion of the integument. This attitude is changing, however, as indicated by Noble-Nesbitt (1967) who states:

> Just as the endoskeletal structures of the vertebrates are known to be in dynamic equilibrium with the metabolic pool, so is the apparently inert extracellular cuticle now becoming to be so regarded. This active state of the major part of the cuticle has implications for the role the cuticle plays in the physiology of the whole insect, changes being associated at various times with changes in shape, state of nutrition, stage of moulting, waterproofing and the capacity to absorb water from sub-saturated atmospheres.

The cuticle is a three-layered structure consisting in general of an endocuticle, an outer exocuticle, and a superficial epicuticle (see Locke, 1964; Noble-Nesbitt, 1967). In some insects a fourth layer, the mesocuticle, occurs between the endocuticle and exocuticle, or between the endocuticle and epicuticle.

The extremely thin (less than 1 μ) epicuticle consists of a protein–lipoprotein complex. Electron microscope observations indicate that the epicuticle is quadripartite with an inner homogeneous electron-dense layer, a very electron-dense cuticulin layer, a wax layer, and a cement layer (Noble-Nesbitt, 1967). The cuticulin layer is tripartite with two dense and one intermediate less dense lamina. At or just before ecdysis, the outermost layer separates to form what is probably the wax layer. The resultant cuticulin layer is perforated by pore canal filaments and small pores 30 Å in diameter during the molting cycle. Immature insects have an epicuticle that is a translucent, colorless layer with no apparent internal structure. In the hardening and darkening process (sclerotization), the epicuticle is tanned; it becomes yellow in color, hard, brittle, hyaline, and highly resistant to chemicals. Cottrell (1964) has discussed in detail the processes associated with the hardening and darkening of the cuticle.

In larvae and soft-bodied insects, the endocuticle forms most of the cuticle. The thickness of the endocuticle is related to the size of the insect and is not uniform from species to species as in the case of the epicuticle. Thus immature insects have a thinner endocuticle than those in later stages, and the endocuticle in large species is more sturdy than that of small species. The hormone bursicon is apparently involved in the deposition of the postemergence endocuticle in adults of *Sarcophaga bullata* (Fogal and Fraenkel, 1969a). Whitten (1969) has studied the fly *S. bullata* with an electron microscope and reports that specific blood cells, in the terminal "blind" area of the developing pretarsus of the fly leg, are involved in some complex way in the intracellular deposition of the endocuticle.

The endocuticle consists principally of a mixture of proteins and one or more glycoproteins of which chitin is invariably one product of chemical degradation. The epidermis secretes the endocuticle as a series of sheets on a flat surface, giving it a characteristic laminated structure that can be seen with light and electron microscopes. The laminae are thin and each layer is firmly bound to its neighbor above and below. Passing through the laminae, from the epidermis to the inner surface of the epicuticle, are minute ducts forming pore canals and gland cell ducts that open on the epicuticular surface.

In those insects undergoing sclerotization to form protective sclerites, the endocuticle forms the mesocuticle and the exocuticle and for this reason becomes very thin. The mesocuticle, external to the endocuticle, comprises at least half of the cuticle. It retains the original laminated structure, pore canals, and colorless appearance of the endocuticle, but is much tougher although still flexible. It differs in staining properties, and presumably in chemical properties, from adjacent regions of the cuticle.

External to the mesocuticle is the exocuticle. Its thickness is directly related to the hardness of the sclerite of which it forms a part. In appearance the exocuticle resembles the epicuticle, being yellow, hard, and brittle. Sclerotization obliterates the original endocuticular structure, although the ducts from the dermal glands are still present. The exocuticle is made up of chitin and quinone-tanned protein. It forms a homogeneous electron-dense matrix, and may comprise one-third or less of the cuticle.

The biochemical process of sclerotization (tanning) of the cuticle has been studied extensively, but the mechanism has not been established (Pryor, 1962; Hackman, 1964; Wyatt, 1968). At least two hormones, ecdysone and bursicon, are involved in sclerotization. Bursicon is active in insects belonging to the orders Orthoptera, Hemiptera, Coleoptera, Lepidoptera, and Diptera (Fraenkel and Hsiao, 1965). In the Diptera, however, tanning of the cuticle of the puparium is induced by ecdysone (Fraenkel, 1935; Butenandt and Karlson, 1954), but in the newly emerged adult flies, tanning is induced by bursicon (Cottrell, 1962; Fraenkel and Hsiao, 1965). Although different hormones may be involved in tanning, the process is considered to be similar, since in each case *N*-acetyl dopamine serves as the tanning precursor (Karlson and

Sekeris, 1962; Sekeris, 1964). In sclerotization of the puparium of *Calliphora erythrocephala*, ecdysone apparently activates the gene, which leads to mRNA synthesis and this directs protein biosynthesis toward the formation of the enzyme dopadecarboxylase, which reacts with tyrosine to form dopamine. Dopamine is acetylated to *N*-acetyldopamine, which interacts with cuticular proteins and results in tanned proteins (Sekeris, 1965; Fogal and Fraenkel, 1969a). Mills *et al.* (1967) studied the conversion of tyrosine in crude homogenates of freshly ecdysed American cockroaches, *Periplaneta americana*. They observed *N*-acetyldopamine and also *N*-acetyltyrosine, and they postulate that these two *N*-acetyl derivatives are precursors of the sclerotization quinones. The hardening and darkening of the cuticle are attributable in part to the formation of indole–melanin (Hackman, 1967; Fogal and Fraenkel, 1969b).

In some flies the integument of the puparium is not hardened by tanning but by calcification, which is also controlled by ecdysone (Fraenkel and Hsiao, 1967).

Secondary secretions are commonly associated with sclerotization. Two thin layers of materials, known collectively as the amphion (Lower, 1964), are deposited over the epicuticle and serve to protect it from abrasion. The inner, or the wax layer, is a mixture of lipids, while overlying this is the cement layer, a plastic material of unknown composition. A continuous secretion of materials keeps the amphion intact and assures the insect of limited water loss, especially in environments with unusually low humidities. Many insect cuticles have no amphion, such as those of purely aquatic forms; abrasion is at a minimum because of the environment.

D. Molting

Because the cuticle is nonliving and cannot be stretched, it must be shed periodically to allow for the growth of the insect. Molting, or ecdysis, involves the entire body wall and its invaginations and is under the control of certain hormones. In some insects, during the molting period, the epidermal cells increase in volume; in others numerous mitoses appear in the cells. Simultaneously, there is a visible loosening of the cuticle from the epidermis. Enzymes are then secreted into the space below the cuticle and begin to dissolve it. While the old cuticle is being dissolved, the epidermal cells begin to secrete the new cuticle; apparently, the epidermis absorbs the materials from the dissolved old cuticle and uses them to produce the new cuticle.

When the new cuticle has been completed, certain enlarged dermal glands discharge a waxy layer over the outside of the new cuticle; this is the outermost layer of the epicuticle. After the new cuticle is completed, the insect ruptures the remaining old cuticle by hydrostatic pressure and squirms free of the old skin. For a short time after molting, the new cuticle is soft and can be stretched. The insect again increases its hydrostatic pressure and enlarges the cuticle as much as possible to allow room for growth. Sclerotization in those parts that are to be hardened occurs shortly after.

There is substantial evidence that molting is governed by hormones. In the "classic scheme" of molting, the neurosecretory cells of the pars intecerebralis of the insect brain secrete a hormone (ecdysiotropin) that stimulates the ecdysial gland (also known as the prothoracic, ventral, or thoracic gland) to secrete a molting hormone (generally considered to be ecdysone). Under the influence of this molting hormone, the molting process is initiated. The combined action of the molting and juvenile hormones, however, determines the type or quality of the molt; a large amount of juvenile hormone results in a larval molt, a decrease in juvenile hormone leads to a pupal molt, and in its absence and in the presence of molting hormone alone, an adult molt is produced. Recently, there has been some amplification and modification of the classic scheme, especially in certain insects. For a detailed description of the molting process and its regulation by hormonal activity, the reader is referred to the publications of Wigglesworth (1964, 1965), Cottrell (1964), Karlson (1966), Herman (1968), and Whitten (1968).

There are innumerable observations on integumental abnormalities resulting from improper molting and metamorphosis. We mention very briefly, if at all, this aspect of epidermal diseases.

III. Free External Microbiota of Healthy Insects

Most insects live in an environment in which their integument is at least somewhat contaminated by microorganisms (see Steinhaus, 1946, 1949). Ordinarily, the kinds of microorganisms involved reflect the nature of the environment. They vary greatly in number as well as in kind. The relationship with the host is usually a fortuitous one. We refer here to those forms that occur freely on the integument, do not attack, and are not firmly attached to it.

The most common types of microorganisms found freely on the external surfaces of insects are bacteria. In most cases the number of different types of bacteria is surprisingly small. Some insects, such as the housefly, may carry relatively large numbers; even this filth-frequenting insect, however, usually harbors more bacteria internally than externally, largely because of the more favorable conditions for bacterial growth that exist in the insect's alimentary tract. In many instances the brushlike appendages of certain insects come in contact with and acquire large numbers of microorganisms as the insects move about in their environments. This is not always the case, however, since the body structure of bees, even though well adapted for the carrying of pollen, has comparatively few bacteria on the external surface.

No thorough study has been made of the external bacterial flora of insects in general, but there are indications that gram-positive spore formers or gram-negative rods probably predominate on most insects. Of course the environment of an insect largely determines the type of microbiota found on it. Soil-inhabiting insects usually harbor soil microorganisms. Of insects living on animals, one might expect to find the types of bacteria usually associated with the skin or fur of the animals. Insects such as houseflies and cockroaches, which frequent filth, carry a flora more or less characteristic of that occurring in their surroundings. In "clean" areas they are likely to have a flora different from that found on the same species of insect living in an area of filth.

The integument of healthy insects frequently carries free spores and bits of fungal hyphae. Representatives of most of the major classes of fungi may be found fortuitously in this location. Most commonly, perhaps, one finds spores or conidia of Fungi Imperfecti. Comparatively few fungi, however, germinate, grow, and reproduce entirely on the external surface of insects. The number of fungal spores found in such a location is usually relatively small but, depending on the habitat or activity of the insect, it is sometimes rather large. Many saprophytic fungi are found growing on dead or weakened insects, or they may assume the role of secondary invaders when death or weakening is brought on by other causes. Fungi are also common on the exuviae of dead insects where they, along with bacteria, undoubtedly play a predominant role in the final disintegration of the bodies of dead insects.

Plant growths on the integument of healthy insects are relatively scarce primarily because of the short life-span, activities, and habitats of the insects. Recently, Gressitt *et al.* (1965, 1968) reported epizoic symbiosis on weevils, especially members of *Gymnopholus*. Gressitt (1966a,b) identified the weevils, many of which were new to science. The weevils feed on the leaves of woody plants in high moss forests or in alpine shrubbery on various New Guinea mountain ranges. They are large, heavily sclerotized, flightless, more or less slow moving, and evidently long-lived. On the bodies of the weevils are fungi, algae, lichens, liverworts, and moss, which in turn support oribatid mites, rotifers, nematodes, diatoms, and other organisms. Some of the plant growths apparently require 3–5 years to develop. The upper surfaces of the weevils are specially modified, having depressions and grooves and specialized scales and hairs; a sticky substance is also apparently produced. According to Gressitt (1966a):

> Explanation of the evolution of the symbiotic relationships involved in the species of *Symbiopholus* requires speculation. Each species has some special modifications related to the encouragement of the plant growth. This involves depressions, pits, etc., on pronotal and elytral surfaces, specially modified scales or hairs, and a sticky secretion. . . .
>
> Presumably the presence of plant growth on the backs of the weevils serves the function of protective resemblance of plants, and thus protection from natural enemies, resulting in natural selection for reproduction of individuals favoring the plant growth. This could account for a general evolutionary trend towards increase in the development of the structural modifications, and the secretion, thus favoring plant growth.

Certain insects, such as ambrosia beetles (mostly Scolytidae), certain ants (Attini), and termites, cultivate special fungi for food. Contact with the fungus gardens often leaves bits of these fungi attached to the external surfaces of the insects.

Yeasts, which occur externally on insects, have been very inadequately studied, but indications are that the number of species present in this location is not great except in certain cases. Wild yeasts may be found occasionally on the exteriors of insects, but usually the association is a chance event. In some cases insects (bees, wasps, ants, mosquitoes, and gnats) have been known to distribute or to carry in nature such yeasts as *Saccharomyces cerevisiae* and *S. ellipsoideus*. *Drosophila* flies may carry yeasts to grapes in vineyards. These yeasts cause a fermentation of the grapes, which provides optimum conditions for the development of the fly larvae.

Very little study of any kind has been made of the protozoa found on the external surfaces of insects. A few reports, such as that on the suctorian *Rhynchophrya palpans*, attached to the water beetle *Hydrophilus piceus*, have been made, but they are few and far between. This protozoan may occur on the beetle in the presence of other Suctoria (*Periacineata linquifera* and *Discophyra ferrum-equinum*), as well as with certain ciliates (*Vorticella*). Undoubtedly, other undescribed species of entomophilic Suctoria exist. Spores and cysts of certain free-living protozoa may occur on the outer covering of insects in nature. Intestinal protozoa of man and other animals are probably acquired, at least temporarily, on the appendages of insects frequenting filth. Similarly, the mouthparts of blood-sucking insects may temporarily be contaminated exteriorly with protozoa from the bloodstream of infected animals. In most cases the insect is used by the protozoan as transportation to richer food supplies.

Possibly the only viruses to be found on exterior surfaces of insects are those that arrive there by accident. Such a circumstance might occur in the case of insect vectors that transmit viruses of plants and animals, in which case the mouthparts or appendages of insects may become temporarily contaminated. Viruses pathogenic for insects may occur on external surfaces of insects that contact the disintegrating bodies of other insects dead of diseases caused by these viruses.

Concerning the relationships of insects and roundworms, particularly nematodes, all types occur, ranging from commensalism to obligate or primary parasitism. Purely mechanical associations are of two kinds, internal and external. Free external association was described by Van Zwaluwenburg (1928) as a relationship in which the insect is merely an external mechanical carrier for species of roundworms which require such a site for undergoing transformations as well as for transportation to new food supplies. For example, *Rhabditis coarctata* in the larval stages attaches itself to, and encysts on, the adults of certain scarabaeid beetles which carry it to fresh manure, whereupon the nematode excysts, leaves the beetle, and proceeds to feed. Also worthy of mention here is the commensal association that many nematodes have with insects, such as those (e.g., beetles, termites, and ants) living in burrows or nests. In many of these cases nematodes may also be found living in the burrows or nests where they feed upon the frass of insects and on other debris which accumulates in the nests. Species of *Rhabditis* and *Diplogaster* associated with certain *Ips* and *Hylobius* are examples.

IV. Microorganisms That Attack or Are Strongly Attached to the Cuticle

A. *Bacteria*

There has been very little work done on bacteria that attack the cuticle. It is remarkable, considering the vast amount of chitinous material derived from insects, that more study has not been made of these microorganisms.

A sizable number of bacteria, as well as other types of microorganisms (actinomycetes, fungi, and protozoa), are known to attack chitin, and apparently are responsible for most of the decomposition of chitin and cuticle in nature. The majority of these bacteria have been isolated from marine sources and, for the most part, have not been named or specifically identified other than to be placed in the genus *Beneckea*. They have been found only on dead aquatic insects; in fact, Benton's (1935) isolation of an unidentified bacterium from exuviae of mayflies is the only report of a chitinivorous bacterium from an entomogenous source that has come to our attention.

Only one instance of a bacterium attached to the cuticle of an insect has been noted by us. Kufferath (1921) has reported that masses of micrococci are found attached to the cuticle of locusts from Greece. The bacteria produce small, floccular, white masses situated primarily on the abdomen of the locusts. The most predominant strain, out of four isolated, is *Staphylococcus acridicida*. The attachment causes no apparent harm to the locust, but if *S. acridicida* is injected or fed *per os*, the locust dies within 48 hours.

B. Fungi

A number of different types of fungi are found living on, and, in a sense, "attacking" the integument of insects. Most of these cause no obvious harm to their insect hosts. Occasionally, because of the location of the fungus, movements may be impeded or made erratic. Thaxter (1896) speaks of "a greater restlessness, owing perhaps to a slight irritation which they [the fungi] may be supposed to produce." Recent investigations indicate that some of these fungi derive nutriment from within the insect. Such parasitism may have a debilitating effect on the host which is not readily recognized.

1. Laboulbeniales

The major group of fungi (about 1500 known species) that grows and multiplies on external surfaces of insects is that designated by the ordinal name Laboulbeniales. These fungi live on the chitinous cuticula of living insects and are transmitted from one individual to another. In some cases, but perhaps more generally than has been realized, they penetrate the body cavity of the insect with extensive rhizoidal processes through which they gain nourishment.

In 1850 Rouget first published a note on these fungi (Rouget, 1850), and two years later Mayr (1852) recorded another species. Neither of these men realized the true nature of these organisms. In 1853 Robin recognized them as fungi, however, and erected the new genus *Laboulbenia* Montagne and C. Robin in honor of Laboulbène, an entomologist (Robin, 1853). This fungus occurs on a species of ground beetle (*Brachinus*) in Europe. In the years following 1853, a few other investigators published accounts of these fungi, but it was not until the monumental work of Thaxter that a real knowledge of the group was obtained. His monograph on the Laboulbeniaceae appeared in five parts (Thaxter, 1896, 1908, 1924, 1926, 1931). Most of our present-day knowledge (especially taxonomic) stems from Thaxter's work. Colla (1934) also presented a detailed account of the group.

The laboulbeniaceous fungi are small, frequently minute, organisms belonging to the class Ascomycetes. On the insect they appear as scattered or as densely crowded bristles or bushy hairs which, on certain areas of the host's integument, form a furry or velvety patch. Their site of attachment is sometimes limited to definite regions on the integument of each host species, that is, the distance of the fungus from the margins of the elytra, for example, is always about the same, and a species usually found living on the left elytron is rarely found living on the right elytron (see Benjamin and Shanor, 1952; Shanor, 1955; Benjamin, 1965).

The main body, or receptacle, of the fungus is fixed to the integument of the insect by means of a blackened base, or foot, and in most cases consists of a very small number of cells differently arranged in different genera. Typically, the perithecia arise directly from the receptacle. The thallus also gives rise to appendages of variable sizes and shapes, which often support the male reproductive organs. The male and female organs occur on the same individual, except in a few cases in which the plants are dioecious. The perithecium, the female reproductive body, or ascocarps, contains asci identical in most respects to the asci of other Ascomycetes.

According to Madelin (1966), a series may be envisaged in the attachment of laboulbeniaceous fungi to the insect cuticle: from forms with the usual blackened foot through *Dimeromyces rhizophorus* having a stout, tapering penetrant filament; *Moschomyces* having a cellular haustorium; *Rhizomyces, Ceraiomyces dahlii,* and *Arthrorhynchus* spp. having copiously branched hyaline and apparently nonseptate filaments; to *Trenomyces histophtorus,* which forms an elaborate system of bulbs and nodular tubes which proliferate in the insect's fat body. He considers the genus *Herpomyces* unique in combining the usual foot with slender rhizoidal threads, but Kamburov *et al.* (1967) have also observed a similar condition in *Hesperomyces virescens.*

In some insects infected with Laboulbeniales, the integument may be pigmented or may have brownish spots (Eichler, 1951).

Transmission of Laboulbeniales from one insect to another occurs through the spores, which at times of direct contact between insects, such as copulation, are discharged or forced out of the asci. In some cases insects become infected by spores present in the soil (Lindroth, 1948). Benjamin and Shanor (1952) believe that in *Laboulbenia odobena* the specific positions of fungi on the bodies of both sexes of the carabid beetle, *Bembidion picipes,* result from the transmission of spores at time of mating. In the little housefly, *Fannia canicularis,* a ratio of at least 1 infected to 10 uninfected flies must be maintained before *Stigmatomyces ceratophorus* can persist in the fly population (Whisler, 1968). Less spreading occurs in cages containing infected and noninfected females than in cages with mixed sexes. In contrast, spreading between infected and noninfected males is equal to the rate of transmission in cages with both sexes. The primary infection, however, is related to transmission at mating. Whisler has not been able to artificially inoculate this fungus into the flies.

The spores of Laboulbeniales are nearly always surrounded by a gelatinous envelope characteristically thickened about its base. This envelope serves as a protective covering and also assists the spore in adhering to the new host insect. Germination of the spore commences with a modification of its lower extremity into an organ of attachment known as the foot. Because of the change that takes place in this end of the gelatinous envelope, the base usually becomes blackened, opaque, and hardened as it attaches the growing plant firmly to the integument of the insect. In some species haustoria enter the body wall at a pore or through the cuticle and become an instrument of food supply to the fungus. According to Chatton and Picard (1909), the haustoria of *Trenomyces* ramify throughout the fat body and other organs of poultry lice (Mallophaga). The infected fat cell degenerates and loses its fat contents; its nuclear chromatin condenses and the cell is finally destroyed. The fat cells become confluent and form a homogeneous and caseous mass.

Some species of the fungus appear to be limited to a certain genus of insects. Most hosts are Coleoptera and Diptera, but some species have been noted in Orthoptera, Dermaptera, Mallophaga, Hymenoptera, and in mites, millipedes, and so on. The species *Laboulbenia formicarum* attacks only those ants of the subfamily Formicinae. All castes of adult ants in a colony may be infected. The fungus shows some preference in location, being found most commonly on the dorsal surface of the head, gaster, and appendages, but has been observed on all parts of the body including the compound eyes.

The distribution of Laboulbeniales apparently is worldwide. Frequently, the distribution of these fungi corresponds to distribution of the genera of insect hosts. For example, *Laboulbenia cristata* occurs on all continents on the large and widespread insect genus *Paederus*. *Laboulbenia pheropsophi* may be found almost wherever its *Pheropsophus* hosts occur in five continents. Others may be restricted to one or a few continents, such as *Laboulbenia variabilis* which occurs on a variety of hosts but has been rarely reported outside the American continent.

In a series of papers, Richards and Smith (1954, 1955a,b, 1956) report on a comprehensive study of *Herpomyces stylopygae*, a laboulbeniaceous fungus found particularly on the antennae of the Oriental cockroach, *Blatta orientalis*. Their study represents one of the most thorough and penetrating ever made of these fascinating fungi; and while it would not be safe to generalize too widely on the basis of their data pertaining to *Herpomyces*, certainly we can now anticipate more clearly some of the relationships existing between all species of Laboulbeniales and their insect hosts. Among their interesting findings are the following.

The fungi grow on large setae or on hard or soft cuticle, but they grow only on a living cockroach, and apparently only on an Oriental cockroach. [Tavares (1966) reports that the spore germinates on a minute or on a large seta.] Infections are heavier on males and on adults, and the fungi are disseminated by contact. The thalli become firmly attached to the insect's cuticle. Development from spore to mature perithecium takes nearly two weeks. Infections on adults persist, but infections on nymphs are completely lost when the nymph molts; the fungus plants are found intact on the shed skin. Apparently, no resistance develops because individuals freed of infection by molting can be readily reinfected. The gross structure and apparent cell lineage are different for female plants growing on large setae in contrast to ones on the body wall; in *H. stylopygae*, cell lineage is fundamentally different for male and female plants.

The Laboulbeniales may increase in volume many thousands of times and therefore must derive considerable nourishment from the insect host. That at least some, if not most, Laboulbeniales penetrate the body wall was recognized by Thaxter (1914), but the histopathology of the association was greatly clarified by Richards and Smith (1956). The structure that penetrates the body wall from the foot is known as the haustorium and exists in many different forms. Thus in the case of *H. stylopygae,* three types have been recognized: fine, filamentous strands 0.1–0.3 μ in diameter; small, distinctly tubular haustoria of 1.5–2.0 μ (associated with male plants); and relatively large haustoria of 2.0–5.0 μ (associated with female plants).

According to Richards and Smith, when a spore germinates it divides into a four-cell stage, develops holdfasts, and then the cells begin to differentiate. By the time the female fungus develops perithecia, a large haustorial tube penetrates a perforation in which it fits snugly. Beneath the cuticle the haustorium (apparently produced by a single cell of the secondary receptacle) expands into a spherical-to-flattened, spheroidal bulb from 30 to 100 μ in diameter. The shape of the bulb varies and does not appear to be a specific character in *Herpomyces.* The haustorium is basophilic and stains a light blue with Mallory's stain, but after extending into a cell of the secondary receptacle, the staining changes either gradually or abruptly to acidophilic, and the end of the cell containing the nucleus stains with the acid fuchsin of Mallory's stain.

The haustorium is limited to the epidermis of the insect. The basement membrane of the integument may bulge inward but it is not penetrated by the fungus. Thus it does not appear that the haustorium penetrates into the body cavity.

Penetration of the cuticle by the haustorium is apparently accomplished by enzyme action. Because the haustorial tube fits the perforation snugly, Richards and Smith presume that the enzymes are bound to the haustorial surface and perhaps only to the tip of the haustorium. There is no depression or distortion of the cuticular laminae, as would probably be the case if penetration were caused largely by mechanical pressure. The dissolution of the cuticle by enzymic action causes the cuticle immediately surrounding the penetrating haustorial tube to become friable. There is also some evidence that the cytoplasm of the epidermal cells undergoes lysis in the region of haustorial penetration.

In heavy infections of *H. stylopygae,* as much as 10% of the total volume of the epidermis may be occupied by haustorial bulbs of the fungus. This seems to involve both the displacement of part of the epidermis and distention of the epidermal volume; sometimes the basement membrane can be seen bulging into the body cavity and, commonly, nearly naked nuclei can be observed more or less engulfed in the haustorial bulb.

Tavares (1965) has presented a detailed description of the development of *Herpomyces paranensis* in the roaches *Blaberus craniifer* and *B. giganteus.* The spores of this fungus germinate on minute setae on the antennae and divide to form a hyaline, four-celled, primary axis with an undifferentiated foot. This investigator observed a direct cytoplasmic connection between the perithecium and the host cuticle.

Although the laboulbeniaceous fungus *S. ceratophorus* produces an obvious penetration hole at the point of thallus attachment to the cuticle of the little housefly, *F. cannicularis,* and may obtain nutrients from the host, this fungus appears not to be particularly injurious to the insect host because the longevities of infected and noninfected fly populations appear to be the same (Whisler, 1968). Kamburov *et al.* (1967) have reported from a limited study, however, that *H. virescens* causes premature mortality of the infected coccinellid beetle, *Chilocorus bipustulatus.* They have observed that the disease is associated with a sudden drop in beetle population in the field but have not been able to establish under laboratory conditions the factors responsible for the decline of the beetle. Gunn and Cosway (1938) have suggested that cockroaches infected with a laboulbeniaceous fungus may react erratically to humidity.

2. Eccrinales

Among the primitive fungi associated with insects, as well as certain other invertebrates, are those commonly known as eccrinids, first reported in 1849 by the American naturalist Leidy (1849a,b). The eccrinids possess unbranched or not extensively branched hyphae attached by a holdfast of callose to the cuticle, especially that lining the hindgut, or to the anal plates, of their hosts. The hyphae are coenocytic at first. Reproduction occurs through the formation of microspores, macrospores, and resting spores. Most investigators who have worked on these fungi consider them to be commensals, but Thaxter (1920) and others felt that the highly specialized cuplike or disclike attachment with which they fasten to their hosts suggests that they may be, to some extent at least, truly parasitic. At the point of attachment of the eccrinid to the host, some physical disturbance to the cuticle may be seen. As pointed out by Lichtwardt (1954), however, this appears to be the result of the strong adhesive properties of the holdfast, and there is no evidence of lysis at or beneath the point of attachment. Moreover, the holdfast does not possess a cytoplasmic core through which nutritive materials are absorbed directly through the hyphal walls. Nevertheless, the fungi live attached to the insect and constitute "growths" that are not present on a typical individual.

Most of the species of eccrinids described are from Europe, and most have been reported by French workers, for example, Lichtenstein (1917a,b), Poisson (1929, 1931), Manier (1950), Tuzet and Manier (1950, 1951, 1952). Of those eccrinids found on insects, a common genus of the first order is *Trichella;* of the second order *Amoebidium* and *Paramoebidium* are frequently found on insects.

3. Other Fungal Epiphytes

Long ago the mycologist Thaxter (1914, 1920) pointed out that living insects are occasionally parasitized externally by fungal parasites of uncertain phylogenetic relationship to each other and to other fungi. Enough examples of similar or related forms have not as yet been described to make clear their relationships or general significance. Although apparently few in number, they appear to have adjusted themselves successfully to what Thaxter calls "the uncertain conditions of life and propagation on rapidly moving living hosts." Just why these fungi, which appear to be similar to Laboulbeniales in their entomogenous habitat, are not found more frequently, and upon other insects closely related to their known hosts, is not clear. They have been placed in the genera *Termitaria, Muiogone, Muiaria, Aposporella,* and others.

As the name implies, *Termitaria* are found on termites and are located on the body or appendages of their hosts. The type species is *Termitaria snyderi* and is found on *Reticulitermes* in the eastern United States and elsewhere. Their general appearance is that of flat, raised, rounded-to-elongate growths. Simple, firmly coherent, parallel sporogenous elements arise vertically, forming an even hymenial surface. Each element forms a single row of endogenous, simple, hyaline spores, which are discharged through a terminal perforation. The peripheral elements are sterile, dark, and indurated, and form a well-defined rim. Apparently, there is no continuous increase of the fungus in diameter after the original proliferation of the primary stage. In section the mature fungus, as it grows on the integument of the host, shows differentiation into several distinct regions (Thaxter, 1920, Fig. 14). A thin, dark layer of cells next to the body wall includes the primary attachment of the fungus. At this point the integument is indented; under the indentation the "cells of the host" (apparently epidermal cells) are hypertrophied, often assume a palisadelike structure, and become somewhat brownish. Thaxter saw no indication of actual penetration by the fungus through the integument. It does not appear to seriously inconvenience the host insect.

The type species of *Muiogone*, *Muiogone chromopteri*, grows on the under surface of the abdomen of a fly (*Chromopterus delicatulum*) in West Africa. Whether or not the fungus penetrates the integument or merely adheres firmly to its surface has not been determined.

Members of the genus *Muiaria* usually grow in dense, more-or-less isolated tufts, each tuft attached by a blackened base and consisting of fertile, or both fertile and sterile, elements. The fertile elements bear solitary terminal spores. In at least one species, *Muiaria repens*, the fungus assumes a creeping, or repent, habit on the wing of its host. The hosts appear to be primarily certain flies (*Leucophenga*, *Drosophila*, *Lonchaea*, *Clasiopa*) in the tropics. The type species, *Muiaria gracilis*, occurs on the legs and inferior surface of the abdomen of *Leucophenga* from West Africa.

Aposporella elegans has been described from a small fly from West Africa. *Hormiscium myrmecophilum* occurs on various body parts of ants (*Pseudomyrmex*) in the Amazon. It is one of several imperfect fungi that have been found on ants. *Chantransiopsis decumbens*, described from undetermined staphylinid beetles collected in Java, is one of several in this genus. *Amphoromorpha entomophila*, which may be related to the Chytridiales has been found on species of staphylinids (e.g., *Diochus conicollis*) and other insects in the Philippines and elsewhere. The individual plants are solitary and occur in small numbers projecting at acute angles from the bristles of the legs, or other parts of the insect's body. The genus *Cantharosphaeria* (of which the type species *Catharosphaeria chilensis* is found on the elytra and appendages of a cucujid beetle in Chile) are true ascomycetes. Since *C. chilensis* may derive its nutriment from the film of foreign matter that covers the surface of its host, Thaxter thought the fungus is probably not truly entomogenous, that is, deriving its nutriment directly from the living insect. This point still remains to be determined.

Another fungus, *Antennopsis gallica*, was discovered growing on termites of the genus *Reticulitermes* by Buchli (1952). This fungus generally grows on the rigid parts of the integument having an exocuticle, such as the head capsule, tergites, and sternites, and is sometimes found on the endocuticle between the segments and pleural membranes. The legs, antennae, and mouthparts carry less fungi than the rest of the body. Buchli proposes that the fungus is spread by direct contact. The fungus affects all castes of the termite colony, including those that work and move the least (king and queen). Although the fungus does not penetrate the integument or cause any internal injury, it does adversely affect the termite and can wipe out a small colony in 4–6 weeks. The harmful effect is caused by a sticky substance produced by the fungus. The heads of the fungi, after producing spores, secrete a sticky substance which spreads over the body of the termite. This substance greatly hinders movement because the antennae stick to the head or mouthparts, the legs become entangled in it, and dirt particles adhere to the termites so that they are weighted down and cannot move. Molting is also hindered because the molted integument sticks and does not come off properly. Termites injured in this way are usually eaten by their fellow workers.

Other genera of undetermined taxonomic location comprised of cuticular fungi include *Coreomycetopsis, Thaxteriola, Endosporella,* and *Laboulbeniopsis.*

C. Protozoa

Of the protozoans found attached to or attacking the cuticle, all are in the class Ciliatea (revised classification by Honigberg *et al.*, 1964). Some doubt surrounds the exact nature of the association between protozoa and insects; most evidence suggests that it is purely physical, and only a few cause harm to their hosts. There has been some suggestion of irritation to the host, but probably only hindrance in feeding and movement occur, and only in heavy infestations.

In the Ciliatea, Welch (1960) found ectozoa of the genera *Vorticella* and *Epistylis* attached to the larvae of *Aedes communis. Vorticella* spp. are found on the surface of the head and thorax and on the abdomen in the intersegmental folds. *Epistylis* spp. are found on the ventral surfaces of the head and anterior thorax. The distribution of these protozoans is probably determined by the food supply available and freedom from host interference.

Elson (1933) reports protozoans of the genus *Epistylis* clinging to various parts of the hydrophylid beetle, *Tropisternus californicus.* They produce no injurious effects to the beetle but act as a distinct handicap in raising the elytra and in movements in general.

A great many other ciliates have been found attached to the cuticle of aquatic insects. Lust (1950) has reported 38 species of the Epistylidae attached to various aquatic Coleoptera and Hemiptera; Nenninger (1948) gives a list of several others. Suctorians found attached to the cuticle are fewer in number than ciliates. Dieter (1956) lists 20 species of the genus *Discophyra* attached to the cuticle of several aquatic

Coleoptera. All suctorians are ectocommensal or ectoparasitic and rarely harm their hosts, but when attached to the respiratory or locomotory organs they hinder the movements of the insects.

V. Pathogens That Attack the Epidermis

Of the pathogens that attack the epidermis of insects, little is known concerning bacteria, fungi, or nematodes. Most of the work in this area is concerned with insect viruses and microsporidians. These two areas are covered extensively in the subsequent discussion, which is followed by a short section on bacteria.

A. *Viruses*

Diseases of insects, now recognized as caused by viruses, have been known to man for several centuries, but the most complete studies have been made on them only during the last 50 years. Several types of viruses have been described. In this chapter we are concerned primarily with two: nuclear polyhedrosis and granulosis viruses, and to a lesser extent cytoplasmic polyhedrosis and nonoccluded viruses. In both nuclear polyhedrosis and granulosis virus diseases of Lepidoptera, the epidermal cells are usually the site of infection along with the fat body and other tissues. There has been no case noted to our knowledge in which the epidermis alone is infected. Although the granulosis virus has not been reported as yet from insects other than the Lepidoptera, the nuclear polyhedrosis virus has been observed in other orders, such as Hymenoptera and Diptera, but in none of these orders does the virus appear to attack the integument.

In a list compiled by Bergold (1963), which was obtained mainly from literature searches by Hughes (1957), Martignoni and Langston (1960), and Krieg (1961), 95 species of Lepidoptera and 12 species of Hymenoptera are known to be susceptible to nuclear polyhedrosis viruses. These same investigators also list 80 species of Lepidoptera susceptible to cytoplasmic polyhedrosis viruses. Findings of recent years have added to these lists.

1. Nuclear Polyhedroses

The first studied and best known group of viruses cause the polyhedroses, so-called because tissues of the infected insect's body become filled with polyhedral-shaped, proteinaceous, crystalline inclusion bodies.[2] Polyhedroses fall into at least two large categories: nuclear, in which the virus first multiplies and then is occluded in a polyhedron inside the cell nucleus (see Bergold, 1958, 1963; Aizawa, 1963); and cytoplasmic, in which the virus multiplies mainly within the cell cytoplasm and is occluded in a polyhedron formed in the cytoplasm (see Smith, 1963). Each type has its own individual characteristics and can be present separately, or simultaneously in the insect's body as a mixed infection.

Nuclear polyhedrosis viruses contain DNA and are generally confined largely to the integument, tracheae, fat bodies, and blood cells of the insect; their effect is to produce a complete liquefaction and disintegration of the affected tissues (see Benz, 1963).

The size and shape of nuclear polyhedra vary considerably from insect to insect and even among members of the same species. They are crystals of many forms, for example, dodecahedra, tetrahedra, and icosahedra; and most of the forms are characteristic for different species of viruses. The size of the polyhedra may range up to 15 μ in diameter, again depending on the species. Morgan *et al.* (1955, 1956) are the first to describe in detail the structure of a polyhedron containing virus particles. The polyhedron has a crystalline lattice of protein molecules, and the virus particles are distributed at random throughout the lattice. The free virus particles of the nuclear polyhedrosis virus are rod-shaped, about 20–50 mμ in diameter (including the developmental membrane), and about 200–400 mμ long.

The virus particle appears to be made up of a dense central core, presumably a DNA helix, surrounded by viral protein and an intimate membrane. Surrounding this is the developmental, or outer, membrane. The particles may occur singly, or in bunches, and scattered at random in the polyhedron. If found in bunches, each virus rod has its own intimate membrane but there is a common developmental membrane surrounding all the rods in a common bunch. The number of rods within a common developmental membrane may be constant, but usually it varies even within the same insect.

Viruses generally infect insects by being ingested by the host. There is no record of invasion through the integument, although the size of the virus particles is small enough to allow passage through some of the "holes" of the cuticle. David (1967) suggests that the presence of polyphenoloxidase in the epicuticle may inactivate insect viruses.

[2] Since Bird (1959), Stairs (1964), and Stairs *et al.* (1966) have shown that polyhedral (cuboidal) inclusion bodies are also produced in granuloses, the use of the term polyhedrosis may become *unsuitable* in the future.

The process of invasion of viruses with inclusion bodies is as follows. After the virus inclusion bodies (polyhedra and capsules) are ingested by the larva, they are dissolved by the action of the gut juice and the virus particles are liberated. Recently, several workers observed in ultrathin sections of the midgut epithelium of larvae exposed to a nuclear polyhedrosis virus (Harrap and Robertson, 1968) and to a granulosis virus (Summers, 1969; Tanada and Leutenegger, 1970) that the virus multiplies initially in the midgut cells, and then passes as a whole particle through the intercellular space and basement membrane into the hemocoel where it infects susceptible tissues. How the virus enters the midgut cell is still not definitely established, but Summers (1969) found virus rods in the microvilli of columnar cells a few hours after virus ingestion. How the infection spreads throughout the tissues of the insect has not been definitely clarified. Since the virus particles within the polyhedra are incapable of causing infection until released from the polyhedra, the infection is presumed to spread from virus particles that have not been occluded and have been set free before or after cellular dissolution.

In the insect integument the virus develops in the nucleus of the epidermal cells. The virus particle is formed in a virogenic stroma and becomes surrounded by polyhedral protein. As the polyhedra increase in size and number, the nucleus swells to an enormous size. After a short time nearly all the chromatin disappears and there remains simply the nuclear membrane enclosing the polyhedra and free virus particles. The nucleus continues to swell until its membrane ruptures. Shortly thereafter, the cell membrane breaks down, releasing the polyhedra and virus particles into the body cavity. The infected integument, including those of virus-infected pupae and adults, is very fragile and easily torn.

The general assumption is that after infection by a nuclear polyhedrosis virus the integument displays the same pathological sequence as the fat, trachea, and other tissues. Watanabe (1968) has shown, however, that in the fall webworm, *Hyphantria cunea*, infection of the larva by a nuclear polyhedrosis virus causes the epidermal cells to proliferate into a multilayered structure at an early stage of the disease. The abnormal proliferation results from amitotic divisions. Subsequently, the cells undergo hypertrophy and polyhedra appear in the nuclei of the multilayered epithelium. At a late stage the multilayered epithelium disintegrates, and the cells are released into the hemocoel. During this period darkly pigmented spots occasionally appear on the body surface of the moribund larva. Sections through these spots show cuticular projections containing muscle tissue, blood cells, fat-body tissue, and disintegrated epidermal cells, and covered with necrotic and melanized scabs. According to Watanabe (1968), the histopathology of other diseased tissues, for example, fat, trachea, and so on, is similar to those described for other nuclear polyhedroses. Harpaz and Zlotkin (1965) have also observed that the epithelium of *Heliothis peltigera* assumes a stratified appearance when it is infected by a nuclear polyhedrosis virus. They have concluded that the stratification is indicative of an increased regenerative activity. On the basis of the observations of these workers, the abnormal cellular proliferation of epithelial cells, somewhat akin to a malignant tumor, may occur commonly in nuclear polyhedroses in insects.

2. Cytoplasmic Polyhedroses

Cytoplasmic polyhedrosis viruses contain RNA and, in lepidopterous insects, are confined to the gut epithelial cells of larvae and adults where they cause cellular breakdown. The virus particles are icosahedral in shape and are usually occluded in proteinaceous polyhedra that develop in the cytoplasm of the midgut cells. The polyhedra, similar to those of nuclear polyhedrosis viruses, differ in shape and size, and the shapes may be characteristic of different strains or species of viruses. In Lepidoptera no cytoplasmic polyhedrosis virus has been reported to attack tissues other than the gut epithelium, but in the mosquito *Culex tarsalis* a cytoplasmic polyhedrosis virus forms polyhedra in the cytoplasm of epidermal cells and in the developing leg, wing, and antennal buds (Kellen *et al.*, 1966).

3. Granuloses

A third group of viruses causes granular diseases or granuloses. In these diseases enormous numbers of very small capsules or granules are found in the cells. The capsules have been described as oval, ellipsoidal, ovoid, or egg-shaped; however, Bird (1959) and Stairs (1964) have reported polyhedral (cuboidal) inclusion bodies in granulosis of the spruce budworm, *Choristoneura fumiferana*, and Stairs *et al.* (1966) in granulosis virus–infected larvae of the codling moth, *Laspeyresia pomonella*. The capsular protein is very similar to polyhedral protein: a macromolecular paracrystalline lattice in a cubic arrangement. Capsule size varies from species to species and ranges anywhere from 300 to 511 mμ in length to 119–350 mμ in width.

Unlike polyhedra, the capsules house only one, or very rarely two at the most, virus particles that contain DNA. The virus particles are rod-shaped, often slightly curved, and are apparently similar in structure to those of the nuclear polyhedrosis virus. They range in width from 36 to 80 mμ and in length from 245 to 411 mμ. Each virus particle, as in the case of the nuclear polyhedrosis virus, is surrounded by two membranes, the intimate and developmental membranes.

Much less is known about the histopathology of granuloses than polyhedroses. It has not been shown in all cases whether the granulosis virus develops in the nucleus, cytoplasm, or in both, but the nucleus appears to be the site of virus rod formation in most of the granuloses investigated with the electron microscope. The virus rods are occluded by the capsular protein while they are in the nucleus or in the cytoplasm. The main tissue affected in granuloses is the fat body, next the epidermis and the tracheal matrix, in one case the Malpighian tubule (Tanada and Leutenegger, 1968), and in two cases the midgut epithelium (Smith *et al.*, 1956; Summers, 1969; Tanada and Leutenegger, 1970). Huger (1963) listed some of the granuloses and the insect tissues that are infected by these viruses. The integument of 7 out of 13 insect species is affected by granuloses. There are distinct pathological changes that each of these tissues undergo; those of the epidermis serve as an example. One of the first reactions that may occur after infection is a mitotic proliferation of the epidermal cells. At the same time the nuclei begin to increase in size and the chromatin material tends to clump together; shortly after, it undergoes degeneration. The nucleus grows to such an extent that it almost fills the entire cell, which has also increased in size. The nuclear membrane begins to break down and the contents of the cytoplasm and nucleus mix; the entire cell is in a state of disintegration at this stage. Just prior to or at about this time, the capsules appear in the nucleus, or the cytoplasm, or both. Thereafter, the cell membrane ruptures, liberating the capsules and virus particles into the body cavity of the insect.

The pathology of the epidermis occurs with more or less delay than that of the fat body, depending on the virus. The infected epidermis often enlarges to 10 or more times the original thickness; numerous internal folds projecting into the body cavity can be observed because of increased thickness. As in the case of the nuclear polyhedroses of Lepidoptera, the integument infected with a granulosis virus becomes very fragile and easily torn.

Tanada (1953b) has reported on the pathology in the epidermal and fat cells of *Pieris rapae* infected with a granulosis virus. The progression of the infection is as stated above, with a more uniform infection in the epidermis than in the fat body. The external symptoms are similar to those of a nuclear polyhedrosis in that the body is bloated but soft and the integument is very fragile; upon rupture of the integument, a milky fluid is released.

Other external symptoms reported by Tanada are a greenish-to-milky-yellow color on the dorsal and lateral surfaces of the larva, while its ventral surface is almost white. Sometimes the integument is mottled and shiny; shortly after death the body darkens rapidly until it is almost black. A marked liquefaction of tissues usually accompanies this darkening.

Paillot, who reported in 1926 the first granulosis disease in an insect (*Pieris brassicae,* the European cabbageworm), also discovered three granuloses, which he calls "pseudo-grasserie," of the cutworm *Euxoa segetum* (Paillot, 1926, 1936, 1937). These three granuloses have been found to be completely distinct from each other, each exhibiting its own symptoms and pathologies. Since granulosis virus 1 affects mainly the fat body and apparently does not involve the integument, we shall not discuss it any further. Granulosis virus 2 infects the fat body, the epidermis, and the tracheal matrix. The epidermis becomes much thicker than that of a healthy insect and internal folds are usually found. Capsules are formed in both the nucleus and the cytoplasm of the cell. The external symptoms of the disease are the same as those caused by granulosis virus 1 except that the body wall usually appears more opaque. Granulosis virus 2 is more contagious than granulosis virus 1.

Granulosis virus 3 also affects the fat body, epidermis, and tracheal matrix. The infected larvae may die without showing a white coloration through the body wall; shortly after death the body darkens and dissolves internally. This disease is much more contagious than granulosis virus 1 or 2.

Martignoni (1957) described the general histopathology of the epidermis of *Eucosma griseana* infected with a granulosis virus. He explains that the epithelial layer, which cannot extend in width, forms invaginations which permit the tissue to grow into the body cavities of the larva. Eventually, the epithelium breaks down and, along with the fat tissue, releases a virus-rich fluid into the body cavity, leaving virtually nothing of the integument other than the cuticle.

In *P. brassicae,* the adults of larvae that have been fed a granulosis virus show aberrant pigmentation that may be related to a granulosis infection in adults (Van de Pol and Ponsen, 1963).

4. Nonoccluded Virus Diseases

In recent years an increasing number of heterogenous viruses that do not occur in inclusion bodies have been reported from insects. Some of them are known to infect the integument. The one that was isolated first by Xeros (1954) from the larva of the leatherjacket, *Tipula paludosa,* has been studied most extensively. This virus is commonly known as *Tipula* iridescent virus, or TIV, and is icosahedral in shape and about 130 mμ in diameter. It contains DNA. Xeros (1954) has reported that in the larva this virus develops in the cytoplasm of cells, primarily of the fat body but also of the muscles and epidermis. The virus has an extremely wide host range, especially when inoculated into the larval hemocoel but infects only a lesser number of insect species when fed to larvae (Smith *et al.*, 1961). When inoculated into the hemocoel of the silkworm larva, according to Hukuhara and Hashimoto (1966), the virus produces a typical iridescence in the silk gland, dermal gland, muscles, dorsal vessel, and trachea, with the iridescence being most pronounced in the silk and dermal glands. They also observed with the electron microscope, in ultrathin sections of the epidermis, masses of electron-dense material and virus particles in the cytoplasm of the epidermal cells.

An iridescent virus has been isolated and described from the larva of the rice stem borer, *Chilo suppressalis,* by Fukaya and Nasu (1966). An infection by this virus produces in the pupal and adult integuments an interesting anomaly that resembles a juvenile hormonelike response (Ono and Fukaya, 1969). When the virus is inoculated into fourth- and fifth-instar silkworm larvae, some larvae molt into pupae which have localized patches of larval cuticle. Such pupae develop into adults that have larval cuticles on the same sites as those observed on the pupae. The larval patches on both the pupal and adult integuments are devoid of pupal characters and adult structures such as scales. The "larval" regions undergo supernumerary molts twice from the fifth larval instar to the adult. Similar results have been obtained when the virus is fed to first-instar larvae for 3–4 hours.

When examined with the electron microscope, the epidermal cells beneath the "larval" patches of the pupal and adult integuments contain virus particles in small groups that are often surrounded by membranes. The virus is absent in epidermal cells beneath the normal integument. Ono and Fukaya (1969) speculate that since the virus is not likely to release a juvenile hormonelike substance there are two possible explanations: (1) The juvenile hormone secreted by the corpus allatum is maintained, especially in virus-infected epidermal cells; and (2) the epidermal cells when infected by the virus become highly sensitive to juvenile hormone, inspite of the fact that the corpus allatum of the silkworm remains inactive from the middle of the last larval instar until the first half of the pupal stage.

Weiser (1965) has reported a new virus in larvae of the mosquitoes *Aedes annulipes* and *A. cantans*. The infected larvae become opaque and opalescent and are usually less motile than uninfected larvae. They are distorted and slightly shortened. Pathological changes are apparent in almost every tissue except the midgut and salivary gland but are most evident in the fat body, epidermis, and muscle. The hemolymph of infected larvae appears pink and contains many minute granules. The nuclei of infected cells become hypertrophied. Irregular stromata form foamy structures in the vacuoles. With the destruction of the cytoplasm by the virus, the nuclei become distended and are finally destroyed. The virus particle is icosahedral in shape and measures 175–185 mμ. It is similar to TIV but differs in size and cross infectivity. No polyhedral inclusions or capsules are formed in the host.

In a blackfly, *Simulium ornatum*, Weiser (1968) also reported an iridescent virus 140–160 mμ in diameter. He observed virogenic stromata in the cytoplasm of the cells of fat body, epidermis, connective tissue, tracheal matrix, and muscle.

In addition to the above iridescent viruses that have been reported to attack the integument, there are other similar viruses on a scarab, *Sericesthis pruinosa* (Steinhaus and Leutenegger, 1963), and the mosquito *Aedes taeniorhynchus* (Clark *et al.*, 1965; Woodard and Chapman, 1968). Detailed histopathological studies of the infections caused by these viruses may reveal that they also attack the integument.

In some species of *Tetranychus*, there appears to be a suppressor agent that prevents the development of certain setae on the forelegs of the mites (Boudreaux, 1959). The suppressor agent is transmitted through the ooplasm and resembles the "integrated virus" transmitted by "cytoplasmic inheritance."

Certain plant viruses are known to cause pathological alterations in their insect vectors. One of them, the wound tumor virus of the leafhopper, *Agallia constricta*, invades the integument in addition to other organs such as the fat body, Malpighian tubules, mycetome, and trachea, and occurs in the cytoplasm but not in the nuclei of the cells of these organs (Shikata and Maramorosch, 1965). In the cytoplasm either crystalline arrangements or clusters of particles are encountered. The frequency of accumulation of virus particles in the epidermal cells is only surpassed by those found in the fat body.

Further studies by Shikata and Maramorosch (1967a) have revealed that virus particles are assembled in accumulations of electron-dense aggregates formed in the cytoplasm of fat body, muscle, midgut, Malpighian tubule, trachea, salivary gland, and epidermal cells. Similar assembly sites occur in the cytoplasm of root tumor cells and of enlarged leaf veinlets of virus-infected plants (*Trifolium incarnatum* and *Melilotus alba*). Shikata and Maramorosch (1967a) designated the virus assembly site viroplasm, a term comparable to virogenic stroma mentioned earlier. The sequential formation of virus development in the cells of the leaf hopper proceeds as follows: (1) formation of a viroplasm in the cytoplasm; (2) appearance of virus particles at the periphery of the viroplasm; (3) formation of increasing numbers of virus particles, not only in the periphery but also in the viroplasm; (4) engulfing of virus particles within multimembranous structures; and (5) formation of virus microcrystals either at the sites of former viroplasms, or at some distance (Shikata and Maramorosch, 1967b).

A bacilliform virus, lettuce necrotic yellows virus, causes a systemic infection in the aphid vector *Hyperomyces lactucae* (O'Loughlin and Chambers, 1967). The virus may exist in two forms within the tissues of the aphid: one type is identical to those found in plant cells, and the other is similar but lacks an outer coat. O'Loughlin and Chambers have seen the uncoated particles ($200–400 \times 32–35$ mμ) in cells of the alimentary canal, salivary gland, muscle, fat body, brain, mycetome, and trachea; and the coated particles (about 45 mμ in diameter) in cells of the alimentary canal, muscle, and epidermis. In the epidermis numerous coated virus particles are commonly found in the basement membrane. O'Loughlin and Chambers do not describe the cytopathology of the virus-infected cells. Apparently, the cells of insect vectors that contain virus particles do not exhibit marked pathologies comparable to those of cells infected with insect-specific viruses.

An animal virus, the Rous sarcoma virus, when added to the medium causes an increased incidence of lethal mutations, visible mutations, chromosome losses, chromosomal nondisjunctions, and tumors in larvae of *Drosophila* (Burdette and Yoon, 1967). In addition, a few mosaics of the eye and translocations are produced. There are slight suggestions that the size of the chromosomal puffs may be reduced by this RNA virus. The virus apparently does not persist in the progeny.

B. Protozoa

Of the phylum Protozoa, the subphyla Sporozoa and Cnidospora contain the most forms pathogenic for insects (revised classification by Honigberg *et al.*, 1964). In the Cnidospora the class Microsporidea is the only one with which this chapter is concerned, for members of this order are known to attack the insect epidermis. Best known of the microsporidia is *Nosema bombycis* which causes pebrine in the silkworm; this disease is discussed later.

Each microsporidian species has several stages in its life cycle, and each stage has a specific function in the infection of an insect. In the first stage, the planont, or amebula, leaves the spore and immigrates into the body of the host; in the second stage the first schizont selects the appropriate tissues for invasion; in the third stage the second schizont produces parasites en masse and penetrates the chosen organ uniformly; and in the fourth stage the diplokaryon produces the sporonts and spores that are the resistant stages (see Weiser, 1961, 1963).

The spores of microsporidians are of great importance; they have distinguishing characteristics used in identification, their formation aids in the study of the infection, and they are highly resistant under certain conditions. The microsporidian spores range from 3 to 6 μ long and 1 to 3 μ wide, and the size varies with the species. The form of the spore also varies considerably, ranging from oval, ovoidal, ovocylindrical, or pyriform to spherical, reniform, tubular, spiral, or crescent-shaped.

Essentially, the spore is made up of a spore membrane surrounding a sporoplasm and a polar filament which is coiled directly in the spore or encased within a polar capsule. The polar filament is extremely fine and long; filaments as long as 500 μ have been reported. The polar filament is a tubular structure that serves to inoculate the planont into the host cell or into the hemocoel.

Spores are transmitted from one host to another perorally or through the ova; ingestion is the most common method of infection. Soon after ingestion, the digestive fluids of the host cause the spore to extrude its filament, which introduces the planont into the midgut cell or into the hemocoel.

After penetration of the intestinal epithelium, the first schizont searches until it finds the proper tissues to invade, but whether or not it invades the epidermis, if this tissue is susceptible, is not known. The second schizonts very likely invade the epidermal cells or other susceptible tissue cells and undergo binary fission to produce daughter schizonts, some of which infect epidermal cells; others form diplokarya. The diplokarya form sporonts which in turn produce spores, and the cycle within the epidermal cell is completed. The multiplication of the microsporidian takes place in the cytoplasm and not in the nucleus.

The external appearance of a microsporidian-infected insect may vary according to the extent of the infection and may result in changes in size, color, form, and activity. One of the most common external symptoms is the change from transparency to opacity of the body, attributable to the accumulation of large numbers of spores in the tissues underlying the insect's integument. The body usually appears dull milky-white. Sometimes, dark mottled spots of a dark brown coloration may appear; a grayish or yellowish color and even a red coloration have been attributed to microsporidian infections.

The body form of the host may change as the result of a microsporidian infection. The insect may be dwarfed, distended, or swollen. Actual abnormalities of the appendages may result, causing the insect's activity to decrease.

In many cases of microsporidian diseases, only a specific tissue is invaded; this is usually the fat body of the insect. The epidermis is also invaded in some insects and, in a few cases, all the tissues of the body become infected. The insect larva is the stage in the insect life cycle most susceptible to infection, as in most other insect diseases, but pupae and adults can also become infected.

Changes in the infected epidermis of an insect occur in the following manner: The cells become enormously enlarged, with the nuclei becoming hypertrophied. Sometimes the nuclei may increase in number. The cytoplasm becomes enlarged mainly because of the increasing number of parasites in this region of the cell. Chromatolysis and karyolysis may occur simultaneously, with the chromatin material gathering in masses at the periphery of the nucleus. The cell membrane usually does not break down during the course of infection, but does so after death of the insect. Infected midgut cells are known to break down as the infection increases in intensity, however.

Pebrine, the name given to the microsporidian disease of *Bombyx mori,* has been known since the early nineteenth century, and has been given this name because of the pepperlike spots on the silkworm's integument. The microsporidian causing pebrine is *N. bombycis.* This particular microsporidian infects several other insects as well as the silkworm. The disease is found mainly in larvae, but infected pupae and adults have been reported.

The characteristic symptom of pebrine is the appearance of dark-brown-to-black spots on the surface of the silkworm's integument. These spots occur principally on the posterior ventral side of the insect, but usually not until the insect is in an advanced stage of the disease. Other symptoms of the disease are irregular growth, particularly in size, sluggishness, and loss of appetite; silk from the cocoons of infected larvae is much inferior in strength and uniformity of thickness.

The fat tissue of the silkworm is the main organ affected, but *N. bombycis* has been reported in nearly every tissue of the insect. Its course in the epidermal cells is as reported above, with the infected cells swelling intensely. The great swelling usually causes the basement membrane to break, thus liberating the spores into the hemocoel. An interesting role of the epidermis in transmitting the causative protozoa of pebrine from one stage of the silkworm to the next has been mentioned by Mitani (1934). Ordinarily, the infected part of the epidermis swells considerably until finally the basement membrane breaks, but sometimes the infected part becomes enclosed by a chitinous layer. When this happens, the infected ecdysial epidermis provides a means of perpetuating the infection. When the schizonts multiply in the epidermal cells, they cause the cells to enlarge; the secondary cuticle just above the infected part also swells. A part of this secondary cuticle enters into the infected part and surrounds the decomposed protoplasm and the microsporidian. Then the entire chitinous layer becomes sac-shaped and completely encloses the pathogen and the decomposed protoplasm. This enclosed mass is at first brownish in color but later turns black; as a result, the well-known characteristic black spot, for which the name pebrine is appropriate, is produced.

Several other microsporidian diseases have been reported in which cells of the epidermis are affected. Tanada (1953a) observed that the imported cabbageworm, *P. rapae,* is infected by *Perezia mesnili* (=*Nosema mesnili*). The epidermis becomes infected in the last stages of the disease; staining shows the infected cells to be vacuolated and to have highly irregular nuclei.

Perezia fumiferanae (=*Glugea fumiferanae*) has been found to be a parasite of the spruce budworm, *C. fumiferana,* by Thomson (1955). He reports that the epidermis becomes infected along with several other tissues, but the epidermal cells retain their shape and show no swelling during the course of the disease.

Paillot (1939) found *Nosema carpocapsae* infecting the larvae of the codling moth. This particular microsporidian parasitizes most of the cells of the host, but those of the silk glands, Malpighian tubules, adipose tissue, muscles, and oenocytes are most commonly found infected. Less frequently, the infections are found in pericardial and epidermal cells, and in the cells at the base of the hairs. In this disease epidermal cells also show no marked swelling, although the cytoplasm is vacuolated and somewhat hypertrophied.

C. Bacteria

In the field of bacterial pathogens that attack the epidermis, there is very little to report. Although certain bacteria are capable of breaking down the cast-off skin and cuticle of dead insects, they do not appear to attack the cuticle of living insects. David (1967) suggests that in living insects epidermal cells supply substances to the cuticle which give it protection. One of the two instances of a bacterium attacking the epidermis of an insect that we have found was reported by Duggar (1896). He observed that *Bacillus entomotoxicon,* at that time a new species, attacks the perivisceral cavity, blood, adipose tissue, cardiac tissue, and epidermis of the squashbug, *Anasa tristis.* The infected squashbug becomes sluggish before death, and at death it becomes darker and softer than in life. After death the body organs are reduced to a mass of "gruel-like fluids." A study of these fluids shows them to be an almost pure culture of the bacillus.

A second bacterium that attacks the epidermis is *Micrococcus nigrofaciens,* which can penetrate the integument of June beetle larvae (*Lachnosterna*), according to Northrup (1914). This bacterium exists in the soil. An infected larva is characterized by the black and shiny aspects of the affected parts, which are sharply circumscribed. The leg joints, spiracles, and dorsal or ventral segments of the white soft portion of the body are the principal sites of infection. Even though the discoloration increases until the insect body seems to be in a state of advanced putrifaction, the insect still shows signs of life. An infected leg turns black segment by segment as the disease progresses, and the segments drop off, leaving the stump shiny, black, and sometimes swollen in appearance. Histological sections of the infected larva show the micrococci embedded in the integumental laminae and in the epidermal cells.

VI. Integument as a Route of Entry and Emergence of Internal Pathogens

We are not aware of any well-authenticated cases of bacteria (except for *M. nigrofaciens*), viruses, or protozoa regularly entering their host by penetrating the unbroken external body wall of the insect. Paillot (1940) has described a new species of spirochete which infects larvae of *P. brassicae,* however. This spirochete does not invade the larvae through the digestive tract, but enters through the integument. Penetration through the integument, however, is not always successful.

Direct penetration through the integument is characteristic of certain entomogenous fungi and nematodes. In spite of the common occurrence of this phenomenon among entomogenous fungi, surprisingly little is known about the mechanisms involved, and only a few specialized studies have been made of it. The presumed enzymic, chemotactic, and mechanical aspects of it are little understood (see David, 1967).

The cuticle of insects contains pore canals and many pathogens, such as bacteria and viruses, are sufficiently small that they would be expected to enter the insect through these pores. However, as pointed out by David (1967), ". . . modern ideas about the form and contents of the canals make it unlikely that entry could occur by this route."

A. *Fungi*

Representatives of the fungi known to penetrate the integument and cause infection and disease in insects are found in the five classes Chytridiomycetes, Zygomycetes, Ascomycetes, Basidiomycetes, and Deuteromycetes (Fungi Imperfecti) [classification after Alexopoulos (1962)]. The classes Zygomycetes, Ascomycetes, and Deuteromycetes contain most of the insect pathogens (see Müller-Kögler, 1965). In the Zygomycetes the order Entomophthorales is the most important since it contains the genera *Entomophthora* and *Massospora,* both composed primarily of entomogenous species (see MacLeod, 1963).

The Ascomycetes and Deuteromycetes cause the most common and well-known fungal infections in insects, namely, *Cordyceps* infections (see McEwen, 1963) and the muscardine disease (see Madelin, 1963), respectively. *Beauveria bassiana* is probably the best-known fungus causing muscardine disease, as it attacks not only a wide range of insect species but is also the first pathogen to be isolated from an insect, the silkworm. Other important and well-known entomogenous fungi of the Deuteromycetes are the green muscardine, *Metarrhizium anisopliae,* and the yellow muscardines, *Paecilomyces farinosa* and *Aspergillus flavus.*

The class Basidiomycetes contains the least number of entomogenous species. The most important belong to the genus *Septobasidium,* which has a complex association of parasitism and mutualism with scale insects. An account of this genus is given later.

Although fungal infections are very common in insects, integument-penetrating fungi do meet with varying degrees of resistance on the part of the cuticle. There is evidence that in addition to the protection afforded by the mechanical structure of the integument some of this resistance is related to the nature and amount of cuticular lipids present in the insect's body wall. For example, in one of a series of papers on the subject, Koidsumi (1957) reports that larvae of the silkworm and the rice stem borer, *C. suppressalis,* become highly susceptible to muscardine fungi when their cuticular lipids are removed either mechanically or chemically. Although the mechanism of the defense provided by the lipids may be either physical or chemical, or both, the lipids present in exuviae of the silkworm show a distinct antifungal action *in vitro* against the growth of *A. flavus*. Free medium-chain saturated fatty acids, presumably caprylic or capric acid, are the most active. In artificial culture germination of fungal spores, elongation of hyphae, size of the colony, and formation of conidia are all affected by the antifungal action of the lipids, which may be fungicidal or fungistatic according to the concentration and duration of exposure to the active constituents. Evlakhova and Chekhourina (1964) obtained results with *B. bassiana* and the insect *Eurygaster integriceps* comparable to those of Koidsumi. An antifungal substance is present in the epicuticle of *Eurygaster* and can be removed by mechanical and chemical treatments. Extracts of the cuticle also inhibit spore germination, mycelial growth, and sporulation of the fungus cultured *in vitro*. Wada (1957) showed a correlation between the resistance of insects to two species of *Spicaria* and the antifungal lipids extracted from the whole bodies of the insect hosts. Just what properties of entomopathogenic fungi characteristically enable them to overcome these and other defense mechanisms of the host insect is not clear; certainly it would be of interest and value to make a comparative study of pathogenic and nonpathogenic fungi from this standpoint.

In contrast to antifungal substances, certain substances present in the cuticle may stimulate spore germination. Notini and Mathlein (1944) have detected such a stimulating factor for the spores of *Metarrhizium anisopliae* in the lipoid layer of the cuticle of certain insects, and the factor is removed by treatment with a fat solvent.

The susceptibility of an insect to invasion by fungi is also associated with the developmental stage of the integument. Rockwood (1950) reports that wireworms appear to be susceptible to infection by the fungus genus *Metarrhizium* only at the time of molting. In *Agriotes obscurus*, Fox (1961) found that the insect is attacked by fungi just before, during, and after pupation, and newly emerged adults also appear to be more susceptible. The newly molted larvae of *Pseudaletia unipuncta* are susceptible to *Entomophthora* spp., but not the fully developed larvae (Gabriel, 1965); and the newly formed pupae of *P. rapae* are susceptible to *B. bassiana* only when 1 day old (Tanada, 1955b). Sussman (1951) has also reported that older pupae of *Platysamia cecropia* are resistant to infection by *A. flavus*.

Except for those instances in which invasion occurs by way of the alimentary tract, a typical entomopathogenic fungus begins its growth and development on the external surface of the insect's body wall. Regardless of the type of fungus concerned (Entomophthorales, *Cordyceps*, Hyphomycetes, and so on), the process is essentially the same. The conidium lands on or becomes attached to the cuticle. Sometimes this attachment is a loose and tenuous one; in other instances it is firm, and the attachment may be facilitated by adhesive properties of the conidium or pellicle surrounding it.

In the presence of adequate atmospheric moisture, the conidium germinates, sending out a conidial hypha. In the case of the resting spore of *Entomophthora*, Schweizer (1947) believes its germination is aided by the action of chitinovorous bacteria which attack the chitinous membranes of the spore making it "viable" when moisture becomes adequate. The chitin-splitting bacteria may be present in the disintegrating body of the host insect, or in the soil, or elsewhere in nature. Perhaps, Schweizer postulates, the outbreak of epizootics is related to the activity of chitin-splitting bacteria at different times of the year. The conidium, however, does not appear to require anything more than appropriate conditions of moisture and temperature to germinate. Germination, once initiated, proceeds rapidly. The conidial hypha usually travels straight and in one direction until a point of penetration is reached. Frequently, this point is one of the thinner areas of the integument, such as an intersegmental fold, but penetration may also take place through more heavily sclerotized parts of the integument. According to Schweizer, the germinating hypha takes the shortest route to the fat tissue (for which it presumably has an affinity) within the body of the fly. However, affinity for the fat body may vary with the fungus species (Prasertphon and Tanada, 1968).

One of the first histological studies attempting to determine just how a conidial hypha penetrates the integument of an insect was that by Wallengren and Johansson (1929) in which they investigated the infection of the European corn borer, *Pyrausta nubilalis* (=*Ostrinia nubilalis*), by the green muscardine fungus, *M. anisopliae*. Of particular interest is their finding that certain structural features of the integument of the corn borer are of significance in the manner in which the conidial hypha pierces the skin of the insect.

Microscopic examination of the integument of a corn borer larva reveals that the areas immediately surrounding the bases of the hairs are darker and brownish and present a granular appearance produced by a number of small, round, dark pigment bodies gathered close to each other immediately under the surface of the exocuticle. The remainder of the skin has similar granules farther apart; here there are similar small, black or dark-brown pigment bodies gathered in small rounded groups, situated at a uniform distance from each other. Between these groups of pigment bodies are pale lines (more or less hexagonal in arrangement), which represent the remaining boundaries between the original epidermal cells. Along these lines are dark, round pigment grains which emphasize the hexagonal shape of the fields. In section the pigment bodies, somewhat elongated, are seen to lie on the outer edge of the cuticle. From each pigment body emanates one or more threads, clustered together, which continue down into the cuticle to about one-third of its thickness. The threads converge so that the entire formation resembles an inverted pyramid. In the areas around the bases of the hairs, however, the threads are not gathered into pyramids but run straight down into the cuticle; they appear to be somewhat shorter than those in the pyramids. The larvae of a number of Lepidoptera, for example, *Psyche* and *Pheosia*, have pigment bodies and the associated threads extending only about one-third of the way down into the cuticle as in the corn borer. In certain other insects, for example, larvae of *Bombyx* and *Smerinthus*, a bundle of diverging threads extends from the peripheral part of each epidermal cell up through the lamellae of the entire cuticle.

With the proper conditions of atmospheric moisture and temperature, the fungus conidia, fastened to the surface of the integument, send out germination hyphae. At those places where the conidia germinate, the cuticle takes on a yellowish color. Under this yellow spot the cuticle assumes a granular appearance, and the pigment bodies become clotted and fall to pieces; the threads also disintegrate. Each conidial hypha pierces the cuticle and begins its entrance into the body wall at a point of one of the thread pyramids, which disintegrates and becomes granular. The outer layer of the cuticle is more or less destroyed, and the area concerned assumes a more yellowish or dark-brown color. These colored spots increase in size as the infection progresses and may fuse or spread over entire segments or parts of the body, turning dark brown or even black. It is possible for the infection to occur without causing brown spots. Also, after the hypha has penetrated the skin, the fungus appears to be able to continue its growth without further discoloring of the integument. Usually, however, in the corn borer, the entire cuticle in the involved area turns dark brown, becomes very brittle and fragile, and breaks easily during sectioning. Incidentally, in the case of *Metarrhizium* infection in the larva of the rhinoceros beetle (*Oryctes*), the discoloration often extends only a short distance into the cuticle, indicating, according to Friederichs (1920), that the fungus has pierced the cuticle but is unable to enter the body cavity and cause a general mycosis.

According to Wallengren and Johansson, the growing conidial hypha appears to secrete some kind of chitin-dissolving substance, possibly an enzyme, which opens or facilitates the way for penetration. Apparently, the hypha also exerts pressure on the substratum. In sections the cuticular lamellae can be seen to be pressed down when the hypha is developing at right angles to them. The hypha often grows for relatively long distances between the lamellae, evidently because growth in this direction offers the least resistance, but sooner or later it turns inward, perforates the endocuticle and epidermis, and enters the body cavity. These observations have been confirmed by Takahashi (1958), Prasertphon and Tanada (1968), and Sannasi (1969).

In another study involving the European corn borer, Lefebvre (1934) observed that conidial hyphae of the white muscardine fungus, *B. bassiana,* can penetrate not only the thin parts of the integument but also the thick sclerotized areas (except the head). Pupae appear to be invaded largely through the thinner intersegmental areas, however. David (1967) has pointed out that the thickness of the cuticle may be a factor in the invasion by fungi.

Takahashi (1958) has found that *B. bassiana* penetrates the cuticula of larvae and pupae of *B. mori* in different ways. Penetration of the larval cuticle by hyphae occurs more readily in the arthrodial membrane than in the sclerite; each hyphal segment penetrates the cuticle separately, causing a little color change during penetration. The area around penetrating hyphae becomes acidophilic (the normal cuticle is basophilic), suggesting that enzymic action is involved in penetration. The fungus penetrates considerably faster when the epicuticular wax layer is removed by rubbing with fine, inert dusts.

Penetration of the pupal cuticle occurs not only in the arthrodial membrane but also in the posterior portion of the sclerite, which is colorless and thinner than the anterior portion. Hyphae do not penetrate singly; rather, they aggregate into spongy masses on the surface and penetrate en masse through the cuticle. In no case do hyphae penetrate through the evenly fully hardened, colored region of the anterior sclerite. Apparently, the fungus is capable of producing enzymes that dissolve and break down the cuticular layer.

In an investigation prior to that of Takahashi's, Katsumata (1931) observed that the germ tubes of *B. bassiana* rarely grow along the surface of the integument but usually penetrate immediately into the cuticle. In penetrating the outermost layer of the cuticle, the hypha becomes constricted but returns to a normal width after passing through this layer. When it reaches the epidermal layer, it usually branches readily. After the fungus kills the insect, the hypha penetrates in a reverse direction to the outside of the body. In doing this it does not constrict in going through the cuticle. From his study, Katsumata has concluded that the penetration of the germ tube through the outermost layer of the cuticle is essentially caused by mechanical pressure exerted by the germ tube; after this penetration the underlying tissues are attacked by the action of enzyme or toxin secreted by the hypha. Mitani and Kawai (1937) assayed hyphae and conidia of *B. bassiana* and detected the presence of chitinase, amylase, raffinase, invertase, maltase, and lactase but found no evidence of cellulase, inulase, pectinase, or glycogenase. Accordingly, these authors conclude that the germ tubes of the fungus perforate the integument of the silkworm by secreting chitinase which dissolves chitin and denatures glucose.

Another Japanese investigator, Aoki (1942), found that when the cuticle, along with other tissues, is infected with *Sterigmatocystis japonica* the cuticle swells and hyphae proliferate in it. The penetration of the integument by growing hyphae is accomplished by "boring" holes in the cuticle of a diameter of that of the hyphae. At this stage of mycosis, black spots can be observed on the surface of the silkworm body.

While studying in the silkworm the infection caused by the fungus *Nomuraea prasina*, Iyoda (1940) observed that the germ tubes do not grow over the surface of the integument but immediately penetrate into the integument. While in the primary cuticle the germ tubes are very thin, in the secondary cuticle they swell, and assume the shape of clubs or are globular. It is interesting that after the germ tubes penetrate the cuticle no conidia connected with them can be seen on the surface of the integument; apparently, the empty conidia are detached soon after germination. When hyphae penetrate the cuticle and invade the epidermis en masse, the epidermis frequently first recedes as a thin layer before being damaged. At times individual hyphae penetrate the epidermal cells, and this usually causes rapid and extensive damage. At the points where the epidermis is damaged, the blood cells of the silkworm usually aggregate, forming a syncytium from which the hyphae eventually break out to invade the body cavity. The cuticle is denatured, does not stain with hematoxylin, and is of a pale brownish color. Hyphae in the denatured cuticle become empty and lose their ability to stain. Interestingly, Iyoda has found that hyphae growing in the integument gradually become a mass, with most of this mass being situated in the epidermis. When the larva molts, the number of remaining hyphae is very small, most of them being removed with the cast-off skin.

Some plant pathogenic fungi produce a flattened, hyphal, pressing organ, the appressorium, from which a minute infection peg usually grows and invades the epidermal cell of the host plant. Several entomopathogenic fungi are known to produce clavate branches *in vitro* whose functions have not been established. Madelin *et al.* (1967) believe that these clavate structures are appressoria as indicated by the circumstances of their formation and their role in the penetration of artificial membranes of paraffin wax. They propose that penetration of the insect integument is accomplished by mechanical pressure and enzymic activity of the clavate branches or appressoria. According to McCauley *et al.* (1968), the green muscardine fungus, *M. anisopliae,* produces appressoria, except where germ tubes gain direct access to the body cavity through pores of sense organs or spiracles, that penetrate the integument of wireworms (Elateridae). They have reported that clusters of appressoria and spherical enlargements usually form "infection cushions," but occasionally a germ tube terminates in a typical appressorium. Zacharuk (1970a,b) believes that the appressoria may utilize the lipoidal covering of the epicuticle of the integument for their nutrition.

On the basis of ultrastructural studies with the electron microscope, Zacharuk (1970a) observed that an enlargement at the tip of the germ tube forms a large cell, the appressorium, which may proliferate to form additional appressoria. The appressorial cells, which are derived from one appressorium, initially are divided from one another by septa, each with a central pore. Some septal pores eventually appear to be closed by a dense plug. Other septa between adjacent appressoria are replaced by double walls to form discrete cells. Zacharuk (1970b) also studied the penetration of the fungus into the host integument on an ultrastructural level. He reports that there is initial mechanical pressure on the epicuticle by the apposed appressoria, and enzymic penetration of the epicuticle by the penetration peg. Although he has not been able to detect any differential zone surrounding the peg as indicated by light microscope studies, nonetheless, ultrastructural evidence suggests a diffusion of histolytic enzymes directly from the appressorium to the integument. He postulates that a typical penetration of the integument of wireworms by *M. anisopliae* occurs in four primary stages: (1) penetration of the epicuticle by penetration pegs and the formation of penetration plates, both derived initially from appressoria; (2) lateral extension of hyphae and production of type-I penetration hyphal bodies, both derived initially from penetration plates; (3) production of type-II hyphal bodies by type-I hyphal bodies, and their proliferation; and (4) vertical penetration of the laminae of the remaining procuticle by vertical penetration hyphae in a stepwise fashion, interspersed by production and proliferation of more type-II hyphal bodies at each step until the vertical penetration hyphae reach the more amorphous inner procuticle, through which they extend into the hypodermis without further production of hyphal bodies.

The production of enzymes capable of dissolving certain components of the integument, such as lipids, chitin, and proteins, has been reported for many entomogenous fungi (see Müller-Kögler, 1965). We have already discussed several studies reporting the production of enzymes by fungi. Gabriel (1968a,b) also investigated these enzymes, and showed by *in vitro* and histochemical studies that *Entomophthora* spp. are capable of producing lipolytic, chitinolytic, and proteolytic enzymes. There have been speculations why an enzyme, such as chitinase, if produced by the fungus, does not dissolve the fungus cell wall which is often largely composed of chitin. This question has not been resolved.

Lefebvre (1934) does not discuss a discoloration of the integument at the site of penetration of the fungus as did Wallengren and Johansson (1929) in the case of *M. anisopliae.* He does, however, observe the infected or freshly dead corn borers to assume the characteristic pink coloration associated with *B. bassiana* infections in the silkworm and other insects. Although discoloration of the integument at the sites of fungal invasion has not been reported by Lefebvre, such discoloration develops in the larval integuments of *P. rapae* (Tanada, 1955b), *Galleria mellonella* (Boczkowska, 1935; Prasertphon, 1963; Gabriel, 1968b), *B. mori* (Kurisu, 1962), *Ostrinia nubilalis* (Toumanoff, 1928), and *Odontotermes obesus* (Sannasi, 1969). Gabriel (1968b) has shown by Lillie's ferrous iron test that the blackening is caused by melanin. Hemocytes accumulate at the point of invasion of the fungus into the hemocoel (Paillot, 1933; Boczkowska, 1935; Tanada, 1955b; Kurisu, 1962; Prasertphon and Tanada, 1968). According to Kurisu (1962), the black-spotted sign and hemocyte accumulation are indications of a defense mechanism by the larva against fungus invasion. Toumanoff (1928), in reporting on studies of the European corn borer infected with *A. flavus* and *Spicaria farinosa* (=*P. farinosa*), states that small black spots appear on the skin and that the filaments of the fungi are found under the dark spots in a kind of "abscess" under the destroyed epidermis.

In the termite *Odontotermes obesus,* the fungus *A. flavus* causes melanin formation in the endocuticle of the intersegmental membrane (Sannasi, 1969). The polyphenols in the esters of acid mucopolysaccharides of healthy endocuticles seem to be liberated in cuticles infected by the fungus. Sannasi also reports that the epidermis is destroyed in the area immediately surrounding the infecting hyphae. The epidermal cells, which have large vacuoles, do not stain as deeply with acid fuchsin as do normal cells. The ascorbic acid–positive granules disappear in the fungus-infected cells.

In *P. rapae* (Tanada, 1955b) and in *G. mellonella* (Prasertphon and Tanada, 1968), the epidermal cells disintegrate when they are penetrated by germinating hyphae of *B. bassiana.* According to Prasertphon and Tanada (1968), the epidermal cells have large vacuoles and hypertrophied nuclei before they disintegrate.

The fungus *Aspergillus clavatus* penetrates the body of *Drosophila* through the stigmata (tubercules), as well as through the articulations of the integument (Blockwitz 1929). Lepesme (1939) observed that *A. flavus* can enter the body of grasshoppers (*Schistocerca* and *Locusta*) through the thoracic stigmata. Working with larvae of the cecropia moth, *P. cecropia,* infected with *A. flavus,* Sussman (1952) obtained clear histological evidence that conidial hyphae can penetrate the integument by way of the membranous portion of the tubercules. Most of the specimens examined, however, appear to have been infected via the alimentary tract. For this reason, probably, he concludes that for direct penetration of the body wall to occur from the exterior surface requires rather special conditions of temperature and humidity; in contrast, these conditions are much more easily met in the digestive tract. Once within the body cavity of the insect, the fungus attacks all tissues except the epicuticular layer. The epidermis and the endocuticle, as well as the chitinous lining of the hindgut, are readily invaded. Similar observations have been made with infected pupae.

Yamaguchi (1961), working with *Aspergillus oryzae, A. flavus,* and *A. ochraceus* infections in silkworms, also has found fungal invasion occurring through the stigmata and cuticle. Hyphae penetrate the cuticle or stigmata immediately after germination, or else they grow on the cuticle and penetrate en masse. If the fungus penetrates the cuticle separately, no change can be observed in the cuticle; if they penetrate en masse, the penetrated area swells 9–14 μ in thickness in comparison with a normal cuticle of 4–5 μ in thickness.

Incipient stages of different fungus infections in the silkworm give different integumental appearances which may have diagnostic significance. According to Aoki (1958), for example, white muscardine (caused by *B. bassiana*) is characterized by "oily, wet, and vague spots" on the integument; green muscardine (*Spicaria pracina*) causes "black, dry, large spots"; yellow muscardine [*Paecilomyces* (=*Isaria*) *farinosa*] is distinguished by numerous black "pin-head like" spots, with those forming on the stigmata being quite large in size; black muscardine (the green muscardine of Europe; *M. anisopliae*) is characterized by spots similar to those of white muscardine, but each spot is distinguished by a black margin; and in the case of the *Aspergillus* muscardines, no obvious spots are formed but the integument takes on a glossy appearance.

In most entomogenous fungi after they develop within the body of the insect, killing it in the process, the hyphae force their way out through the body wall and appear on the surface of the integument. This penetration from the interior to the exterior of the insect has not been well studied, but apparently it occurs somewhat in the fashion in which the original penetration into the body occurred. As a result of the general mycosis, however, it is possible that the body wall of the insect has been weakened so that the emergence of the conidiophores and other hyphal strands is not as difficult and occurs more or less at random. In some insects, and with some mycoses, it is clear that because the cuticle is thinner at such places as the intersegmental folds emerging hyphae appear at these locations first, or exclusively. Lefebvre (1934) thinks that there probably is a great deal of mechanical action involved, for the hyphae seem to be under much pressure and their diameters are greatly decreased when forcing their way through the hard, striated cuticle. He also feels that since the hyphae swell as they are about to break through the exocuticle this indicates a mechanical action to some extent at least. Such swollen hyphae can be seen in the process of pushing pigment granules outward. In the larva of *G. mellonella* infected with *Entomophthora coronata*, the hyphal tips of the fungus emerging from the host are stopped momentarily in the exocuticle, and the tips become blunt and increase in size (Prasertphon, 1967). The conidiophores emerge singly or in groups. Sawyer (1933), for example, has observed histologically that the hyphae of *Entomophthora sphaerosperma* burst through the cuticle of the black-headed fireworm, *Rhopobota vacciniana*, in coalescing groups.

Whatever the mechanisms involved in aiding the hyphae and conidiophores to emerge through the body wall to the exterior of the insect, once the fungus has emerged it matures and forms fruiting bodies. Thus, allowing for those fungi that sporulate within the body of the host, the integument becomes the structure on which the fungus completes its development. As is expected, there is a great deal of variation in the exact manner in which the hyphae emerge and in the development and form of the fungus after it has emerged. Some fungi form scattered tufts of hyphae or conidiophores on the body surface, others appear at intersegmental folds, others cover the body entirely, and still others appear only as a stroma arising from a sclerotium formed within the body of the insect. Those fungi that cover the insect's body may appear as a soft, downy fluff, as a powdery or mealy covering, or as a hard crust, or a mixture of these.

In the case of *B. bassiana* infection in the European corn borer, Lefebvre (1934) observed that after emerging from the body wall a septum is formed across the hypha, thus producing a terminal cell which becomes an oval-shaped conidium that is soon budded off. The hypha continues to grow out from the body of the insect and soon develops conidia on zigzag phialides borne in whorls along the hyphal strands. These whorls or heads of conidium-bearing phialides increase in size and in number until the larva is completely covered with a fluffy or a powdery, mealy mat.

In the case of *Massospora,* which attacks cicadas, the conidiophores do not emerge through the insect integument but remain within the posterior segments of the insect's abdomen where they form hymenium-like layers around cavities of various sizes (Speare, 1921; Goldstein, 1929). A conidium is formed at the free end of each conidiophore which projects into the cavity. The conidiophores eventually shrink and collapse and are crushed by other hyphae. The mature conidia lie free in groups or clusters within the global pockets. As each successive body segment of the insect becomes filled with the fungus spores, the segment breaks away because of the pressure of the swelling mass of fungus hyphae. The exposed spore clusters then crumble or fall out in a single piece. Progressively more and more segments slough off until the insect, which is still living, flies about with head and thorax only.

Another similarly unusual type of fungus infection has been described in the adult seed-corn maggot, *Hylemya cilicrura,* by Strong *et al.* (1960). The fungus occurs in the hemocoel and causes a round hole in the integument on the midventral surface of the fly's abdomen. The diameter of the hole is usually one-third to one-half the maximum width of the abdomen. The fungus produces complete sterility in the fly; no ill effects are seen other than the sterility and the large hole from which the conidia drop out. Batko and Weiser (1965) have placed this fungus in a new genus, *Strongwellsea,* and they consider it to be related to *Massospora.*

One of the more unusual relationships between fungi and insects is that of the fungus *Septobasidium* (Basidiomycetes) with scale insects. The relationship is a mutualistic one; the fungus provides a home and shelter for the insect, while the insect provides the food for the fungus. The young scale insect is infected by the basidiospores of the fungus while creeping around trying to find a place to settle down on the host plant. The basidiospores germinate on the insect's integument and send numerous coiled hyphae through the integument into the body cavity. As the insect attaches itself to the host plant, the fungus grows and forms a hyphal mat over the insect. This mat, two or more layers in height, is traversed by tunnels and chambers. The tunnels with openings to the surface serve as exits for the young insects.

The hyphal mat may house a whole colony of scale insects, some of which may or may not be parasitized by the fungus. The parasitized insect is dwarfed and rendered sterile. Those not parasitized by the fungus are able to reproduce normally. The young scale insects do not always remain under the mat of fungus but instead may crawl out from one of the tunnels and find a new place to settle. Usually, they carry on their bodies basidiospores which germinate and a new plant–insect–fungus relationship is established.

B. Nematodes

Nematode infections in insects are not uncommon; in fact, Van Zwaluwenburg (1928) published a list showing that at that time at least 759 insect species (in 16 orders) were infected by nematodes. The majority of these nematode infections are in Lepidoptera, but some are in the Coleoptera, Orthoptera, and Diptera. Today this number has probably doubled or even tripled as more work is being done on the subject. More recently, Welch (1963, 1965) reviewed the nematodes associated with insects.

Christie (1941) divided nematodes associated with invertebrates into three groups: those that live in the alimentary tract of the invertebrate; those that are more or less closely related to free-living species; and those that parasitize the body cavity or tissues of their host. The first two categories mentioned are of little importance to this discussion, as the insect becomes infected through the ingestion of the nematode. The nematodes that are parasitic in the body cavity or the tissues of an insect are of interest here, for they gain entrance to the insect through ingestion or by penetration of the integument.

No complete study has been made on the penetration of the integument, but it has been noted that only those nematodes with stylets or odontostyles can penetrate the cuticle. According to Christie (1941), the stylet is "probably aided by the dissolving action of a chitin solvent secreted by one or more of the most anterior esophageal glands." In

1932 Bovien noted the jabbing of the stylet and the flow of a digestive enzyme. Welch (1959) confirmed the flow of such an enzyme from the dorsal esophageal gland in his studies of a species of *Howardula* parasitizing Drosophilidae.

The point of entrance and emergence through the integument has been observed by several investigators. Bovien (1932) found that *Scatonema wulkeri* penetrates any part of the body, and Christie (1936) noted that *Agamermis decaudata* usually penetrates its grasshopper host under the edges of the pronotum, between the abdominal segments, or at other locations where the integument is thin. Bovien observed that when the females of *S. wulkeri* emerge from the larva of *Scatopse fuscipes* [Diptera], they penetrate the cuticle at almost any point of the insect's body. The lack of preference as to the point of entrance and emergence may possibly be explained by Dickinson's (1959) observations that the larvae of *Heterodera* pierce hydrophobic better than hydrophilic surfaces because of an apparent response to a physical rather than a biological stimulus. Since insect cuticle is uniformly waxy and hydrophobic, this may explain the lack of preference.

The nematode *Tripius sciarae* attacks the larvae and pupae of the fly *Bradysia paupera*. According to Poinar and Doncaster (1965), the female nematode attaches herself to the host by an adhesive mass which is produced by digesting the front part of the unshed, last, larval cuticle. After attachment the nematode uses its spear and possibly also enzymes for penetration into the host.

Different nematodes are parasitic in different stages. Mermithids, which are the main nematode parasites of insects, are parasitic only during their larval stages. The eggs may be ingested by the insect or they may hatch in the open and the larvae penetrate the integument. After four molts the adult form is attained, and copulation occurs within the insect. The female adult then emerges through the body wall to lay her eggs in the soil.

Other nematodes may be parasitic in insects only in the adult stage. The eggs hatch in the soil and the larvae live their first three stages outside the insect. The third-stage larva penetrates the integument and enters the insect and molts to become a preadult parasitic larva. This larva develops into a parasitic adult; copulation occurs within the insect and the eggs are usually passed out the anus.

Continuous parasitism is less common, but it has been noted in *S. fuscipes* by the nematode *S. atonema wulkeri*. The eggs are laid in the body cavity of the host; they hatch and the larvae grow to the adult stage. The adults copulate within the body cavity and remain there. A free-living stage has been observed, but it is of a very short duration (Bovien, 1932).

Emergence of a nematode from the body of the insect can occur through the anus, gonopore, or integument. Mermithids generally emerge through the intersegmental folds, and upon emergence cause the death of their hosts. If death is not immediate, the insect usually dies in a few days as a result of the loss of vital tissues consumed by the mermithid. Other nematodes that emerge through the body wall do not cause the death of the insect; instead, they cause some permanent damage to the insect's growth, reproductive abilities, and flight mechanisms, to name a few. Also, the formation of intersexes is an interesting effect of nematode parasitism.

C. Entry through Wounds and Entry by Means of Vectors

Once the integument has been damaged in any way, one of the main defenses of the insect is broken and disease may result. Bacteria in particular can be secondary invaders of an insect through a wound caused by fungi, nematodes, or parasitic and predaceous insects. Some bacteria pass through a wound produced mechanically and are the sole cause of an insect's disease.

Although the bacterium *M. nigrofasciens* can pass through the integument of a June beetle larva without the aid of wounds, an injury to the integument greatly increases the likelihood of infection (Northrup, 1914). This same micrococcus is also pathogenic to the cockroach *P. americana* if the insect is wounded, but it only affects the legs of the insect.

Stutzer and Wsorow (1927) have found that a "Spring disease" among caterpillars of *E. segetum* is partially caused by the entrance of *Pseudomonas septica* through the damaged integument of the insect.

Many bacteria cause disease only after a fungus has invaded the insect's body through the integument. *Pseudomonas aeruginosa* has been found by Lepesme (1937) to be a secondary invader after *A. flavus* has invaded the grasshopper *Schistocerca gregaria.* This same bacterium is highly pathogenic to larvae of the wax moth, *G. mellonella,* if it enters through a wound in the integument.

Insects that are predaceous or parasitic on other insects also transmit pathogens by biting through the integument or puncturing it with a contaminated stinger or ovipositor. Infection by this route is not common but it has been reported in some instances for virus, bacteria, protozoa, and fungi (see Tanada, 1963, 1967; Müller-Kögler, 1965). Some predators and parasites are also susceptible to the same pathogen that infects the insect host, and they serve in the multiplication, distribution, and transmission of the pathogen. For example, microsporidian-infected parasites, such as *Apanteles* sp. or *Pteromalus* sp., may transmit the microsporidian to their host insect after ovipositing in the host (Blunck, 1952; Tanada, 1955a; Weiser, 1961; Laigo and Tamashiro, 1967). This mode of transmission is uncommon, for usually the parasitic insect is not diseased itself; the ovipositor is merely contaminated.

The mechanical transmission of bacteria on the ovipositor of insect parasites has been reported by Metalnikov and Metalnikov (1935), Toumanoff (1959), and Vago and Kurstak (1965). When the ovipositor of the parasite *Nemeritis canescens* is contaminated with spores of *Bacillus thuringiensis,* the parasite transmits the bacterium as it stings its host, the larva of *Ephestia kuhniella* (Vago and Kurstak, 1965). Although insect parasites themselves are not susceptible, they are able to transmit viruses to their hosts (Thompson and Steinhaus, 1950; Bird, 1953, 1961; Laigo and Tamashiro, 1966). In tests conducted by Thompson and Steinhaus (1950), the parasite *Apanteles medicaginis,* after exposure to larvae of *Colias eurytheme* infected with a nuclear polyhedrosis virus, transmits the virus to a progressively fewer number from the first to the third series of larvae. Laigo and Tamashiro (1966) report, however, that *Apanteles marginiventris* transmits the virus from infected larvae of *Spodoptera mauritia acronyctoides* to other larvae not in a logical order but at random, that is, the sequence of transmission does not occur chronologically in the order in which the larvae are stung. The viruses used in these studies infect the integument and so they may be transmitted by the parasites to this tissue in addition to other susceptible host tissues.

Smirnoff (1959) has reported an interesting case of transmission by the sucking mouth parts of a predaceous bug, *Pilophorus uhleri,* which can transmit a nuclear polyhedrosis virus when it feeds on the larvae of a sawfly, *Neodiprion swainei.*

VII. Noninfectious Diseases and Abnormalities of the Integument

A. *Physical Injuries*

Physical injuries to the integument can occur in many ways and cause various amounts of harm to the integument and the insect itself (see

Day and Oster, 1963). The force of gravity, percussion, mechanical stimulation, air pressure, and sound upon the integument may cause little or no injury, or a great amount of injury. Other physical forces that can be brought to play against the integument are temperature, high-frequency electric fields, radiation, desiccation, and wounds. Little is known about the effects of many of these forces; what is known is discussed below.

1. Gravity

Sullivan and McCauley (1960) found that most insects possess an overall resistance to the forces of acceleration and deceleration during space flight. The integument, particularly that of small, hard-bodied insects, can apparently withstand great stresses. Tests on *Tribolium confusum* have revealed that at 20,600 $\times$ g it takes 73 minutes to produce 50% mortality. The large, hard-shelled Japanese beetle, *Popillia japonica,* has proved to be the least resistant to the forces of gravity; 2 minutes at 10,000 $\times$ g produce about 85% mortality.

Sullivan and McCauley have shown that the differences in resistance are attributable to differences in mass and in the nature of the exoskeleton. Male houseflies, *Musca domestica,* although they have relatively thin integuments, are small and can withstand multiple g values much better than the larger Japanese beetle. Those insects killed during the centrifuging period have shattered integuments and are eviscerated.

2. Percussion

The effects of percussion on the integument are similar to those of gravity: a shattering of the integument leading to evisceration and death of the insect. In a comparison of the effects of percussion on adult and immature stages of the granary weevil, *Sitophilus granarius,* Bailey (1962) found that adults are killed at velocities much lower than those needed to kill the soft-bodied immature stages. Bailey explains this by the degree of flattening that an insect undergoes. Any flattening causes an increase in internal body pressure; since immature insects have soft cuticles, they undergo extreme flattening and a large internal pressure, and the cuticle bursts easily. Adult insects withstand flattening much better and therefore the cuticle does not rupture as easily at lower velocities. When the immature stages are present in grains, intense forces that cause excessive breakage of the grains are necessary to kill the insects.

3. Desiccation

Desiccation is described as the rapid passage of water out of an insect's body at an abnormal rate and usually results in the death of the insect. It can occur under a variety of conditions: (1) when a certain percentage of the molecules in the wax layer of the epicuticle has been removed; (2) by the removal of wax the entire distance down to the lipid–protein interface by abrasion; (3) by an increase in temperature to the extent that the molecules of the lipid-protein layer become disorganized; (4) by the application of oil or solvents, thus removing the wax layer; and (5) by the application of a wide variety of insecticides. Of these, desiccation through abrasion by inert dusts and other particles is the only physical force mentioned.

The action of inert dusts is to cause abrasion of the thin lipid layer of the epicuticle, thus breaking down the protective layer which prevents rapid water loss. Several investigators (Alexander *et al.*, 1944; Wigglesworth, 1945; Beament, 1945; Hurst, 1948) found that inert dusts do not cause water loss in dead or motionless insects and have concluded that these dusts cause abrasion of the epicuticle as the insect moves over them. Alexander *et al.* report that adult beetles and beetle larvae are affected differently by inert dusts. Among the adult beetles tested, they observed that abrasion of the epicuticle increases with the hardness of the particles and with the angular surface of the particles; effectiveness also increases with decreasing particle size.

Some inert dusts remove lipoid material from the epicuticle through absorption rather than abrasion (Wigglesworth, 1945; Hurst, 1948; Jones, 1955; Ebeling and Wagner, 1959; Ebeling, 1964). Dusts that are the least abrasive and the most sorptive are the most effective. Ebeling (1961) found that the effective dusts are silica aerogels, silica gels, activated carbon, sorptive clays, sand, and carborundum. They produce very rapid desiccation and quick death of the insect involved.

4. Wounds

Wounds to the integument can be caused by anything sharp such as glass, stones, and sticks. One interesting cause of a wound to an insect has been reported by Johnson (1953) to be the epidermal hairs of a plant. French bean plants (*Phaseolus vulgaris*) have small, hooked epidermal hairs that are extremely injurious to aphids frequenting the plants. These hairs cover the petioles, stems, and undersurfaces of the leaves and are most dense on growing shoots. As the aphids move across a leaf or move their legs while feeding, the hairs may puncture the intersegmental membranes of the legs or even the integument. The hooks become securely embedded as the aphids try to free themselves. Often the hooks slide out when the aphids cease to struggle, but more frequently the legs are pulled off. Becoming caught on more than one hook can lead to bleeding, starvation, exhaustion, and even death of the aphids.

In general, more important than the wound itself is the healing of the wound and the abnormalities that can result in the integument. In the healing process, the epidermal cells surrounding the wound are activated and migrate toward the wound opening where there is a simultaneous aggregation of hemocytes. Mitoses begin in the peripheral area where the cells have been depleted because of this migration. As the cells build up in number, they spread over the wound until the cellular continuity has been restored and then a new cuticle is secreted.

When an insect is wounded, a darkening generally develops around the wounded tissues. Phenolases, which are responsible for hardening and darkening of the cuticle, are also involved in darkening of the wounded tissues in most insects. Lai-Fook (1966) investigated these phenolases in *Calpodes ethlius, Sarcophaga bullata, Musca autumnalis, Tenebrio* larvae, and *Rhodnius* adults. In *C. ethlius,* the phenolase associated with wounds is produced by the activation of a proenzyme and both the proenzyme and activator are localized in the epicuticle. The cuticle of *S. bullata* contains both a phenolase used in puparium formation and prophenolase which is activated on injury. The phenolase produced from the prophenolase in *Sarcophaga* during wounding differs in substrate specificity from the phenolase already present in the cuticle for puparium formation. According to Lai-Fook (1966), phenolase activity is limited by the availability of substrate molecules whose concentration and types are controlled by the epidermis. The wounded dark cuticle appears to be analogous to a partial exocuticle by reducing permeability of the integument when the epicuticle is damaged. The phenolase, however, may not be present in all insect cuticle. Lai-Fook has found that phenolase is lacking in the larval cuticle of *M. autumnalis,* which has a hard but colorless puparium.

Wigglesworth (1937) observed several abnormalities occurring in the integument as healing takes place. He reports that as the epidermal cells spread over a wound they do not always come directly together but instead one layer overlays another. In this case it is not always the uppermost layer that becomes the new epidermis. The innermost layer becomes the basement membrane and this begins producing the epidermis, but sometimes the layer above the new epidermis becomes a mass of more-or-less disorganized cells resembling the basement membrane. Even after the new cuticle has been formed, this layer of cells can still be detected on the outer surface of the integument.

Another common abnormality in wound healing is the occurrence of irregular mitoses, polyploidy, and giant cell formation among the epidermal cells covering the wound. The nuclei of the cells may attain enormous sizes, multipolar mitotic figures are frequent, or the dividing cells may show equatorial plates containing 100 or more chromosomes. Eventually all these abnormal nuclei disintegrate and disappear, and a normal-appearing epidermis remains with no sign of the wound or the abnormal cells.

Wigglesworth (1940) has shown another abnormality in the integument of a *Rhodnius* larva wounded by burning. When the cells surrounding the burn begin to migrate in and repair the wound, they carry with them the potentiality to form the type of cuticle characteristic of the region from which they came. Thus, at the next molt, the integumental pattern shows a centripetal displacement. These migrating cells also carry with them their latent adult capacities, so that upon metamorphosis they show a corresponding displacement of the adult pattern. Because of this, what may be a black zone in the larva may be a pale zone in the adult, but the displacement causes a new, striking, integumental pattern.

The reaction of the insect integument to grafts is apparently associated with the presence of a gradient in the integument. Barbier (1966) successfully introduced homologous grafts from corresponding segments of donors even when the two individuals were not of the same sex. The implantation of a graft obtained from a segment other than the one on which it is placed (heterologous homograft) produces abnormal reactions, however.

B. Chemical Injuries

There are few, if any, chemicals that are free in nature and are capable of producing damage to the insect integument. An antibiotic, griseofulvin, that apparently interferes with the biosynthesis of chitin in fungus cell wall, affects the normal molting of larvae of the mosquito *Aedes atropalpus* (Anderson, 1966). Mosquito larvae reared in a medium containing griseofulvin (1) develop gross anatomical changes in the cuticle, (2) undergo detachment of somatic muscles from the integument, and (3) undergo a prolonged molting cycle. With the exception of the last-mentioned effect, all the anomalies become apparent during an instar subsequent to the one initially exposed to the compound. The anomalous development of the cuticle causes detachment of the muscles from the integument rather than an effect on the muscles themselves.

The steroid hormone ecdysone is known to function in the process of molting and cuticle sclerotization. Hora *et al.* (1966) found several sterol derivatives that inhibit postecdysial hardening and sclerotization of the cuticle of *Pyrrhocoris.* These compounds are derivatives of cholestane and $24\beta_F$-methylcholestane. They assume that these compounds may have ecdysone-antagonistic action. When high dosages of ecdysone and 20-hydroxyecdysone are injected into the hemocoel of diapausing European corn borers, *O. nubilalis,* they cause apolysis, a separation of the epidermal cells from the cuticle (Beck and Shane, 1969). The apolytic response appears to be pathological because Beck and Shane have obtained only moribund larvae-pupal mosaics after treatment with the hormones. The apolysis is an abortive molting cycle in which the insects show a variety of responses, including (1) complete absence of pupal characteristics, (2) mosaics of larval and pupal cuticular patches, or (3) a partially tanned nearly pupal form. Madhavan and Schneiderman (1968) also have caused apolysis in *Cecropia* and *Cynthia* moths when they injected crystalline ecdysone and an inhibitor (mitomycin C) of DNA synthesis into the pupae or into the ligated abdomens of the adults.

Man-made chemicals, such as insecticides, produce damage not only to the integument but to the entire insect as well. Although man has made insecticides and seen them work, it is generally stated that insecticide penetration is relatively little understood (Hoskins, 1940; Shepard, 1951; Richards, 1951, 1953; Ebeling, 1964).

Insecticides have been divided into two basic groups according to their action: stomach and contact poisons. Stomach poisons are used primarily on chewing insects. Contact poisons are generally used on sucking insects and can act in two ways; they can kill by contact and penetration of the integument, or they can close the spiracles and cause suffocation of the insect. Some insecticides, however, may function as either a stomach or a contact poison. We are interested only in contact insecticides in this section.

Contact insecticides have been divided into different categories by many workers. Shepard (1951) breaks them down into direct contact insecticides, sprays killing insects in flight, and residual contact insecticides which are effective even though the insects are not directly contacted. Richards (1951) classifies contact insecticides according to their penetration powers; one group is made up of those compounds and mixtures that destructively affect the cuticle composition, while the other group consists of those mixtures and toxins that penetrate the cuticle without producing detectable alteration. He then places dry, residual insecticides in the second group except when they are abrasives, and insecticides with an oil base in the first group.

In order for most contact insecticides to do their job, they must first penetrate the integument. As already stated, the waxy or lipoid layer and tectocuticle (the cement layer) of the epicuticle serve as protection for the insect against just such occurrences (Wigglesworth, 1942). Insecticides are commonly made up of two or more compounds, one that disrupts or penetrates this barrier and one that is the actual insecticide. Most insecticides are oil or water based although some contain detergents.

Lipids act as solvents, and any oil probably mixes more or less thoroughly with the waxes of the epicuticle and partially disrupts them. Once the waxes have been removed, the toxic half of the insecticide penetrates the rest of the integument and kills the insect. Oils cannot usually penetrate the tectocuticle but several detergents can, so insects with the cement layer over the waxy layer are treated with detergent-based insecticides. Often an oil and a detergent together serve as a very effective base.

Examples of water-based insecticides are arsenic trioxide and sodium fluoride; those soluble in fats or fat solvents are the pyrethrins; and nicotine and hydrogen cyanide are soluble in both water and fats. All insecticides need not be in liquid form to penetrate the cuticle; nicotine, pyridine, and piperidine in the gaseous state pass through the integument of certain insects quite readily.

Penetration of insecticides occurs more readily through some parts of the integument than others. For example, pyrethrins penetrate very readily, particularly through the articular membranes. They then pass into the trichogen cells and the hypodermis. DDT penetrates the thin tarsal cuticle of *Musca* much more readily than in any other area of its body. Therefore a fly standing on a surface treated with DDT may be killed merely by standing in the poison (Hayes and Liu, 1947).

Reports of specific injury to the integument by insecticides and other chemicals have been made by several investigators. Wigglesworth (1945) reports that the wax layer of the cuticle of whole insects is disrupted by chloroform, thus allowing increased evaporation through the cuticle. Ludwig (1948), in testing the effects of peanut oil and ether, also has found that the wax layer is disrupted and water loss is increased.

A study of diptheria toxin by Pappenheimer and Williams (1952) has revealed that the toxin affects the integument of diapausing pupae in two ways. (1) The epithelium gradually loses its normal intimate attachment to the overlying pupal cuticle and undergoes a process of retraction throughout the insect. This is accompanied, in certain instances, by degenerative changes in the region of the legs and antennae. (2) The toxin also blocks wound healing at sites where transparent plastic windows have been placed. The usual development of connective tissue and outgrowth of hypodermis fail to occur and the defect in the integument is never repaired.

Heavy metals have also been found to damage the integument. Mercuric chloride, when applied to bedbugs or other soft-bodied insects, precipitates the hypodermal protein (Shafer, 1911). 4,6-Dinitro-*o*-cresol (DNOC) has been found to stain the epidermal cells after passing through the cuticle, presumably also precipitating the proteins (Stellwaag and Staudenmayer, 1940).

An example of an insect with an integument specialized to withstand exaggerated environmental conditions and conditions under which insecticides act is the petroleum fly, *Psilopa petrolii.* This fly develops in the shallow pools of waste petroleum (tar pits) of Southern California. The larva breathes through posterior spiracles positioned at the surface of the pool. The cuticle of the larva is highly impermeable to the oil, and the insect leads a good life, obtaining its food from bacteria and other animals caught in the oil. As specialized as the integument is, the larva can only survive in oil that has lost its more volatile, less viscous materials (Thorpe, 1930; Shepard, 1951).

For an account of the general pathological changes induced in insects by chemicals, the reader is referred to the review by Brown (1963).

Colchicine, a classic mitotic inhibitor, has been shown to modify the postembryonic differentiation of insect antennae (Vogt, 1947), wings (Sláma, 1962), and pupae (Ilan and Quastel, 1966). Ilan and Quastel report that colchicine effects the DNA and RNA synthesis of the pupae of *T. molitor.*

The discovery that juvenile hormone is essential for the growth and metamorphosis of insects, and at the same time may result in their death when present in excess at critical periods in insect development, has led to proposals that it be used as an insecticide (Williams, 1967). This idea has assumed practicability when topical application of the juvenile hormone has been found to cause lethal effects (Williams, 1956; Vinson and Williams, 1967; Srivastava and Gilbert, 1968, 1969); when this hormone and substances with related activity have been synthesized

(Braun *et al.*, 1968; Bowers, 1968; Srivastava and Gilbert, 1969); and when substances extracted from plants have shown juvenile hormonelike activity (Sláma and Williams, 1965, 1966; Saxena and Williams, 1966; Carayon and Thouvenin, 1966). The molting hormone (ecdysone) and plant extracts containing hormonal activity also cause larvae to attain pupal characteristics when the hormones are applied topically (Sato *et al.*, 1968; Robbins *et al.*, 1968).

Cecropia oil, when injected subcuticularly into newly formed pupae of *T. molitor,* produces juvenilized cuticle in a high proportion of adults, but when injected into middle-aged pupae does not cause this effect (Zlotkin and Levinson, 1968). Juvenilized cuticle differs anatomically from normal pupal cuticle (Zlotkin and Levinson, 1969). Moreover, juvenilized cuticle of the adult does not resemble the cuticle of any developmental stage and is considered an abnormality. Its distinguishing features are a lack of differentiation into exo- and endocuticle, a loose stratification, an absence of pore canals, and an increased thickness. The structure and stain reactions of juvenilized cuticle strongly resemble pupal endocuticle.

Derivatives of farnesoic acid are known to have juvenile hormonelike activity in the silkworm. Spielman and Skaff (1967) showed that these derivatives, when placed in water in which larvae of the mosquitoes *Aedes aegypti* and *Culex pipiens* are living, cause inhibition of the metamorphosis and ecdysis of the larvae. Some of the individuals retain larval characters in the pupal stage, others fail to undergo adult ecdysis and instead become hardened within the pupal skin, and still others develop into adult males with unrotated terminalia caused by abnormal hardening of the cuticle.

Topical applications of fatty acids, fatty alcohols (axerophthol, nerolidol, and farnesol), and colchicine suppress the normal development of immature nymphs of *Pyrrhocoris apterus* to adults (Sláma, 1962). Farnesol, when applied topically to rice stem borer larvae in the last stage, produces a high degree of metathetely and mortality. When it is applied to last-stage nymphs of *Periplaneta,* it leads to the appearance of short-winged adults (Fukaya, 1962).

C. Nutritional Diseases

Although many studies have been done on nutrition in insects, few observations have been made other than those concerning the effects of deficiencies on growth and metamorphosis. Since in most insects a deficiency in any of the essential nutrients merely causes a cessation of growth and prolonged survival, detailed histopathological studies have been slighted by most workers. Much of the work involving nutrition has been done on *Drosophila, Aedes, Tribolium,* and *Tenebrio,* with everyone reporting many of the same effects. Those reports concerning nutrition and the integument are mentioned below.

In a chapter on nutritional diseases in *Insect Pathology, An Advanced Treatise,* House (1963) presents a charted summary of the histopathological effects of nutritional factors on insects. Under causes of abnormalities of the integument, he places proteins, vitamins, and starvation. We have found no references to integumental abnormalities attributable to carbohydrates, minerals, or water. Fatty acids and sterols, however, may affect wing development in adult Lepidoptera (Fraenkel and Blewett, 1946a,b).

Haydak (1937) reports that newly emerged honeybees, *Apis mellifera,* when fed on pure sugar and deprived of protein, show significant abnormalities of the integument. Butler (1943) also studied honeybees fed protein-deficient diets in which he also noted several abnormalities. The adult bees, especially the nurse bees, use their integumental nitrogenous supplies in order to make up for the deficiency. As a result, the chitin becomes very brittle, hair is lost, and the wings break off.

Vitamins are generally important in the tanning and coloring of the insect integument. Fraenkel and Chang (1954) observed the effects of vitamin B_T (carnitine) deficiency in *T. molitor.* They report three main types of symptoms: (1) The larva dies almost immediately after the molt and the integument becomes soft and light in color; (2) the larva dies sometime after the molt, and the cuticle usually shows black spots although otherwise normal; and (3) the larva dies in a stage intermediate between one and two and the cuticle is soft but a little darker. Naton (1961) also found that carnitine is essential in coloring and tanning of the new cuticle in several beetles. The cuticle of aposymbiotic insects is often unnaturally light colored (Brooks, 1963). This is apparently associated with a deficiency in the nutrients provided to the host insect by the symbionts. In Section II,A it has already been pointed out that in addition to nutrition, hormones, light, and genetic factors may affect the color of the integument.

Starved insects usually show a loss of nutrient reserves. As glycogen, fats, proteins, and so on, are depleted from the tissues, the cells begin to degenerate and abnormalities appear. In a study based on starvation, Lower (1959) reports that there is a permanent and often lethal deformation in the cuticle of the New Zealand armyworm, *Persectania ewingii.* Chemical and structural changes occur that prevent the close union of the layers of endocuticle secreted during the pre- and poststarvation periods.

With the advent of artificial diet or medium for the rearing of many Lepidoptera, evidence has accumulated that a deficiency of fatty acids and sterols in the diet causes abnormal wing development. This has been shown in the cercropia and other saturniid moths (Riddiford, 1968).

D. Physiological and Metabolic Diseases

Diseases that result from deranged physiology and metabolism may arise from diverse causes, such as physical, chemical, nutritional, and biotic factors. Some of the diseases of the integument described previously can also be included in this category. Other abnormalities, such as genetic diseases, teratologies, and neoplastic diseases are discussed in succeeding sections, but they can also be included here. Accordingly, we wish to cite only a few examples that have not been included in these other sections.

Roussel (1967) found that pigmentation of the integument of *Gryllus bimaculatus* is controlled strictly by the corpus allatum, the absence of which induces black pigmentation. The control by the corpus allatum is a direct one and acts on the integument. Color changes in adults of *Schistocerca gregaria* are also affected by allatectomy and sectioning of the nerves of corpora allata (Pener, 1967). In the roach *P. americana*, cuticular tanning stops when the ventral nerve cord is cut (Mills, 1967). Control stimulus seems to pass through the nerve cord because when it is stimulated *in vivo* the terminal ganglion releases the tanning hormone, bursicon.

According to Madhavan and Schneiderman (1968), ecdysone causes apolysis, separation of pupal cuticle from the epidermis, when it is inoculated into *Polyphemus* pupae and ligated abdomens of adult *Cercropia* and *Cynthia* moths. Apolysis occurs even when DNA synthesis is blocked by an inhibitor, mitomycin C, which inhibits pupal–adult transformation. The response of pupal epidermal cells of *Polyphemus* to ecdysone differs before and after DNA synthesis, however. Prior to DNA synthesis pupal epidermal cells respond to ecdysone only by apolysis, but after DNA synthesis they respond by secreting a cuticle. Adult epidermal cells, however, can secrete a cuticle without DNA synthesis. Beck and Shane (1969) also noted that ecdysone and 20-hydroxyecdysone, when inoculated into diapausing larvae of the European corn borer, induce apolysis that appears to be pathological.

E. Genetic Diseases and Aberrations

Insects, similar to all other forms of life, are not immune to the spontaneous occurrence of mutation. Because they are so short-lived and the power of selection is so great, however, very few mutations occur en masse in a population. Work that has been done in this field is almost totally limited to studies on *B. mori, A. mellifera, Drosophila, C. pipiens, Ephestia kuhniella, Bracon hebetor,* and *Tribolium* spp. Of these insects, probably the work with *Drosophila* is the most published.

Melanosis is a common hereditary diease in *Drosophila.* It is characterized by pigmented spots appearing on the integument of the fly. Rizki (1953) has reported in strain 42P of *Drosophila willistoni* that dark-brown or black pigmented spots appear on the hardened regions of the sclerites of the larvae. 42P is a recessive lethal with 100% penetrance in the homozygous condition. Death of the larvae usually occurs in the third instar; about 30% of the larvae develop spots in the cuticle.

"Tumorous head" is another condition found in *Drosophila.* Gardner and Woolf (1949) used the term in a broad sense to describe abnormal growths or enlargements on the head of *Drosophila melanogaster.* It is a hereditary trait and is not related to neoplasia. The trait is characterized in a variety of ways by growths on the head region showing all gradations of size and no localized region. There are growths that cover a few facets of the eye as well as massive growths that cover the whole head. They usually show evidence of tissue destruction in the integument. This particular condition is an interaction between a recessive, sex-linked gene and a semidominant, autosomal gene, and is not seen unless both genes are present.

Another mutant of *D. melanogaster* has been designated X20. It is a lethal mutant producing four types of embryos: (1) no blastoderm formation and no cellular differentiation, (2) malformation of blastoderm and an irregular germ band, (3) complete hypodermis formation but little or no formation of nervous tissue, and (4) no hypodermis formation in the ventral region and therefore the gut is allowed to protrude through the body wall (Ede, 1956). The fundamental process of differentiation is affected so that a proper blastoderm is not formed. In the normal blastoderm ventral ectoderm cells become part epidermis and part neuroblasts; while in the mutants, it forms either epidermis [type (3)] or nervous tissue [type (4)] but not both.

According to Barigozzi (1963), the manifestation of melanotic tumors in *Drosophila,* with which a cytoplasmic activity is associated, is controlled by a complex genotype. There seems to exist an exogenous factor which acts persistently upon the second chromosome. Barigozzi suggests that a particulate episome-like factor may be involved.

Tanaka (1953) observed several mutations in *B. mori* that involve the color and shape of the body. The color patterns depend largely on distribution of pigments in the dermal cells and the primary cuticle. There is a large range of patterns, all determined genetically. In fact, Tanaka lists 51 different patterns ranging from plain (white over whole body), striped, black, eye-spotted, to brown.

Several body shapes can also be attributed to genetic abnormalities of the integument. In the *elongate* shape, the first and second abdominal segments are unusually elongated as the result of a stretching of the intersegmental folds. The mutant *stick* appears as a slender, hard body; it affects the hardness of the cuticle and allows little flexibility to the larvae. The mutant *knobbed* expresses itself as dermal protuberances on several segments of the insect.

Translucent skin is another hereditary factor in *B. mori.* This phenotype is attributable to several genes relating to the quantity of urate crystals in the epidermal cells. A few of the translucent mutants are lethal, and all are recessive characters. In the translucent skin of the mutant larva, smaller amounts of crystalline uric acid are found than in the skin of normal larvae, and the amounts vary proportionally with the transparency of the skin (Shimizu, 1943). From his studies, Shimizu concludes that the genetic factors for translucent skin play important physiological roles in the quantitative changes in uric acid, namely, the amount precipitated in the skin at the larval stage, the amount excreted at the mature larval stage, and the quantity produced at the pupal stage.

The factor *lemon-lethal* in *B. mori* affects the hardening of the chitinous parts of the embryo and the larva. At high expressivity the mouthparts of the fully developed embryo are so soft that they cannot bite through the egg shell. Other mutants may be able to hatch but are unable to eat and die of starvation (Tsujita, 1953).

Aruga (1939, 1940) has also reported on a genetically based pigmentation in *B. mori.* The gene *brown ursa* in a heterozygous condition produces numerous dark-brown dots on a reddish-brown ground color of the skin of the mutant larva. In a homozygous condition (U^{br}/U^{br}), the young larva dies during the fourth molt because it cannot cast off its old skin.

T. Hukuhara of the University of Tokyo summarized the genetic diseases that affect the integument of the silkworm in a personal communication. The hereditary traits in *B. mori* amount to 211. Most of the mutants can be distinguished from the normal silkworm by structural and color changes. In this sense they can be said to be abnormal or malformed. However, there is difficulty in defining a normal silkworm because no wild type of this insect exists. At present the normal characters of *B. mori* are only tentatively determined by silkworm geneticists, so a discussion of the definition of malformation or deformity would not be very fruitful. Hereditary abnormalities appear in such external organs as the integument, segments, thoracic legs, abdominal legs, ocelli, spiracles, caudal horn, as well as in such internal organs as muscles, ganglions, dorsal vessels, tracheae, silk glands, and Malpighian tubules.

Hukuhara stated further that one of the most extensively studied hereditary deformities in the silkworm is controlled by *E* pseudoallelic genes. *E* genes are arranged in close sequence at the end (0.0) of chromosome VI. At present 20 genes are known to belong to the *E* complex loci. They have similar pleiotropic action on several tissues and organs of ectodermal origin. For example, the E^N/E^N embryo, which dies before blastokinesis, has a pair of thoracic legs on each segment from the first to the eighth abdominal segments, two caudal horns, only three pairs of rudimentary spiracles, and a poorly developed tracheal system. In $E^N/—$ larvae a pair of extra crescents are often present on the third abdominal segment and the star spots are always absent. Larvae with malformed segments sometimes appear among *E* mutants. The appearance of malformed segments and the incidence of malformation are characteristic of each *E* gene. For example, in 0.3% of $E^{Ca}/—$ larvae, the fourth abdominal segment is fused with the fifth, or the fifth with the sixth, while in 5% of $E^D/+$ larvae, the third thoracic segment is fused with the abdominal segment, or the first with the second abdominal segment. When the E^{Ca} and E^D genes are combined, 15.7% of E^{Ca}/E^D larvae have malformed segments from the third thoracic to the sixth abdominal segments. The body wall of the silkworm larva has its origin in a dorsal extension of the lateral margins of the germ band, that is, the extensions from either side of the germ band meet and fuse along the median line on the dorsal side, forming a continuous wall. If the extensions are asymmetrical, the fusion on the dorsal side becomes irregular; a part of the extension remains free in a segment or fuses with the extension in the neighboring segment. *E* genes seem to act in the course of wall formation.

For detailed information on genetic abnormalities in the silkworm, we refer the reader to the text by Yokoyama (1959).

In a volume on the genetics of *Tribolium* and related species, Sokoloff (1966) lists the results of extensive investigations into the genetics of abnormal structures in various Coleoptera, especially *Tribolium confusum* and *T. castaneum.* He attributes certain elytral variations in *T. castaneum* to the action of specific genes, for example: (1) *Due*—a sex-linked, incomplete recessive expressed in *Tribolium* as divergent elytra, with occasional blisters on the wing; (2) *Te*—an incomplete recessive, sex-linked, and lethal or semilethal in *Tribolium;* the phenotypic expression of this gene is truncated or bent-down elytra; (3) *Ble*—a recessive gene expressed as blistered elytra; the blisters can appear either at metamorphosis or may be visible in the pupa; (4) *Sh*—gene of linkage group VII and expressed as short elytra; (5) *Pe*—a recessive gene expressed as divergent and narrow elytra coming to a sharp point at the distal ends.

F. Nongenetic Teratologies

There is currently so much confusion as to which teratological abnormalities are truly genetic in origin and which are nongenetic that any attempt at this point in time to distinguish them is frustrating. This is especially the case with the so-called nongenetic teratologies. There are in the literature many reports of teratologies caused by environmental influences which later are found to have their origin in genetic causes or in a combination of genetic and environmental causes.

Among the teratologies that have been reported to arise from nongenetic causes are the following examples that occur in beetles: development of rudimentary wings in larvae, partial fusion of body segments, variation in number and position of spines on the last segment, absence of an eye, variations in size, shape, and position of the elytra, occurrence of blisters on the cuticle, numerous abnormalities and distortions of the appendages, anomalies of wing venation, and so on. A comprehensive study on the teratologies of the beetle *T. molitor,* has been completed by Steinhaus and Zeikus (1968a,b; 1969) and Zeikus and Steinhaus (1968, 1969). Although they have described some of the teratologies listed above, most of their detailed study has been confined to the teratology designated as pupal-winged adult, in which the adult retains the wings and elytra of the pupal stage.

Similar teratologies may occur in other insect orders and invertebrates (Vago and Sauvezon, 1969). These teratologies are caused by physical factors such as temperature, humidity, and radiation; nutritional factors, for example, vitamins and fatty acids; chemical factors, for example, toxins and chemical insecticides; and infectious microorganisms. Apparently, in most cases these adverse factors affect the hormones involved in metamorphosis. There are innumerable examples of these factors causing teratologies and we shall not discuss them except for the effect of toxins of *B. thuringiensis* and of entomophthorous fungi, since these pathogens are important in the microbial control of insect pests.

Burgerjon and Biache (1967) found that the thermostable toxins from different serotypes of *B. thuringiensis,* when fed at sublethal doses to several species of Lepidoptera and to the housefly, produce teratologies in pupae and adults. In Lepidoptera the pupae may lack the palp and proboscis, and in the fly the adult has atrophied mouthparts caused by a reduction in the labrum epipharynx. Further studies have shown that the thermostable toxin also produces teratological effects in the Colorado potato beetle, *Leptinotarsa decemlineata,* and these effects are comparable to those in the Lepidoptera (Burgerjon *et al.*, 1969). The effects involve mainly the buccal parts, eyes, and antennae, and are evidenced by the atrophy of these organs. In the beetle, however, modifications other than atrophy may also occur, such as an abnormal antenna in the form of a club or claw, protuberances on the eyes and palps, and the transformation of a paired to an unpaired part of the labial palp.

Two entomophthorous fungi, *Entomophthora coronata* and *E. apiculata,* produce substances that are toxic to lepidopterous larvae when inoculated into larval hemocoels (Prasertphon and Tanada, 1969). These toxins generally cause larvae to turn black prior to their death. In the corn earworm, *Heliothis zea,* which is somewhat resistant to the toxin, a massive dose of the mycotoxin, when inoculated into the larva a few days prior to pupation, causes the formation of an abnormal pupa whose ventral integument remains larval in character. Such an abnormal pupa has an enlarged abdomen, with a head and a thorax of larval character, and retains the prolegs but lacks adult wings, antennae, or legs.

Needless to say, whether the cause of a teratology is genetic or nongenetic, if the abnormality is apparent from external examination of the insect, the integument is almost certainly involved. Therefore, to the extent that the integument is abnormal, we may consider the teratology as representative of a disease of the integument as well as perhaps other structures or organ systems of the insect. As to the precise cause of the majority of nongenetic teratologies, we are in a sea of ignorance. Such environmental or external factors as temperature, humidity, and nutrition have been implicated by some authors, but these conclusions are usually based more on conjecture or casual observation than on precise and accurate experimental proof (see Arendsen Hein, 1920, 1924; Singh-Pruthi, 1924; Balazuc, 1948; Fyg, 1964). In some cases, however, these physical and chemical factors produce teratologies by their effect on the hormonal metabolism in insects. This aspect has already been considered in the various sections pertaining to the effect of hormones on integumental development.

G. Neoplastic Diseases

Neoplasms in insects are almost totally unknown. The primary barrier to their discovery is the difficulty in evaluating the status of "growths" or swellings. Harker (1963) treats the subject with caution, stating that even the general definition of neoplasms—"proliferations in which the cells grow in a new and different way"—may not be applicable to insects because of the versatility of their cells. She also states that the five basic characteristics seen in vertebrate tumors are present in insect cells in several instances, such as wound healing or in tissues affected by hormones, and therefore cannot be used as a basis for tumors in insects.

Considering the number of insects that are examined each year, it is surprising that more naturally occurring neoplasms have not been described. Again, *Drosophila* is the leader in tumor studies, with only two instances of tumors in other insects having been reported in recent years (Harker, 1963). We have found five reports of "tumors" in the integument and these are discussed, although the reader must decide for himself whether or not they are designated correctly.

Federley (1936) studied sex-linked hereditary cancer in the larvae of the lepidopteran *Pygaera*. He postulates that although the occurrence of the cancer is sex-linked (appearing only in males), it is not a result of gene action but a result of the division of the polar nuclei in the formation of the egg. He presents evidence for his hypothesis by listing the localization and histological structure of the tumors, including those of the hypodermis. Briefly, he has found that in the larvae tumors in the epidermis are common although not unusually large. If the tumors are located in the glands of the epidermis, however, they are very large and made up of large cells of the same type as the gland cells.

Another incidence of a tumor has been reported by Hukuhara (1964). He states that TIV causes epidermal tumors in the silkworm larva. The first sign of this virus disease is the appearance of white spots on the larval skin, which becomes abnormally translucent. Hukuhara showed that under the white spots on the skin are whitish masses of cells or tumors caused by the abnormal proliferation of the epidermal cells. The epidermis near the tumor region is many layered as compared to the single-layered epidermis of uninfected larva. This multilayered region is thrown into folds or is swollen, forming rounded nodes. The cells of the tumors are much smaller than normal epidermal cells.

In the larva of *Hyphantria cunea* infected with a nuclear polyhedrosis virus, the integumental epithelium undergoes hyperplasia and hypertrophy to form a multilayered structure (Watanabe, 1968). This condition, which has been described previously, may be considered a malignant neoplasm.

The fourth instance of tumors in the epidermis has been reported by Stark (1937). She states that pigmented areas occur on the skin epithelium of *Drosophila* and that these are hereditary, lethal tumors. The cells of the pigmented areas become loaded with pigment and form uniformly shaped patches. Cross sections of the areas show that the pigment is confined to the epithelial cells.

The fifth report of tumors concerns an oncogenic virus of vertebrates (Bryan high-titer strain of Rous sarcoma virus), which apparently interacts with the genome of *D. melanogaster* to cause an increased incidence of lethal mutation, visible mutation, chromosomal losses, chromosomal nondisjunctions, and tumors when the larvae are placed in media containing the virus (Burdette and Yoon, 1967). The absence of one leg or wing and a few eye mosaics are among the visible mutants that appear. The tests for the persistence of the virus in the progeny have been negative so far. Kirk *et al.* (1970) also produced melanotic lesions with the same vertebrate virus in *D. melanogaster*, but they believed that the lesions were not analogous to mammalian neoplasia and should be called lesions rather than tumors.

H. Injuries Caused by Parasites and Predators

One feature of the class Insecta is that its members may be parasitic upon each other. Insects are also parasitized by nematodes. As a rule, the insect is eventually killed by its parasite. This can happen upon entry of the parasite or upon its exit. In the case of the latter, the host and parasite may have gone through several stages together and become intimately associated with the functions of each other (see Doutt, 1963).

Many parasitic species puncture the integument of the host insect in order to oviposit. This usually causes slight mechanical damage to the host. The effect, however, is usually negligible and the wound heals normally. Occasionally, a female parasite does not puncture the integument to oviposit but rather to feed on the material that exudes from the wound. In such cases death of the insect may result. Flanders (1942) has reported on the extensive probing of the black scale by its parasite *Metaphycus helvolus*. After probing, the body contents of the scale turn pink and the parasite feeds at the wound site until the scale dies.

Some parasitic species hatch from externally placed eggs and then enter the host's body to begin an endoparasitic existence. Most of them do not cause much injury at the site of entry; others, however, utilize the entry hole for respiratory purposes. The tachinid *Dexia ventralis*, which parasitizes scarabaeid grubs, somehow develops a funnel-shaped structure at the point of entry into the grub. The structure is attached to the caudal, spiracle-bearing portion of the parasite (Clausen *et al.*, 1927; Clausen, 1952). How the funnel-shaped structure is developed is not definitely known, although it has been suggested that this "respiratory tube" is an ingrowth of the epidermis resulting from a defense reaction on the part of the host to the irritation caused by the parasite.

Nemestrinid fly larvae, *Neorhynchocephalus sackenii*, parasitic on grasshoppers, enter the body through a puncture on the soft lateroventral abdominal surface just below the row of spiracles (Prescott, 1961). Complete penetration of the host occurs in 1–10 minutes, depending on the difficulty in cutting through the integumentary membrane. Once this is accomplished, complete penetration is relatively fast. Upon entry the puncture hole immediately closes, with no trace being evident.

Prescott noted that after penetration into the host the first-instar larva enters the tracheal system and wanders around for some time. Subsequently, it reappears under the integument, usually some distance from the point of entry, and begins to cut a respiratory pore in the integument. This takes about 4 or 5 hours, after which the larva reverses itself to plug the pore with the posterior, spiracle-bearing segment. After 1 or 2 days, a respiratory pore develops, connecting the larva with the pore. The tube is apparently a defense reaction on the part of the integument of the host.

When parasites leave the body of a still-living host, either to pupate or to begin feeding from an external position, some mechanical injury occurs at the point of exit. Often the insect is killed as its parasite emerges or there is no apparent effect at all on the insect. Thompson (1915) reports that when planidia of *Perilampus* leave the pupa of the tachinid *Ernestia*, the effect is all out of proportion to the mechanical injury inflicted upon entry into the host. The pupa takes on a distinctive translucent appearance, especially in the head and thoracic regions. The head attains only half its normal size and the eyes and appendages develop only slightly. Thompson suggests that the minute emergence wound at this critical time brings about an upset in the equilibrium of the body fluids, resulting in almost complete cessation of development.

The manner in which tachinid larvae emerge from their hosts is dependent on the stage of the host and whether it is alive or dead. In larval hosts tachinids usually make an incision in the thinnest portion of the ventral abdominal integument. This is accomplished by use of their mouth hooks or by pressure of the tachinid's caudal end and is aided by the solvent action of body secretions.

If the host is still alive, the tachinid will leave the body either through the anal opening or the nearby intersegmental membrane. The maggot of *Minella chalybeata* exits from its host, the beetle *Cassida* sp., through an aperture dorsally situated between the first and second abdominal segments. The maggot of *Thrixion* emerges from the body of its phasmid host through a wound at the side of the thorax which had previously been used for respiratory purposes. In this case mechanical injury is relatively slight (Clausen, 1940).

Slight mechanical injury is produced in the integument of *Simulium vittatum* when its nematode parasites leave the body. The parasites become entwined around some nearby object, possibly even the insect, and pull themselves free of their host (Anderson and DeFoliart, 1962).

Certain parasitic nematodes are known to cause intercastes and intersexes in insects, and parasites of the family Stylopidae produce abnormality in adult bees known as stylopization. These derangements may affect not only the gonads of the parasitized insects but also secondary sexual characters, some of which are apparent in alterations, such as markings and pilosity, of the integument.

Kaya and Tanada (1969) observed that the presence of dead parasite eggs within the larva of the armyworm *Pseudaletia unipuncta* may prevent the latter from pupating normally and produce an abnormal pupa as described in Section VII,F. The eggs of the insect parasite *Apanteles militaris* are killed when the armyworm larva in which they occur is reared at 35°C for 1–2 days and returned to 23°C. Nonparasitized armyworm larvae pupate normally when held at 35°C for 1 day or even several days and then returned to 23°C.

VII. Concluding Remarks

The integument, primarily because it is the major barrier against injurious biotic and abiotic factors, merits considerable attention from the standpoint of the diseases that afflict it. An important objective of this chapter is to bring out the broadness and extensiveness of the nature and scope of the diseases that develop in the insect integument. Our review clearly reveals the serious lack of knowledge in many aspects of integumental diseases resulting from biotic and abiotic causes. We have attempted to cover the subject extensively, but major emphasis has been placed on the diseases associated with microorganisms, especially pathogens. The treatment of the diseases caused by abiotic factors, including genetic diseases, is far from complete, and we do not wish to imply that they are less important than those caused by biotic factors. In fact, under certain environmental conditions, some of these diseases may be very serious and important in the life of an insect. For example, under very high temperature or unfavorable nutritional conditions, teratologies may develop during molting and metamorphosis.

Our aim is to enhance interest and to encourage and stimulate research on the diseases of the integument. Moreover, we wish to point out that an important area of insect pathology that has been neglected is the interaction of factors, biotic and abiotic, that cause diseases of the integument for the control of insect pests.

ACKNOWLEDGMENTS

The authors are pleased to acknowledge the invaluable help of Faylla Chapman and Harry K. Kaya who assisted in the literature search and to express our appreciation to Dr. Isabelle Tavares for reviewing the section on the Laboulbeniales.

REFERENCES

Aizawa, K. (1963). The nature of infections caused by nuclear-polyhedrosis viruses. *In* "Insect Pathology, An Advanced Treatise" (E. A. Steinhaus, ed.), Vol. 1, pp. 381–412. Academic Press, New York.

Alexander, P., Kitchener, J. A., and Briscoe, H. V. A. (1944). Inert dust insecticides. Pt. I. Mechanism in action. Pt. II. The nature of effective dusts. Pt. III. The effect of dusts on stored products pests other than *Calanara granaria*. *Ann. Appl. Biol.* **31**, 143–159.

Alexopoulos, C. J. (1962). "Introductory Mycology," 2nd Ed., 613 pp. Wiley, New York.

Anderson, J. F. (1966). Anomalous development of the cuticle of mosquitoes induced by griseofulvin. *J. Econ. Entomol.* **59**, 1476–1482.

Anderson, J. R., and DeFoliart, G. R. (1962). Nematode parasitism of black fly (Diptera: Simuliidae) larvae in Wisconsin. *Ann. Entomol. Soc. Amer.* **55**, 542–546.

Aoki, K. (1942). On new fungous parasites of *Sturmia sericariae* C. and *Bombyx mori* L. II. *Sterigmatocystis japonica* Aoki sp. nov. *Sanshi Shikensho Hokoku* **11**, 1–21.

Aoki, K. (1958). Control of the muscardines. *J. Silkworm,* **10**, 295–314.

Arendsen Hein, S. A. (1920). Studies on variation in the mealworm *Tenebrio molitor.* I. Biological and genetical notes. *J. Genet.* **10,** 227–264.

Arendsen Hein, S. A. (1924). Studies on variation in the mealworm *Tenebrio molitor.* II. Variations in tarsi and antennae. *J. Genet.* **14,** 1–38.

Aruga, H. (1939). Genetical studies on mutants obtained from silkworms treated with X-rays. I–IV. *Sanshi Shikensho Hokoku* **9,** 295–352.

Aruga, H. (1940). Genetical studies on mutants obtained from silkworms treated with X-rays. V. *Sanshi Shikensho Hokoku* **9,** 495–520.

Bailey, S. W. (1962). The effects of percussion on insect pests of grain. *J. Econ. Entomol.* **55,** 301–304.

Balazuc, J. (1948). La teratologie des coléoptères et expériences de transplantation sur *Tenebrio molitor* L. *Mem. Mus. Nat. Hist. Natur.* (*Paris*) **25,** 1–293.

Barbier, R. (1966). Étude de l'hypoderme de *Galleria mellonella* L. (Lépidoptère Pyralidae) à l'aide d'homogreffes larvaires. *C. R. Acad. Sci., Ser. D* **262,** 2073–2076.

Barigozzi, C. (1963). Relationship between cytoplasm and chromosome in the transmission of melanotic tumours in *Drosophila. In* "Biological Organization at the Cellular and Supercellular Level" (R. J. C. Harris, ed.), pp. 73–89. Academic Press, New York.

Batko, A., and Weiser, J. (1965). On the taxonomic position of the fungus discovered by Strong, Wells, and Apple: *Strongwellsea castrans* gen. et. sp. nov. (Phycomycetes; Entomophthoraceae). *J. Invertebr. Pathol.* **7,** 455–463.

Beament, J. W. L. (1945). The cuticular lipoids of insects. *J. Exp. Biol.* **21,** 115–131.

Beck, S. D., and Shane, J. L. (1969). Effects of ecdysones on diapause in the European corn borer, *Ostrinia nubilalis. J. Insect Physiol.* **15,** 721–730.

Benjamin, R. K. (1965). Study in specificity. Minute fungi parasitize living arthropods. *Natur. Hist.* **74,** 42–49.

Benjamin, R. K., and Shanor, L. (1952). Sex of host specificity and position specificity of certain species of *Laboulbenia* on *Bembidion picipes. Amer. J. Bot.* **39,** 125–131.

Benton, A. G. (1935). Chitinovorous bacteria. *J. Bacteriol.* **29,** 449–465.

Benz, G. (1963). Physiopathology and histochemistry. *In* "Insect Pathology, An Advanced Treatise" (E. A. Steinhaus, ed.), Vol. 1, pp. 299–338. Academic Press, New York.

Bergold, G. H. (1958). Viruses of insects. *In* "Handbuch der Virusforschung" (C. Hallauer and K. F. Meyer, eds.), Vol. 4, pp. 60–142. Springer, Vienna.

Bergold, G. H. (1963). The nature of nuclear-polyhedrosis viruses. *In* "Insect Pathology, An Advanced Treatise" (E. A. Steinhaus, ed.), Vol. 1, pp. 413–456. Academic Press, New York.

Bird, F. T. (1953). The use of a virus disease in the biological control of the European pine sawfly, *Neodiprion sertifer* (Geoffr.). *Can. Entomol.* **85,** 437–446.

Bird, F. T. (1959). Polyhedrosis and granulosis viruses causing single and double infections in the spruce budworm, *Choristoneura fumiferana* Clemens. *J. Insect Pathol.* **1,** 406–430.

Bird, F. T. (1961). Transmission of some insect viruses with particular reference to ovarial transmission and its importance in the development of epizootics. *J. Insect Pathol.* 3, 352–380.

Blockwitz, A. (1929). Schimmelpilze als Tierparasiten. *Ber. Deut. Bot. Ges.* **47,** 31–34.

Blunck, H. (1952). Ueber die bei *Pieris brassicae* L., Ihren Parasiten und Hyperparasiten Schmarotzenden Mikrosporidien. *Trans. 9th Int. Congr. Entomol., Amsterdam, 1951* **1**, 432–438.

Boczkowska, M. (1935). Contribution à l'étude de l'immunité chez les chenilles de *Galleria mellonella* L., contre les champignons entomophytes. *C. R. Soc. Biol.* **119**, 39–40.

Boudreaux, H. B. (1959). A viruslike transovarian factor affecting morphology in spider mites. *J. Insect Pathol.* **1**, 270–280.

Bovien, P. (1932). On a new nematode, *Scatonema wülkeri* gen. et sp. n. parasitic in the body-cavity of *Scatopse fuscipes* Meig. (Diptera nematocera). *Vidensk. Medd. Naturhist. Foren. Kjobehavn* **94**, 13–32.

Bowers, W. S. (1968). Juvenile hormone: activity of natural and synthetic synergists. *Science* **161**, 895–897.

Braun, B. H., Jacobson, M., Schwarz, M., Sonnet, P. E., Wakabayashi, N., and Waters, R. M. (1968). A convenient synthesis of mixed isomers of juvenile hormone. *J. Econ. Entomol.* **61**, 866–869.

Brooks, M. A. (1963). Symbiosis and aposymbiosis in arthropods. *Soc. Gen. Microbiol.* **13**, 200–231.

Brown, A. W. A. (1963). Chemical injuries. *In* "Insect Pathology, An Advanced Treatise" (E. A. Steinhaus, ed.), Vol. 1, pp. 65–131. Academic Press, New York.

Buchli, H. H. R. (1952). *Antennopsis gallica,* a new parasite on termites. *Trans. 9th Int. Congr. Entomol., Amsterdam, 1951* **1**, 519–524.

Bückmann, D. (1959). Die Auslösung der Umfärbung durch das Häutungshormon bei *Cerura vinula* L. (Lepidoptera, Notodontidae). *J. Insect Physiol.* **3**, 159–189.

Burdette, W. J., and Yoon, J. S. (1967). Mutations, chromosomal aberrations, and tumors in insects treated with oncogenic virus. *Science* **155**, 340–341.

Burgerjon, A., and Biache, G. (1967). Effects tératologiques chez les nymphes et les adultes d'insectes, dont les larves ont ingéré des doses subléthales de toxine thermostable de *Bacillus thuringiensis* Berliner. *C. R. Acad. Sci., Ser. D* **264**, 2423–2425.

Burgerjon, A., Biache, G., and Cals, P. (1969). Teratology of the Colorado potato beetle, *Leptinotarsa decemlineata,* as provoked by larval administration of the thermostable toxin of *Bacillus thuringiensis. J. Invertebr. Pathol.* **14**, 274–278.

Butenandt, A., and Karlson, P. (1954). Über die Isolierung eines Metamorphose-Hormons der Insekten in Kristallisierter Form. *Z. Naturforsch. B* **9**, 389–391.

Butler, C. G. (1943). Bee paralysis, May-sickness disease, etc. *Bee World* **24**, 3–7.

Carayon, J., and Thouvenin, M. (1966). Emploi d'une substance mimétique de l'hormone juvénile pour la lutte contre les *Dysdercus,* Hémiptères nuisibles au contonnier. *C. R. Hebd. Seances Acad. Agr. Fr.* **52**, 340–346.

Chatton E., and Picard, F. (1909). Contribution à l'étude systèmatique et biologique des Laboulbéniacées: *Trenomyces histophtorus* Chatton et Picard, endoparasite des poux de la poule domestique. *Bull. Soc. Mycol. Fr.* **25**, 147–170.

Christie, J. R. (1936). Life history of *Agamermis decaudata,* a nematode parasite of grasshoppers and other insects. *J. Agr. Res.* **52**, 161–198.

Christie, J. R. (1941). Life history (Zooparasitica). Parasites of invertebrates. *In* "Introduction to Nematology" (B. G. Chitwood and M. B. Chitwood, eds.), Sect. 2, Pt. 2, Ch. 5, pp. 246–266. Monumental Printing Co., Baltimore, Maryland.

Clark, T. B., Kellen, W. B., and Lum, P. T. M. (1965). A mosquito iridescent virus (MIV) from *Aedes taeniorhynchus* (Wiedemann). *J. Invertebr. Pathol.* **7**, 519–521.

Clausen, C. P. (1940). "Entomophagous Insects," 688 pp. McGraw-Hill, New York.

Clausen, C. P. (1952). Respiratory adaptations in the immature stages of parasitic insects. *Arthropoda* **1**, 197–224.

Clausen, C. P., King, J. L., and Teranishi, C. (1927). The parasites of *Popillia japonica* in Japan and Chosen (Korea) and their introduction into the United States. *U.S. Dep. Agr. Bull.* **1429**, 56 pp.

Colla, S. (1934). Laboulbeniales Peyritschiellaceae, Dimorphomycetaceae, Laboulbeniaceae Heterothallicae, Laboulbeniaceae Homothallicae, Ceratomycetaceae. *Flora Italica Cryptogama* (*Societa Botanica Italiana*), *Fasc.* **16**, 1–157.

Cottrell, C. B. (1962). The imaginal ecdysis of blowflies. Detection of the blood-borne darkening factor and determination of some of its properties. *J. Exp. Biol.* **39**, 413–430.

Cottrell, C. B. (1964). Insect ecdysis with particular emphasis on cuticular hardening and darkening. *Advan. Insect Physiol.* 3, 175–218.

Dahlman, D. L. (1969). Cuticular pigments of tobacco hornworm (*Manduca sexta*) larvae: effects of diet and genetic differences. *J. Insect Physiol.* **15**, 807–814.

David, W. A. L. (1967). The physiology of the insect integument in relation to the invasion of pathogens. *In* "Insects and Physiology" (J. W. L. Beament and J. E. Treherne, eds.), pp. 17–35. Oliver & Boyd, Edinburgh and London.

Day, M. F., and Oster, I. I. (1963). Physical injuries. *In* "Insect Pathology, An Advanced Treatise" (E. A. Steinhaus, ed.), Vol. 1, pp. 29–63. Academic Press, New York.

Delachambre, J. (1966). Remarques sur l'histophysiologie des oenocytes épidermiques de la nymphe de *Tenebrio molitor* L. (Col. Tenebrionidae). *C. R. Acad. Sci., Ser. D* **263**, 764–767.

Dickinson, S. (1959). The behaviour of larvae of *Heterodera schachtii* on nitrocellulose membranes. *Nematologica* **4**, 60–66.

Dieter, M. (1956). Säugeninfusorien auf Wasserkafern. *Orion* **11**, 369–373.

Doutt, R. L. (1963). Pathologies caused by insect parasites. *In* "Insect Pathology, An Advanced Treatise" (E. A. Steinhaus, ed.), Vol. 2, pp. 393–422. Academic Press, New York.

Duggar, B. M. (1896). On a bacterial disease of the squash-bug (*Anasa tristis* DeG.). *Ill. State Lab. Natur. Hist., Bull.* **4**, 340–379.

Ebeling, W. (1961). Physicochemical mechanisms for the removal of insect wax by means of finely divided powders. *Hilgardia* **30**, 531–564.

Ebeling, W. (1964). The permeability of insect cuticle. *In* "The Physiology of Insecta" (M. Rockstein, ed.), Vol. 3, pp. 507–556. Academic Press, New York.

Ebeling, W., and Wagner, R. E. (1959). Rapid desiccation of drywood termites with inert sorptive dusts and other substances. *J. Econ. Entomol.* **52**, 190–207.

Ede, D. A. (1956). Studies on the effects of some genetic lethal factors on the embryonic development of *Drosophila melanogaster*. IV. An analysis of the mutant *X20*. *Wilhelm Roux' Arch. Entwicklungsmech. Organismen* **149**, 101–104.

Eichler, W. (1951). Laboulbeniales bei Mallophagen und Laüsen. I. Die Gattung *Trenomyces*. *Feddes Repertorium Specierum Novarum Regni Vegetabilis* **54** (2/3), 185–206.

Elson, J. A. (1933). Protozoans and beetles. *Amer. Natur.* **67**, 283–285.

Evlakhova, A. A., and Chekhourina, T. A. (1964). L'activité de défense de la cuticule de la punaise des céréales (*Eurygaster integriceps* Put.) contre les micro-organismes végétaux. Coll. Int. Pathol. Insectes, Paris, 1962. *Entomophaga, Mem. Hors* Ser. **2**, 137–141.

Federley, H. (1936). Sex-limited hereditary cancer in lepidopterous larvae. *Hereditas* **22**, 193–216.

Flanders, S. E. (1942). *Metaphycus helvolus,* an encyrtid parasite of the black scale. *J. Econ. Entomol.* **35**, 690–698.

Fogal, W., and Fraenkel, G. (1969a). The role of bursicon in melanization and endocuticle formation in the adult fleshfly, *Sarcophaga bullata. J. Insect Physiol.* **15**, 1235–1247.

Fogal, W., and Fraenkel, G. (1969b). Melanin in the puparium and adult integument of the fleshfly, *Sarcophaga bullata. J. Insect Physiol.* **15**, 1437–1447.

Fox, C. J. S. (1961). The incidence of green muscardine in the European wireworm, *Agriotes obscurus* (Linnaeus), in Nova Scotia. *J. Insect Pathol.* **3**, 94–95.

Fraenkel, G. (1935). A hormone causing pupation in the blowfly, *Calliphora erythrocephala. Proc. Roy. Soc. (London), Ser. B* **118**, 1–12.

Fraenkel, G., and Blewett, M. (1946a). The dietetics of the caterpillars of three *Ephestia* species, *E. kuehniella, E. elutella,* and *E. cautella,* and of a closely related species, *Plodia interpunctella. J. Exp. Biol.* **22**, 162–171.

Fraenkel, G., and Blewett, M. (1946b). Linoleic acid, vitamin E and other fat-soluble substances in the nutrition of certain insects, *Ephestia kuehniella, E. elutella, E. cautella,* and *Plodia interpunctella* (Lep.). *J. Exp. Biol.* **22**, 172–190.

Fraenkel, G., and Chang, P.-I. (1954). Manifestations of a vitamin B_T (Carnitine) deficiency in the larvae of the mealworm, *Tenebrio molitor* L. *Physiol. Zool.* **27**, 40–52.

Fraenkel, G., and Hsiao, C. (1965). Bursicon, a hormone which mediates tanning of the cuticle in the adult fly and other insects. *J. Insect Physiol.* **11**, 513–556.

Fraenkel, G., and Hsiao, C. (1967). Calcification, tanning, and the rôle of ecdyson in the formation of the puparium of the facefly, *Musca autumnalis. J. Insect Physiol.* **13**, 1387–1394.

Friederichs, K. (1920). On the pleophagy of the insect-attacking fungus *Metarrhizium anisopliae* (Metsch.) Sor. *Zentralbl. Bakteriol., Parasitenk., Infektionskr. Hyg., Abt. 2* **50**, 335.

Fukaya, M. (1962). The inhibitory action of farnesol on the development of the rice stem borer in post-diapause. *Nippon Oyo Dobutsu Konchu Gakkai-Shi* **6**, 298.

Fukaya, M., and Nasu, S. (1966). A *Chilo* iridescent virus (CIV) from the rice stem borer, *Chilo suppressalis* Walker (Lepidoptera: Pyralidae). *Appl. Entomol. Zool.* **1**, 69–72.

Fyg, W. (1964). Anomalies and diseases of the queen honey bee. *Annu. Rev. Entomol.* **9**, 207–224.

Gabriel, B. P. (1965). A biochemical and histochemical study of the penetration of the insect cuticle by *Entomophthora coronata* (Costantin) Kevorkian. 129 pp. Ph.D. Thesis, Univ. of California, Berkeley, California.

Gabriel, B. P. (1968a). Enzymatic activities of some entomophthorous fungi. *J. Invertebr. Pathol.* **11**, 70–81.

Gabriel, B. P. (1968b). Histochemical study of the insect cuticle infected by the fungus *Entomophthora coronata. J. Invertebr. Pathol.* **11**, 82–89.

Gardner, E. J., and Woolf, C. M. (1949). Maternal effect involved in the inheritance of abnormal growths in the head region of *Drosophila melanogaster*. *Genetics* **34**, 573–585.

Girardie, A. (1967). Contrôle neuro-hormonal de la métamorphose et de la pigmentation chez *Locusta migratoria cinerascens* (Orthoptère). *Bull. Biol. Fr. Belg.* **101**, 79–114.

Goldstein, B. (1929). A cytological study of the fungus *Massospora cicadina*, parasitic on the 17-year cicada, *Magicicada septendecim*. *Amer. J. Bot.* **16**, 394–401.

Gressitt, J. L. (1966a). Epizoic symbiosis: the Papuan weevil genus *Gymnopholus* (*Leptopiinae*) symbiotic with cryptogamic plants, oribatid mites, rotifers and nematodes. *Pacific Insects* **8**, 221–280.

Gressitt, J. L. (1966b). Epizoic symbiosis: cryptogamic plants growing on various weevils and on a colydiid beetle in New Guinea. *Pacific Insects* **8**, 294–297.

Gressitt, J. L., Sedlacek, J. A., and Szent-Ivany, J. J. H. (1965). Flora and fauna on backs of large Papuan moss-forest weevils. *Science* **150**, 1833–1835.

Gressitt, J. L., Samuelson, G. A., and Vitt, D. H. (1968). Moss growing on living Papuan moss-forest weevils. *Nature* (*London*) **217**, 765–767.

Gunn, D. L., and Cosway, C. A. (1938). The temperature and humidity relations of the cockroach. V. Humidity preference. *J. Exp. Biol.* **15**, 555–563.

Hackman, R. H. (1964). Chemistry of the insect cuticle. *In* "The Physiology of Insecta" (M. Rockstein, ed.), Vol. 3, pp. 471–506. Academic Press, New York.

Hackman, R. H. (1967). Melanin in an insect, *Lucilia cuprina* (Wied.). *Nature* (*London*) **216**, 163.

Harker, J. E. (1963). Tumors. *In* "Insect Pathology, An Advanced Treatise" (E. A. Steinhaus, ed.), Vol. 1, pp. 191–214. Academic Press, New York.

Harpaz, I., and Zlotkin, E. (1965). A nuclear-polyhedrosis virus of the safflower leaf worm *Heliothis peltigera* Schiff. [Lep., Noctuidae]. *Ann. Soc. Entomol. Fr.* **1**, 963–972.

Harrap, K. A., and Robertson, J. S. (1968). A possible infection pathway in the development of a nuclear polyhedrosis virus. *J. Gen. Virol.* **3**, 221–225.

Haydak, M. H. (1937). The influence of a pure carbohydrate diet on newly emerged honeybees. *Ann. Entomol. Soc. Amer.* **30**, 258–262.

Hayes, W. P., and Liu, Y.-S. (1947). Tarsal chemoreceptors of the housefly and their possible relation to DDT toxicity. *Ann. Entomol. Soc. Amer.* **40**, 401–416.

Herman, W. S. (1968). Control of hormone production in insects. *In* "Metamorphosis, a Problem in Developmental Biology" (W. Etkin and L. I. Gilbert, eds.), pp. 107–141. Appleton-Century-Crofts, New York.

Hidaka, T., and Ohtaki, T. (1963). Éffet de l'hormone juvénile et du farnésol sur la coloration tégumentaire de la nymphe de *Pieris rapae crucivora* Boisd. *C. R. Soc. Biol.* **157**, 928–930.

Honigberg, B. M., Balamuth, W., Bovee, E. C., Corliss, J. O., Gojdics, M., Hall, R. P., Kudo, R. R., Levine, N. D., Loeblich, A. R., Jr., Weiser, J., and Wenrich, D. H. (1964). A revised classification of the phylum Protozoa. *J. Protozool.* **11**, 7–20.

Hora, J., Lábler, L., Kasal, A., Černý, V., Šorm, F., and Sláma, K. (1966). On steroids C111. Molting deficiencies produced by some sterol derivatives in an insect (*Pyrrhocoris apterus* L.). *Steroids* **8**, 887–914.

Hoskins, W. M. (1940). Recent contributions of insect physiology to insect toxicology and control. *Hilgardia* **13**, 307–386.

House, H. L. (1963). Nutritional diseases. *In* "Insect Pathology, An Advanced Treatise" (E. A. Steinhaus, ed.), Vol. 1, pp. 133–160. Academic Press, New York.

Huger, A. (1963). Granuloses of insects. *In* "Insect Pathology, An Advanced Treatise" (E. A. Steinhaus, ed.), Vol. 1, pp. 531–575. Academic Press, New York.

Hughes, K. M. (1957). An annotated list and bibliography of insects reported to have virus diseases. *Hilgardia* **26**, 597–629.

Hukuhara, T. (1964). Induction of epidermal tumor in *Bombyx mori* (Linnaeus) with *Tipula* iridescent virus. *J. Insect Pathol.* **6**, 246–248.

Hukuhara, T., and Hashimoto, Y. (1966). Development of *Tipula* iridescent virus in the silkworm, *Bombyx mori* L. (Lepidoptera: Bombycidae). *Appl. Entomol. Zool.* **1**, 166–172.

Hurst, H. (1948). Asymmetrical behaviour of insect cuticle in relation to water permeability. *Discuss Faraday Soc.* **3**, 193–210.

Ilan, J., and Quastel, J. H. (1966). Effects of colchicine on nucleic acid metabolism during metamorphosis of *Tenebrio molitor* L. and in some mammalian tissues. *Biochem. J.* **100**, 448–457.

Iyoda, S. (1940). Studies on green muscardine of the silkworm. III. On the course of multiplication of *Nomuraea prasina* Maubl. in the silkworm larva with special reference to histopathological observations. *Aichi-Ken Sangyo Shikensho Iho* **11**, 49–75.

Johnson, B. (1953). The injurious effects of the hooked epidermal hairs of French beans (*Phaseolus vulgaris* L.) on *Aphis craccivora* Koch. *Bull. Entomol. Res.* **44**, 779–788.

Jones, G. D. G. (1955). The cuticular waterproofing mechanism of the worker honey-bee. *J. Exp. Biol.* **32**, 95–109.

Kamburov, S. S., Nadel, D. J., and Kenneth, R. (1967). Observations on *Hesperomyces virescens* Thaxter (Laboulbeniales), a fungus associated with premature mortality of *Chilocorus bipustulatus* L. in Israel. *Israel J. Agr. Res.* **17**, 131–134.

Karlson, P. (1966). Ecdyson, das Häutungshormon der Insekten. *Naturwissenschaften* **53**, 445–453.

Karlson, P., and Sekeris, C. E. (1962). N-acetyldopamine as sclerotizing agent of the insect cuticle. *Nature (London)* **195**, 183–184.

Katsumata, F. (1931). On the penetration of *Beauveria bassiana* into the host. *Sanshigaku Zasshi* **3**, 168–171.

Kaya, H. K., and Tanada, Y. (1969). Responses to high temperature of the parasite *Apanteles militaris* and of its host, the armyworm, *Pseudaletia unipuncta*. *Ann. Entomol. Soc. Amer.* **62**, 1303–1306.

Kellen, W. R., Clark, T. B., Lindegren, J. E., and Sanders, R. D. (1966). A cytoplasmic-polyhedrosis virus of *Culex tarsalis* (Diptera: Culicidae). *J. Invertebr. Pathol.* **8**, 390–394.

Kirk, H. D., Ewen, A. B., and Emson, H. E. (1970). Melanotic lesions in two insect species: *Drosophila melanogaster* (Diptera) and *Melanoplus sanguinipes* (Orthoptera). *J. Invertebr. Pathol.* **15**, 351–355.

Koidsumi, K. (1957). Antifungal action of cuticular lipids in insects. *J. Insect Physiol.* **1**, 40–51.

Krieg, A. (1961). "Grundlagen der Insektenpathologie Viren-, Rickettsien- und Bakterien-Infektionen," 304 pp. Steinkopff, Darmstadt.

Kufferath, M. H. (1921). Microbe pathogene pour les sauterelles et d'autres insectes. *Ann. Gembloux* **27**, 253–257.

Kurisu, K. (1962). Histopathological studies on the muscardines in silkworm larvae. *Kyoto Kogei Sen'i Daigaku Sen'igakubu Gakujutsu Hokoku* 3, 392–420.

Lai-Fook, J. (1966). The repair of wounds in the integument of insects. *J. Insect Physiol.* **12**, 195–226.

Laigo, F. M., and Tamashiro, M. (1966). Virus and insect parasite interaction in the lawn-armyworm, *Spodoptera mauritia acronyctoides* (Guenée). *Proc. Hawaii. Entomol. Soc.* **19**, 233–237.

Laigo, F. M., and Tamashiro, M. (1967). Interactions between a microsporidian pathogen of the lawn-armyworm and the hymenopterous parasite *Apanteles marginiventris. J. Invertebr. Pathol.* **9**, 546–554.

Lefebvre, C. L. (1934). Penetration and development of the fungus, *Beauveria bassiana,* in the tissues of the corn borer. *Ann. Bot.* (*London*) **48**, 441–454.

Leidy, J. (1849a). Descriptions of new genera and species of entophyta. *Proc. Acad. Natur. Sci. Philadelphia* **4**, 249–250.

Leidy, J. (1849b). On the existence of entophyta in healthy animals, as a natural condition. *Proc. Acad. Natur. Sci. Philadelphia* **4**, 225–233.

Lepesme, P. (1937). Sur la présence du *Bacillus prodigiosus* chez le criquet pèlerin (*Schistocerca gregaria Forsk.*) *Bull. Soc. Hist. Natur. Afr. Nord* **28**, 406–411.

Lepesme, P. (1939). Influence de la température et de l'humidité sur la pathogénie de l'Aspergillose des Acridiens. *C. R. Acad. Sci.* **208**, 234–236.

Lichtenstein, J. L. (1917a). Sur un *Amoebidium* à commensalisme interne du rectum des larves d'*Anax imperator* Leach: *Amoebidium fasciculatum* n. sp. *Arch. Zool. Exp. Gen.* **56**, 49–62.

Lichtenstein, J. L. (1917b). Sur un mode nouveau de multiplication chez les Amoebidiacées. *Arch. Zool. Exp. Gen.* **56**, 95–99.

Lichtwardt, R. W. (1954). Three species of eccrinales inhabiting the hindguts of millipeds, with comments on the eccrinids as a group. *Mycologica* **46**, 564–585.

Lindroth, C. H. (1948). Notes on the ecology of Laboulbeniaceae infesting carabid beetles. *Sv. Bot. Tidskr.* **42**, 34–41.

Locke, M. (1964). The structure and formation of the integument in insects. *In* "The Physiology of Insecta" (M. Rockstein, ed.), Vol. 3, pp. 379–470. Academic Press, New York.

Lower, H. F. (1959). Some effects of starvation on the larval cuticle of *Persectania ewingii* (Wwd.) (Lepidoptera: Noctuidae). *Amer. Midl. Natur.* **61**, 390–398.

Lower, H. F. (1964). The arthropod integument. *Stud. Gen.* **5**, 275–288.

Ludwig, D. (1948). Relation between lipid content of cuticle, duration of diapause, and resistance of desiccation of pupae of the Cynthia moth. *Physiol. Zool.* **21**, 252–257.

Lust, S. (1950). Symphorionte Peritrichen auf Käfern und Wanzen. *Zool. Jahrb. Abt. Syst. Oekol. Geogr. Tiere* **79**, 353–436.

McCauley, V. J. E., Zacharuk, R. Y., and Tinline, R. D. (1968). Histopathology of green muscardine in larvae of four species of Elateridae (Coleoptera). *J. Invertebr. Pathol.* **12**, 444–459.

McEwen, F. L. (1963). Cordyceps infections. *In* "Insect Pathology, An Advanced Treatise" (E. A. Steinhaus, ed.), Vol. 2, pp. 273–290. Academic Press, New York.

MacLeod, D. M. (1963). Entomophthorales infections. *In* "Insect Pathology, An

Advanced Treatise" (E. A. Steinhaus, ed.), Vol. 2, pp. 189–231. Academic Press, New York.

Madelin, M. F. (1963). Diseases caused by hyphomycetous fungi. *In* "Insect Pathology, An Advanced Treatise" (E. A. Steinhaus, ed.), Vol. 2, pp. 233–271. Academic Press, New York.

Madelin, M. F. (1966). Fungal parasites of insects. *Annu. Rev. Entomol.* **11,** 423–448.

Madelin, M. F., Robinson, R. K., and Williams, R. J. (1967). Appressorium-like structures in insect-parasitizing Deuteromycetes. *J. Invertebr. Pathol.* **9,** 404–412.

Madhavan, K., and Schneiderman, H. A. (1968). Effects of ecdysone on epidermal cells in which DNA synthesis has been blocked. *J. Insect Physiol.* **14,** 777–781.

Manier, J.-F. (1950). Recherches sur les Trichomycètes. *Ann. Sci. Natur., Bot. Biol. Vegetale, Ser. 11* **11,** 53–162.

Martignoni, M. E. (1957). Contributo alla conoscenza di una granulosi di *Eucosma griseana* (Hübner) (Tortricidae, Lepidoptera) quale fattore limitante il pullulamento dell'insetto nella Engadina alta. *Swiss Forest Research Institute, Memoirs* **32,** 371–418.

Martignoni, M. E., and Langston, R. L. (1960). Supplement to an annotated list and bibliography of insects reported to have virus diseases. *Hilgardia* **30,** 1–40.

Mayr, G. (1852). Abnorme Haargebilde an Nebrien und einige Pflanzen Krains. *Verhandl. Zool. Bot. Verein Wien* **2,** 75–77.

Metalnikov, S., and Metalnikov, S. S. (1935). Utilisation des microbes dans la lutte contre les insectes nuisibles. *Ann. Inst. Pasteur* **55,** 709–760.

Mills, R. R. (1967). Control of cuticular tanning in the cockroach: bursicon release by nervous stimulation. *J. Insect Physiol.* **13,** 815–820.

Mills, R. R., Lake, C. R., and Alworth, W. L. (1967). Biosynthesis of N-acetyl dopamine by the American cockroach. *J. Insect Physiol.* **13,** 1539–1546.

Mitani, K. (1934). "Modern Silkworm Pathology," 2nd Ed., Vol. II, 480 pp. Meibundo, Tokyo.

Mitani, K., and Kawai, K. (1937). Enzymatic studies on *Beauveria bassiana.* I. On the carbohydrase and chitinase. *Gunze Sanshi Kenkyu Yoho* **2,** 226.

Morgan, C., Bergold, G. H., Moore, D. H., and Rose, H. M. (1955). The macromolecular paracrystalline lattice of insect viral polyhedral bodies demonstrated in ultrathin sections examined in the electron microscope. *J. Biophys. Biochem. Cytol.* **1,** 187–190.

Morgan, C., Bergold, G. H., and Rose, H. M. (1956). Use of serial sections to delineate the structure of *Porthetria dispar* virus in the electron microscope. *J. Biophys. Biochem. Cytol.* **2,** 23–28.

Müller-Kögler, E. (1965). "Pilzkrankheiten bei Insekten Anwendung zur biologischen Schädlingsbekämpfung und Grundlagen der Insektenmykologie," 444 pp. Parey, Berlin.

Naton, E. (1961). Über die Entwicklung des schwarzbraunen Mehlkäfers, *Tribolium destructor* Uyttenb. III. Die Aufzucht in "synthetischen," carnitinunterdosierten Diäten und die darauf beruhenden Schädigungen. *Z. Angew. Entomol.* **48,** 58–74.

Nenninger, U. (1948). Die Peritrichen der Umgeben von Erlangen mit besonderer Berücksichtigung ihrer Wirtsspezifität. *Zool. Jahrb. Abt. Syst. Oekol. Geogr. Tiere* **77,** 169–266.

Noble-Nesbitt, J. (1967). Aspects of the structure, formation and function of some insect cuticles. *In* "Insects and Physiology" (J. W. L. Beament and J. E. Treherne, eds.), pp. 3–16. Oliver & Boyd, Edinburgh and London.

Northrup, Z. (1914). A bacterial disease of June beetle larvae, *Lachnosterna* spp. *Mich. Agr. Coll. Exp. Sta., Tech. Bull.* **18**, 37 pp.

Notini, G., and Mathlein, R. (1944). Grönmykos förorsakad av *Metarrhizium anisopliae* (Metsch.) Sorok. I. Grönmykosen som biolgiskt insektbekämpningsmedel. *Statens Vaextskyddsanstalt Meddelande* **43**, 1–58.

Ohtaki, T. (1960). Humoral control of pupal coloration in the cabbage white butterfly, *Pieris rapae crucivora. Annot. Zool. Jap.* **33**, 97–103.

O'Loughlin, G. T., and Chambers, T. C. (1967). The systemic infection of an aphid by a plant virus. *Virology* **33**, 262–271.

Ono, M., and Fukaya, M. (1969). The juvenile-hormone-like effect of *Chilo* iridescent virus (CIV) on the metamorphosis of the silkworm, *Bombyx mori* L. (Lepidoptera: Bombycidae). *Appl. Entomol. Zool.* **4**, 211–212.

Paillot, A. (1926). Sur une nouvelle maladie du noyau ou grasserie des chenilles de *Pieris brassicae* et un nouveau groupe de micro-organismes parasites. *C. R. Acad. Sci.* **182**, 180–182.

Paillot, A. (1933). "L'Infection chez les Insectes," 535 pp. Patissier, Trévoux, France.

Paillot, A. (1936). Contribution à l'étude des maladies à ultravirus des insectes. *Ann. Epiphyt. Phytogenet.* **2**, 341–379.

Paillot, A. (1937). Nouveau type de pseudo-grasserie observé chez les chenilles d'*Euxoa segetum. C. R. Acad. Sci.* **205**, 1264–1266.

Paillot, A. (1939). Le carpocapse dans la règion lyonnaise et les règions limitrophes. *Ann. Epiphyt. Phytogenet.* **5**, 199–211.

Paillot, A. (1940). Existence d'une septicémie à spirochètes chez les chenilles de *Pieris brassicae. C. R. Acad. Sci.* **210**, 615–616.

Pappenheimer, A. M., Jr., and Williams, C. M. (1952). The effects of diphtheria toxin on the *Cecropia* silkworm. *J. Gen. Physiol.* **35**, 727–740.

Pener, M. P. (1967). Effects of allatectomy and sectioning of the nerves of the corpora allata on oöcyte growth, male sexual behaviour, and color change in adults of *Schistocerca gregaria. J. Insect Physiol.* **13**, 665–684.

Philogène, B. J. R., and McFarlane, J. E. (1967). The formation of the cuticle in the house cricket, *Acheta domesticus* (L.), and the role of oenocytes. *Can. J. Zool.* **45**, 181–190.

Poinar, G. O., Jr., and Doncaster, C. C. (1965). The penetration of *Tripius sciarae* (Bovien) (Sphaerulariidae: Aphelenchoidea) into its insect host, *Bradysia paupera* Tuom. (Mycetophilidae: Diptera). *Nematologica* **11**, 73–78.

Poisson, R. (1929). Recherches sur quelques Eccrinides parasites de crustacés, amphipodes et isopodes. *Arch. Zool. Exp. Gen.* **69**, 179–216.

Poisson, R. (1931). Recherches sur les Eccrinides. Deuxième contribution. *Arch. Zool. Exp. Gen.* **74**, 53–68.

Prasertphon, S. (1963). Pathogenicity of different strains of *Entomophthora coronata* (Costantin) Kevorkian for larvae of the greater wax moth. *J. Insect Pathol.* **5**, 174–181.

Prasertphon, S. (1967). Circulation of hyphal bodies in the insect host and mycotoxin production in entomophthoraceous fungi. 205 pp. Ph.D. Thesis, Univ. of California, Berkeley, California.

Prasertphon, S., and Tanada, Y. (1968). The formation and circulation, in *Galleria*, of hyphal bodies of entomophthoraceous fungi. *J. Invertebr. Pathol.* **11**, 260–280.

Prasertphon, S., and Tanada, Y. (1969). Mycotoxins of entomophthoraceous fungi. *Hilgardia* **39**, 581–600.

Prescott, H. W. (1961). Respiratory pore construction in the host by the nemestrinid parasite *Neorhynchocephalus sackenii* (Diptera), with notes on respiratory tube characters. *Ann. Entomol. Soc. Amer.* **54**, 557–566.

Pryor, M. G. M. (1962). Sclerotization. *Comp. Biochem.* **4**, 371–396.

Richards, A. G. (1951). "The Integument of Arthropods," 411 pp. Univ. of Minnesota Press, Minneapolis, Minnesota.

Richards, A. G. (1953). The penetration of substances through the cuticle. *In* "Insect Physiology" (K. D. Roeder, ed.), pp. 42–54. Wiley, New York.

Richards, A. G., and Smith, M. N. (1954). Infection of cockroaches with *Herpomyces* (Laboulbeniales). III. Experimental studies on host specificity. *Bot. Gaz.* (*Chicago*) **116**, 195–198.

Richards, A. G., and Smith, M. N. (1955a). Infection of cockroaches with *Herpomyces* (Laboulbeniales). I. Life history studies. *Biol. Bull.* **108**, 206–218.

Richards, A. G., and Smith, M. N. (1955b). Infection of cockroaches with *Herpomyces* (Laboulbeniales). IV. Development of *H. stylopygae* Spegazzini. *Biol. Bull.* **109**, 306–315.

Richards, A. G., and Smith, M. N. (1956). Infection of cockroaches with *Herpomyces* (Laboulbeniales). II. Histology and histopathology. *Ann. Entomol. Soc. Amer.* **49**, 85–93.

Riddiford, L. M. (1968). Artificial diet for cecropia and other saturniid silkworms. *Science,* **160**, 1461–1462.

Rizki, M. T. M. (1953). A histochemical study of hereditary melanosis in *Drosophila willistoni. Genetics* **38**, 685–686.

Robbins, W. E., Kaplanis, J. N., Thompson, M. J., Shortino, T. J., Cohen, C. F., and Joyner, S. C. (1968). Ecdysones and analogs: effects on development and reproduction of insects. *Science* **161**, 1158–1160.

Robin, C. (1853). "Histoire Naturelle des Végétaux Parasites qui Croissent sur l'Homme et sur les Animaux Vivants," 702 pp. Baillière, Paris.

Rockwood, L. P. (1950). Entomogenous fungi of the genus *Metarrhizium* on wireworms in the Pacific Northwest. *Ann. Entomol. Soc. Amer.* **43**, 495–498.

Rouget, A. (1850). Notice sur une production parasite observée sur le *Brachinus crepitans. Ann. Soc. Entomol. Fr.* **19**, 21–24.

Roussel, J. P. (1967). Fonctions des corpora allata et contrôle de la pigmentation chez *Gryllus bimaculatus* de Geer. *J. Insect Physiol.* **13**, 113–130.

Sannasi, A. (1969). Studies of an insect mycosis. I. Histopathology of the integument of the infected queen of the mound-building termite *Odontotermes obesus. J. Invertebr. Pathol.* **13**, 4–10.

Sato, Y., Sakai, M., Imai, S., and Fujioka, S. (1968). Ecdysone activity of plant-oriented molting hormones applied on the body surface of lepidopterous larvae. *Appl. Entomol. Zool.* **3**, 49–51.

Sawyer, W. H. (1933). The development of *Entomophthora sphaerosperma* upon *Rhopobota vacciniana. Ann. Bot.* (*London*) **47**, 799–808.

Saxena,, K. N., and Williams, C. M. (1966). "Paper factor" as an inhibitor of the metamorphosis of the red cotton bug, *Dysdercus koenigii* F. *Nature* (*London*) **210**, 441–442.

Schweizer, G. (1947). Über die Kultur von *Empusa muscae* Cohn und anderen Entomophthoraceen auf kalt sterilisierten nährböden. *Planta* **35**, 132–176.

Sekeris, C. E. (1964). Sclerotization in the blowfly imago. *Science* **144**, 419–420.

Sekeris, C. E. (1965). Action of ecdysone on RNA and protein metabolism in the blowfly, *Calliphora erythrocephala. In* "Mechanisms of Hormone Action" (P. Karlson, ed.), pp. 149–167. Academic Press, New York.

Shafer, G. D. (1911). How contact insecticides kill. I. On the effects of certain gases and insecticides upon the activity and respiration of insects. II. Some properties of lime-sulphur wash that make it effective in killing scale-insects. *Mich. Agr. Exp. Sta., Tech. Bull.* **11**, 65 pp.

Shanor, L. (1955). Some observations and comments on the Laboulbeniales. *Mycologia* **47**, 1–12.

Shepard, H. H. (1951). "The Chemistry and Action of Insecticides," 504 pp. McGraw-Hill, New York.

Shikata, E., and Maramorosch, K. (1965). Electron microscopic evidence for the systemic invasion of an insect host by a plant pathogenic virus. *Virology* **27**, 461–475.

Shikata, E., and Maramorosch, K. (1967a). Electron microscopy of the formation of wound tumor virus in abdominally inoculated insect vectors. *J. Virol.* **1**, 1052–1073.

Shikata, E., and Maramorosch, K. (1967b). Electron microscopy of wound tumor virus assembly sites in insect vectors and plants. *Virology* **32**, 363–377.

Shimizu, S. (1943). Studies on the excretive function of the Malpighian tube in the silkworm. IV. On the excretion of uric acid in translucent skin mutants. *Sanshi Shikensho Hokoku* **11**, 379–385.

Singh-Pruthi, H. (1924). Studies on insect metamorphosis. I. Prothetely in mealworms (*Tenebrio molitor*) and other insects. Effects of different temperatures. *Proc. Cambridge Phil. Soc.* (*Biol. Sci.*) **1**, 139–147.

Sláma, K. (1962). The juvenile hormone like effect of fatty acids, fatty alcohols, and some other compounds in insect metamorphosis. *Acta Entomol. Bohemoslov.* **59**, 323–340.

Sláma, K., and Williams, C. M. (1965). Juvenile hormone activity for the bug *Pyrrhocoris apterus*. *Proc. Nat. Acad. Sci. U.S.* **54**, 411–414.

Sláma, K., and Williams, C. M. (1966). "Paper factor" as an inhibitor of the embryonic development of the European bug, *Pyrrhocoris apterus*. *Nature* (*London*) **210**, 329–330.

Smirnoff, W. A. (1959). Predators of *Neodiprion swainei* Midd. (Hymenoptera: Tenthredinidae) larval vectors of virus diseases. *Can. Entomol.* **91**, 246–248.

Smith, K. M. (1963). The cytoplasmic virus diseases. *In* "Insect Pathology, An Advanced Treatise" (E. A. Steinhaus, ed.), Vol. 1, pp. 457–497. Academic Press, New York.

Smith, K. M., Hills, G. J., and Rivers, C. F. (1961). Studies on the cross-inoculation of the *Tipula* iridescent virus. *Virology* **13**, 233–241.

Smith, O. J., Hughes, K. M., Dunn, P. H., and Hall, I. M. (1956). A granulosis virus disease of the western grape leaf skeletonizer and its transmission. *Can. Entomol.* **88**, 507–515.

Sokoloff, A. (1966). "The Genetics of *Tribolium* and Related Species," 212 pp. Academic Press, New York.

Speare, A. T. (1921). *Massospora cicadina* Peck a fungous parasite of the periodical cicada. *Mycologia* **13**, 72–82.

Spielman, A., and Skaff, V. (1967). Inhibition of metamorphosis and ecdysis in mosquitoes. *J. Insect Physiol.* **13**, 1087–1095.

Srivastava, U. S., and Gilbert, L. I. (1968). Juvenile hormone: effects on a higher dipteran. *Science* **161**, 61–62.

Srivastava, U. S., and Gilbert, L. I. (1969). The influence of juvenile hormone on the metamorphosis of *Sarcophaga bullata*. *J. Insect Physiol.* **15**, 177–189.

Stairs, G. R. (1964). Selection of a strain of insect granulosis virus producing only cubic inclusion bodies. *Virology* **24**, 520–521.

Stairs, G. R., Parrish, W. B., Briggs, J. D., and Allietta, M. (1966). Fine structure of a granulosis virus of the codling moth. *Virology* **30**, 583–584.

Stark, M. B. (1937). The origin of certain hereditary tumors in *Drosophila*. *Amer. J. Cancer* **31**, 253–267.

Steinhaus, E. A. (1946). "Insect Microbiology," 763 pp. Cornell Univ. Press (Comstock), Ithaca, New York.

Steinhaus, E. A. (1949). "Principles of Insect Pathology," 757 pp. McGraw-Hill, New York.

Steinhaus, E. A. (1963). "Insect Pathology, An Advanced Treatise," Vol. 1, 661 pp. and Vol. 2, 689 pp. Academic Press, New York.

Steinhaus, E. A., and Leutenegger, R. (1963). Icosahedral virus from a scarab (*Sericesthis*). *J. Insect Pathol.* **5**, 266–270.

Steinhaus, E. A., and Marsh, G. A. (1962). Report of diagnoses of diseased insects 1951–1961. *Hilgardia* **33**, 349–490.

Steinhaus, E. A., and Zeikus, R. D. (1968a). Teratology of the beetle *Tenebrio molitor*. I. Gross morphology of certain abnormality types. *J. Invertebr. Pathol.* **10**, 190–210.

Steinhaus, E. A., and Zeikus, R. D. (1968b). Teratology of the beetle *Tenebrio molitor*. III. Ultrastructural alterations in the flight musculature of the pupal-winged adult. *J. Invertebr. Pathol.* **12**, 40–52.

Steinhaus, E. A., and Zeikus, R. D. (1969). Teratology of the beetle *Tenebrio molitor*. IV. Ultrastructure of the necrotic fat body and foregut associated with the pupal-winged adult. *J. Invertebr. Pathol.* **13**, 337–344.

Stellwaag, F., and Staudenmayer, T. (1940). Wie wirkt Dinitro-ortho-kresol auf Insekten? Ein Beitrag zum Mechanismus der Giftwirkung. *Anz. Schaedlingskunde* **16**, 37–39.

Strong, F. E., Wells, K., and Apple, J. W. (1960). An unidentified fungus parasitic on the seed-corn maggot. *J. Econ. Entomol.* **53**, 478–479.

Stutzer, M. J., and Wsorow, W. J. (1927). Über Infektionen der Raupen der Wintersaateule (*Euxoa segetum* Schiff). *Zentralbl. Bakteriol., Parasitenk., Infektionskr., Abt. 2* **71**, 113–129.

Sullivan, W. N., and McCauley, T. R. (1960). Effect of acceleration force on insect mortality. *J. Econ. Entomol.* **53**, 691–692.

Summers, M. D. (1969). Apparent in vivo pathway of granulosis virus invasion and infection. *J. Virol.* **4**, 188–190.

Sussman, A. S. (1951). Studies of an insect mycosis. I. Etiology of the disease. *Mycologia* **43**, 338–350.

Sussman, A. S. (1952). Studies of an insect mycosis. IV. The physiology of the host-parasite relationship of *Platysamia cecropia* and *Aspergillus flavus*. *Mycologia* **44**, 493–505.

Takahashi, Y. (1958). Studies on the cuticle of the silkworm, *Bombyx mori* L. XI. Penetration of hyphae of the fungus, *Beauveria bassiana* (Bals.) Vuill., through the larval and pupal cuticles. *Annot. Zool. Jap.* **31**, 13–21.

Tanada, Y. (1953a). A microsporidian parasite of the imported cabbageworm in Hawaii. *Proc. Hawaii. Entomol. Soc.* **15**, 167–175.

Tanada, Y. (1953b). Description and characteristics of a granulosis virus of the imported cabbageworm. *Proc. Hawaii. Entomol. Soc.* **15**, 235–260.

Tanada, Y. (1955a). Field observations on a microsporidian parasite of *Pieris rapae* (L.) and *Apanteles glomeratus* (L.). *Proc. Hawaii. Entomol. Soc.* **15**, 609–616.

Tanada, Y. (1955b). Susceptibility of the imported cabbageworm to fungi: *Beauveria* spp. *Proc. Hawaii. Entomol. Soc.* **15**, 617–622.

Tanada, Y. (1963). Epizootiology of infectious diseases. *In* "Insect Pathology, An Advanced Treatise" (E. A. Steinhaus, ed.), Vol. 2, pp. 423–475. Academic Press, New York.

Tanada, Y. (1967). Microbial pesticides. *In* "Pest Control: Biological, Physical, and Selected Chemical Methods" (W. W. Kilgore and R. L. Doutt, eds.), pp. 31–88. Academic Press, New York.

Tanada, Y., and Leutenegger, R. (1968). Histopathology of a granulosis-virus disease of the codling moth, *Carpocapsa pomonella. J. Invertebr. Pathol.* **10**, 39–47.

Tanada, Y., and Leutenegger, R. (1970). Multiplication of a granulosis virus in larval midgut cells of *Trichoplusia ni* and possible pathways of invasion into the hemocoel. *J. Ultrastruct. Res.* **30**, 589–600.

Tanaka, Y. (1953). Genetics of the silkworm, *Bombyx mori. Advan. Genet.* **5**, 239–317.

Tavares, I. I. (1965). Thallus development in *Herpomyces paranensis* (Laboulbeniales). *Mycologia* **57**, 704–721.

Tavares, I. I. (1966). Structure and development of *Herpomyces stylopygae* (Laboulbeniales). *Amer. J. Bot.* **53**, 311–318.

Thaxter, R. (1896). Contribution towards a monograph of the Laboulbeniaceae, Part I. *Mem. Amer. Acad. Arts Sci.* **12**(3), 187–439.

Thaxter, R. (1908). Contribution toward a monograph of the Laboulbeniaceae, Part II. *Mem. Amer. Acad. Arts Sci.* **13**(6), 217–469.

Thaxter, R. (1914). On certain peculiar fungus-parasites of living insects. *Bot. Gaz.* (*Chicago*) **58**, 235–253.

Thaxter, R. (1920). Second note on certain peculiar fungus-parasites of living insects. *Bot. Gaz* (*Chicago*) **69**, 1–27.

Thaxter, R. (1924). Contribution towards a monograph of the Laboulbeniaceae, Part III. *Mem. Amer. Acad. Arts Sci.* **14**(5), 309–426.

Thaxter, R. (1926). Contribution towards a monograph of the Laboulbeniaceae, Part IV. *Mem. Amer. Acad. Arts Sci.* **15**(4), 427–580.

Thaxter, R. (1931). Contribution towards a monograph of the Laboulbeniaceae, Part V. *Mem. Amer. Acad. Arts Sci.* **16**(1), 1–435.

Thomson, H. M. (1955). *Perezia fumiferanae* n. sp., a new species of microsporidia from the spruce budworm *Choristoneura fumiferana* (Clem). *J. Parasitol.* **41**, 416–423.

Thompson, C. G., and Steinhaus, E. A. (1950). Further tests using a polyhedrosis virus to control the alfalfa caterpillar. *Hilgardia* **19**, 411–445.

Thompson, W. R. (1915). Contribution à la connaissance de la larve *Planidium* (Hymenoptera Chalcidoidea). *Bull. Sci. Fr. Belg.* **48**, 319–349.

Thorpe, W. H. (1930). The biology of the petroleum fly (*Psilopa petrolii,* Coq.). *Trans. Entomol. Soc. London* **78**, 331–344.

Toumanoff, C. (1928). On the infection of *Pyrausta nubilalis* Hb. by *Aspergillus flavus* and *Spicaria farinosa. Int. Corn Borer Invest., Sci. Rept.* **1**, 74–76.

Toumanoff, C. (1959). Observation concernant le role probable d'un prédateur dans la transmission d'un bacille aux chenilles de *Pieris brassicae. Ann. Inst. Pasteur* **96**, 108–110.

Tsujita, M. (1953). Maternal inheritance of "lethal yellow." *Annu. Rep., Nat. Inst. Genet. (Japan)* 3, 24–27.

Tuzet, O., and Manier, J.-F. (1950). Les Trichomycètes. Revision de leur diagnose. Raisons qui nous font y joindre les *Asellariées. Ann. Sci. Natur. Zool. Biol. Anim. (Ser. 11)*, **12**, 15–23.

Tuzet, O. and Manier, J.-F. (1951). Le cycle de l'*Amoebidium parasiticum* Cienk. Revision du genre *Amoebidium. Ann. Sci. Natur., Zool. Biol. Anim. (Ser. 11)*, **13**, 351–364.

Tuzet, O., and Manier, J.-F. (1952). Trichophytes commensaux de l'intestin postérieur de Diplopodes du Brésil. Quelques considérations sur les Trichophytes déjà décrits infestant les Diplopodes. *Ann. Sci. Natur., Zool. Biol. Anim. (Ser. 11)*, **14**, 249–262.

Vago, C., and Kurstak, E. (1965). Mécanisme d'action de *Bacillus thuringiensis* introduit par un parasite Hyménoptère dans l'hémolymphe d'un Lépidoptère. *Antonie van Leeuwenhoek; J. Microbiol. Serol.* **31**, 282–294.

Vago, C., and Sauvezon, J.-L. (1969). Les tumeurs chez les invertébrés. *Ann. Zool. Ecol. Anim.* **1**, 15–38.

Van de Pol, P. H., and Ponsen, M. B. (1963). Pathologische verschijnselen bij vlinders van *Pieris brassicae* L., verband houdend met een granula- (virus) infectie van rupsen. *Entomol. Ber. (Amsterdam)* **23**, 106–108.

Van Zwaluwenburg, R. H. (1928). The interrelationships of insects and roundworms. *Hawaiian Sugar Planters' Ass., Entomol. Ser., Exp. Sta. Bull.* **20**, 68 pp.

Vinson, J. W., and Williams, C. M. (1967). Lethal effects of synthetic juvenile hormone on the human body louse. *Proc. Nat. Acad. Sci. U.S.* **58**, 294–297.

Vogt, M. (1947). Beeinflussung der Antennendifferenzierung durch Colchicin bei der *Drosophila* mutante *Aristopedia. Experientia* 3, 156–157.

Wada, Y. (1957). Studies on the antimicrobial function of insect lipids. VI. Difference in susceptibility of field insects to fungal diseases. *Jap. J. Ecol.* **7**, 90–93.

Wallengren, H., and Johansson, R. (1929). On the infection of *Pyrausta nubilalis* Hb. by *Metarrhizium anisopliae* (Metsch.). *Int. Corn Borer Invest., Sci. Rept.* **2**, 131–145.

Watanabe, H. (1968). Abnormal cell proliferation in the epidermis of the fall webworm, *Hyphantria cunea,* induced by the infection of a nuclear-polyhedrosis virus. *J. Invertebr. Pathol.* **12**, 310–315.

Weiser, J. (1961). Die Mikrosporidien als Parasiten der Insecten. *Monogr. Angew. Entomol.* **17**, 149 pp.

Weiser, J. (1963). Sporozoan infections. *In* "Insect Pathology, An Advanced Treatise" (E. A. Steinhaus, ed.), Vol. 2, pp. 291–334. Academic Press, New York.

Weiser, J. (1965). A new virus infection of mosquito larvae. *Bull. W. H. O.* **33**, 586–588.

Weiser, J. (1968). Iridescent virus from the blackfly *Simulium ornatum* Meigen in Czechoslovakia. *J. Invertebr. Pathol.* **12**, 36–39.

Welch, H. E. (1959). Taxonomy, life cycle, development, and habits of two new species of *Allantonematidae* (Nematoda) parasitic in drosophilid flies. *Parasitology* **49**, 83–103.

Welch, H. E. (1960). Effects of protozoan parasites and commensals on larvae of the mosquito *Aedes communis* (DeGeer) (Diptera: Culicidae) at Churchill, Manitoba. *J. Insect Pathol.* **2**, 386–395.

Welch, H. E. (1963). Nematode infections. *In* "Insect Pathology, An Advanced Treatise" (E. A. Steinhaus, ed.), Vol. 2, pp. 363–392. Academic Press, New York.

Welch, H. E. (1965). Entomophilic nematodes. *Annu. Rev. Entomol.* **10**, 275–302.
Whisler, H. C. (1968). Experimental studies with a new species of *Stigmatomyces* (Laboulbeniales). *Mycologia* **60**, 65–75.
Whitten, J. (1968). Metamorphic changes in insects. *In* "Metamorphosis, a Problem in Developmental Biology" (W. Etkin and L. I. Gilbert, eds.), pp. 43–105. Appleton-Century-Crofts, New York.
Whitten, J. M. (1969). Haemocyte activity in relation to epidermal cell growth, cuticle secretion, and cell death in a metamorphosing cyclorrhaphan pupa. *J. Insect Physiol.* **15**, 763–778.
Wigglesworth, V. B. (1933). The physiology of the cuticle and of ecdysis in *Rhodnius prolixus* (Triatomidae, Hemiptera); with special reference to the function of the oenocytes and of the dermal glands. *Quart. J. Microsc. Sci.* **76**, 269–318.
Wigglesworth, V. B. (1937). Wound healing in an insect (*Rhodnius prolixus* Hemiptera). *J. Exp. Biol.* **14**, 364–381.
Wigglesworth, V. B. (1940). Local and general factors in the development of "pattern" in *Rhodnius prolixus* (Hemiptera). *J. Exp. Biol.* **17**, 180–200.
Wigglesworth, V. B. (1942). Some notes on the integument of insects in relation to the entry of contact insecticides. *Bull. Entomol. Res.* **33**, 205–218.
Wigglesworth, V. B. (1945). Transpiration through the cuticle of insects. *J. Exp. Biol.* **21**, 97–114.
Wigglesworth, V. B. (1948). The structure and deposition of the cuticle in the adult mealworm, *Tenebrio molitor* L. (Coleoptera). *Quart. J. Microsc. Sci.* **89**, 197–217.
Wigglesworth, V. B. (1956). The haemocytes and connective tissue formation in an insect, *Rhodnius prolixus* (Hemiptera). *Quart. J. Microsc. Sci.* **97**, 89–98.
Wigglesworth, V. B. (1964). The hormonal regulation of growth and reproduction in insects. *Advan. Insect Physiol.* **2**, 247–336.
Wigglesworth, V. B. (1965). "The Principles of Insect Physiology," 6th Ed., 741 pp. Methuen, London.
Williams, C. M. (1956). The juvenile hormone of insects. *Nature (London)* **178**, 212–213.
Williams, C. M. (1967). Third-generation pesticides. *Sci. Amer.* **217**, 13–17.
Woodard, D. B., and Chapman, H. C. (1968). Laboratory studies with the mosquito iridescent virus (MIV). *J. Invertebr. Pathol.* **11**, 296–301.
Wyatt, G. R. (1968). Biochemistry of insect metamorphosis. *In* "Metamorphosis, a Problem in Developmental Biology" (W. Etkin and L. I. Gilbert, eds.), pp. 143–184. Appleton-Century-Crofts, New York.
Xeros, N. (1954). A second virus disease of the leatherjacket, *Tipula paludosa*. *Nature (London)* **174**, 562.
Yamaguchi, K. (1961). Histological observations on the infection of silkworms by *Aspergillus*. *Kenkyu Yoho Saitama-Ken Sanshi Shikensho* **33**, 70–76.
Yokoyama, T. (1959). "Silkworm Genetics," 185 pp. Japan Soc. Promotion Sci., Tokyo.
Zacharuk, R. Y. (1970a). Fine structure of the fungus *Metarrhizium anisopliae* infecting three species of larval Elateridae (Coleoptera). II. Conidial germ tubes and appressoria. *J. Invertbr. Pathol.* **15**, 81–91.
Zacharuk, R. Y. (1970b). Fine structure of the fungus *Metarrhizium anisopliae* infecting three species of larval Elateridae (Coleoptera). III. Penetration of the host integument. *J. Invertebr. Pathol.* **15**, 372–396.
Zeikus, R. D., and Steinhaus, E. A. (1968). Teratology of the beetle *Tenebrio*

molitor. II. The development and gross description of the pupal-winged adult. *J. Invertebr. Pathol.* **11**, 8–24.

Zeikus, R. D., and Steinhaus, E. A. (1969). Teratology of the beetle *Tenebrio molitor*. V. Ultrastructural changes and viruslike particles in the foregut epithelium of pupal-winged adults. *J. Invertebr. Pathol.* **14**, 115–121.

Zlotkin, E., and Levinson, H. Z. (1968). Influence of cecropia oil on the epidermis of *Tenebrio molitor*. *J. Insect. Physiol.* **14**, 1719–1723.

Zlotkin, E., and Levinson, H. Z. (1969). Influence of cecropia oil on the cuticle of *Tenebrio molitor*. *J. Insect Physiol.* **15**, 105–110.

Neoplasia in Fish: A Review

Lionel E. Mawdesley-Thomas

HUNTINGDON RESEARCH CENTRE,
HUNTINGDON, ENGLAND

Omnis cellula e cellula.
—Rudolf Virchow (1821–1902)

I. Introduction

Neoplasia or tumor formation in fish may not appear at first sight to be a very profitable field of study for the pathologist, yet there is a wealth of widely scattered literature to be found on the subject (Hofer, 1904; Bean, 1907; Plehn, 1924; Schäperclaus, 1954; Schlumberger, 1958; Finkelstein, 1960; Lombard, 1962; Gusseva, 1963; McGregor, 1963; Reichenbach-Klinke and Elkan, 1965; van Duijn, 1967; Dawe and Harshbarger, 1968; Mawdesley-Thomas, 1969; Wellings, 1969).

Definition

A fundamental problem for the pathologist, especially the comparative pathologist, is one of definition and nomenclature. In many instances pathological conditions observed in nonhuman species are not considered on their own merits but are related back to man, thus promoting a misinformed and ill-understood "specialty." It cannot be overstated that any disease in an animal, be it fish, mammal, or bird, should be treated on its own merit and not related to a pseudosimilar human condition. In bacterial infections of fish, the term "furunculosis" still persists as the reminder of a misleading nomenclature.

The word "neoplasm" is a combination of French and Greek words which, according to the *Shorter Oxford English Dictionary*, was first used in 1864 to describe "a new formation of tissue in some part of the body: a tumour." This is perhaps a useful starting definition. In this paper, however, the term "tumor" is used in its specific sense—that of a neoplasm—and not nonspecifically to mean a swelling in a general sense. As with any definition, it is limited in its application. Virchow (1821–1902), the father of cellular pathology, concluded after a lifetime of study: "I do not think that a living human being can be found that even under torture could actually say what tumours really are." Nicholson (1926) maintained that it was impossible to define a tumor, and while one can only agree with such authorities, it is helpful if some kind of working definition can be applied. Willis (1967) defined a tumor as "an abnormal mass of tissue, the growth of which exceeds and is uncoordinated with that of the normal tissue, and persists in the same excessive manner after cessation of the stimuli which evoked the change." It is to this working definition that most pathologists are committed.

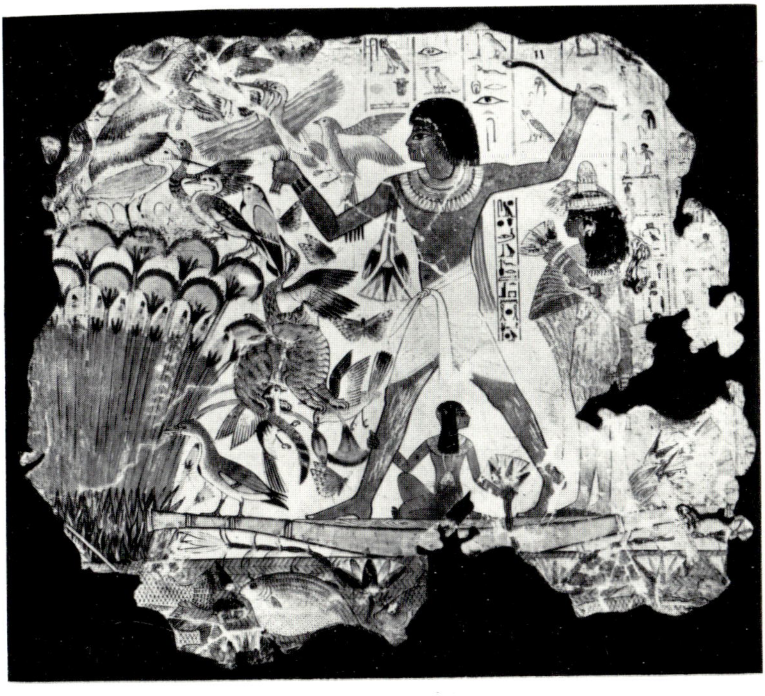

Fig. 1. Fowling scene from Egyptian tomb (Thebes, 1450 B.C.). Note fish (*Tilapia?*) with abdominal enlargement. (By courtesy of the Trustees of the British Museum.)

CONRADI GESNERI
medici Tigurini Historiæ Animalium
Liber IIII. qui est de Piscium &
Aquatilium animantium
natura.

CVM ICONIBVS SINGVLORVM AD
VIVVM EXPRESSIS FERE OMNIB. DCCVI.

Continentur in hoc Volumine, GVLIELMI RONDELETII *quoq;*
medicinæ professoris Regij in Schola Monspeliensi, *&* PETRI BEL-
LONII *Cenomani, medici hoc tempore Lutetiæ eximij, de*
Aquatilium singulis scripta.

AD INVICTISSIMVM PRINCIPEM, DIVVM FERDINAN-
dum Imperatorem semper Augustum, &c.

Μωμήσεταί τις ῥᾷον, ἢ μιμήσεται.

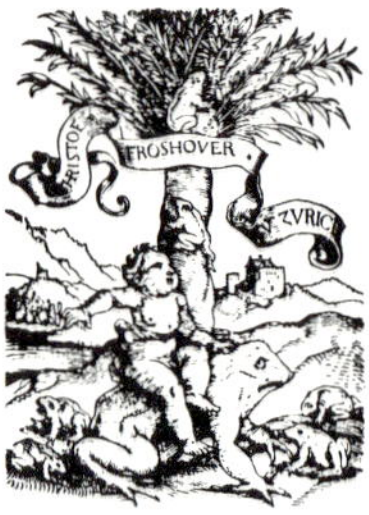

CVM Priuilegijs S. Cæsareæ Maiestatis ad octennium, & poten-
tissimi Regis Galliarum ad decennium.

TIGVRI APVD CHRISTOPH. FROSCHOVERVM,
ANNO M. D. LVIII.

2

MUSEUM WORMIANUM.
SEU
HISTORIA
RERUM RARIORUM,
Tam Naturalium, quam Artificialium, tam Domesticarum,
quam Exoticarum, quæ Hafniæ Danorum in
ædibus Authoris servantur.

Adornata ab

OLAO WORM, MED. DOCT.
&, in Regiâ Hafniensi Academiâ, olim
Professore publico.

Variis & accuratis Iconibus illustrata.

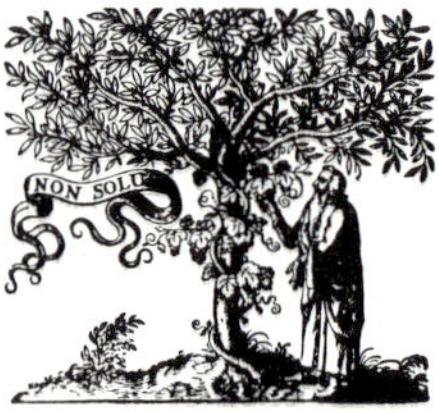

LUGDUNI BATAVORUM,
Apud IOHANNEM ELSEVIRIUM, Acad. Typograph.
CIↃ IↃC LV.

3

Gottorffische
Kunst-Kammer/
Worinnen
Allerhand ungemeine Sachen / So
theils die Natur/ theils künstliche Hände her-
vor gebracht und bereitet.
Vor diesem
Aus allen vier Theilen der Welt
zusammen getragen/
Und
Vor einigen Jahren beschrieben/
Auch mit behörigen Kupffern gezieret
Durch
Adam Olearium, Weil. Bibliothecarium
und Antiquarium auff der Fürstl. Resi-
dentz Gottorff.
Anjetzo aber übersehen/ und zum andern mal
gedruckt/

Auff Gottfriedt Schultzens Kosten. 1674.

In dessen Buchladen zu Schleßwig solche zu finden ist.

4

II. Historical Review

"There is no new thing under the sun." So it is with tumors of fish. A survey of the classic literature is disappointing, for while Thompson (1947) in his excellent *Glossary of Greek Fishes* gives much information concerning fish as described by the classic authors, no written or illustrated reference to any tumor or tumorlike formation is to be found. This fact is also confirmed by the British Museum's Department of Greek and Roman Antiquities. Similarly, Gaillard (1923) in his "Researches into Fish Represented on Egyptian Tombs" fails to reveal any reference

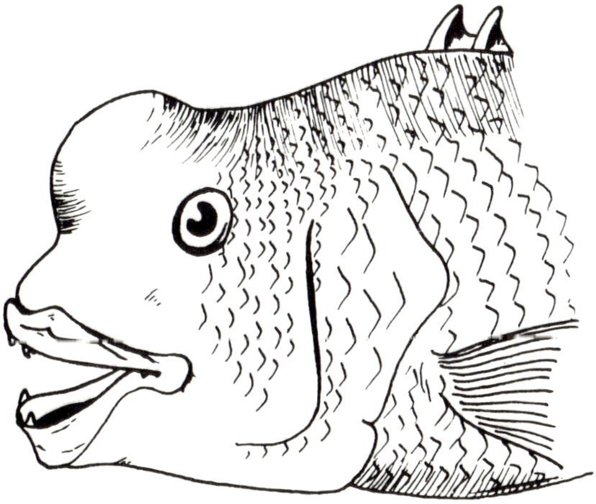

Fig. 5. *Dentex vulgaris*, showing a "gibbosity" on the forehead (Aldrovandi, 1613). (Drawing by Peter Healey.)

in the Egyptian literature. On one tomb painting from Thebes (1450 B.C.) in the British Museum, however, a fish (*Tilapia* ?) which appears to have an abdominal tumor can be seen (Fig. 1), although the differential diagnosis of a gravid hen fish must be considered the most likely. While much of the medieval literature is well illustrated (Gessner, 1558; Worm, 1655) (Figs. 2 and 3), only Olearius (1674) (Fig. 4) makes reference to any anomaly and notes the presence of exostoses in various fish. The obscurity of some of the medieval Latin makes this statement

Fig. 2. Frontispiece from *Historiae Animalium* of Conrad Gessner (1558), concerning fish and aquatic animals.

Fig. 3. Frontispiece from *Historia Rerum Rariorum* of Olao Worm (1655).

Fig. 4. Frontispiece of the work of Adam Olearius (1674).

far from absolute, however. In the sixteenth century the Italian Aldrovandi (1522–1605), one of the great naturalists of his century (Gudger, 1934, 1936), described a gibbous (humped) sea perch (Fig. 5) in his book *De Piscibus* (1613). Whether or not this represented a true tumor

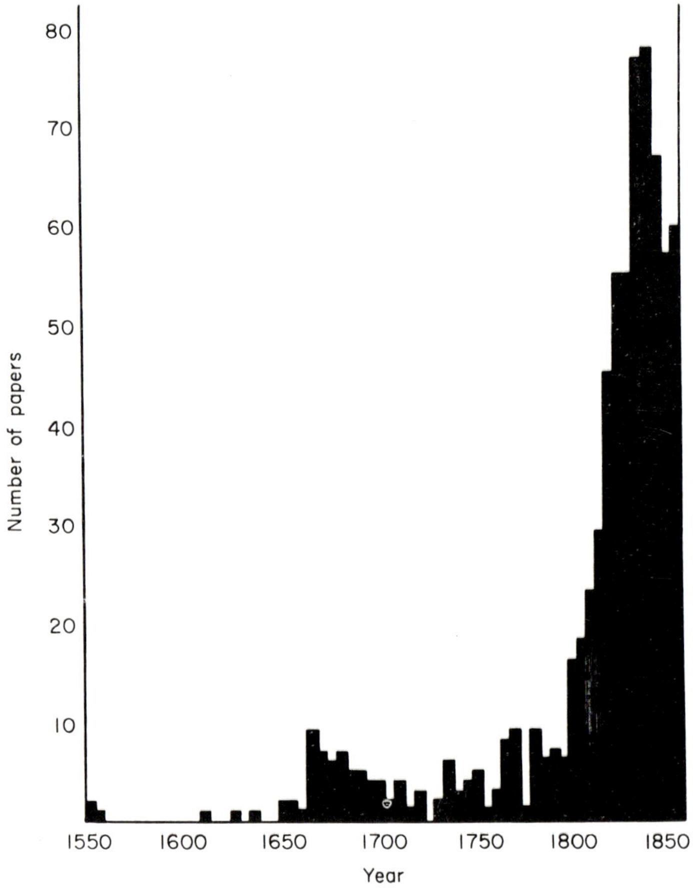

Fig. 6. Analysis of scientific papers written concerning fish over three centuries (1550–1850). (Modified after Cole and Eales, 1917.)

such as a lipoma is uncertain, and the possibility of a fat storage organ cannot be excluded. These tumors, still to be seen in members of the families Cichlidae, Labridae, and Sparidae, show some sexual dimorphism and age association. Historical surveys are often disappointing owing to the scarcity of precise documentation from earlier times. It

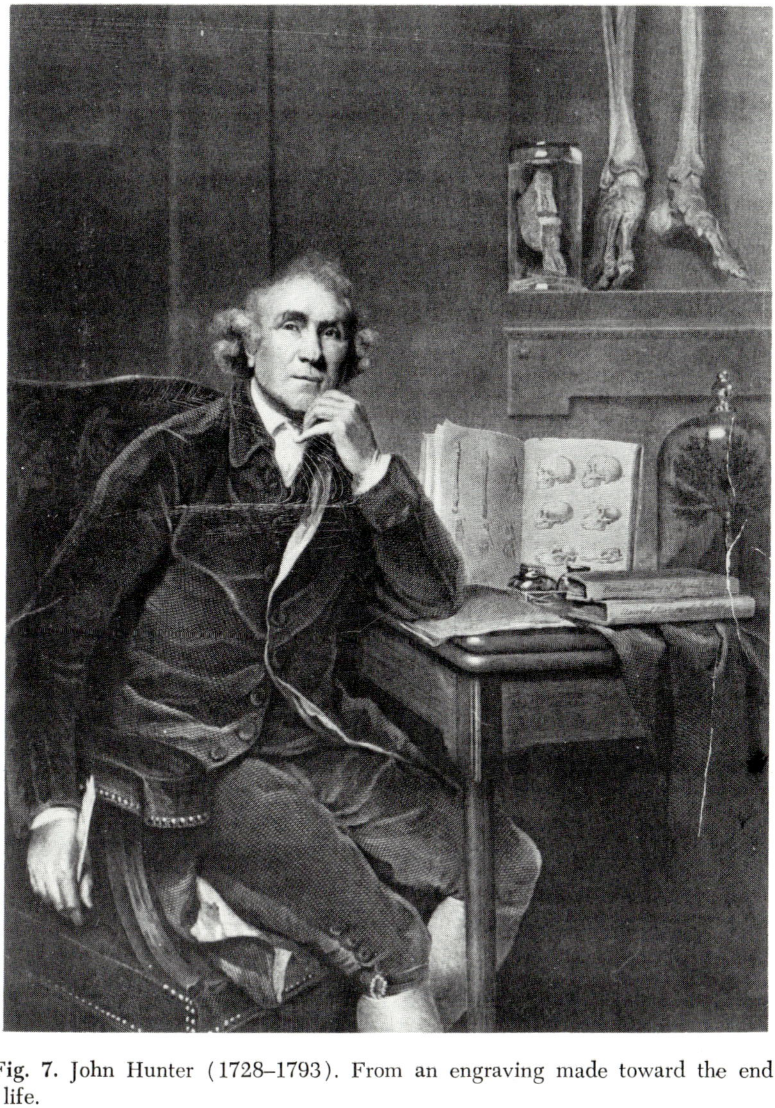

Fig. 7. John Hunter (1728–1793). From an engraving made toward the end of his life.

is interesting to note the statistical evaluation of the literature by Cole and Eales (1917) (Fig. 6), which indicates the numbers of papers written on fish over three centuries. One factor contributing more than any other to this lack of documentation is that while abnormal fish must have been seen by many observers the means for preserving them for

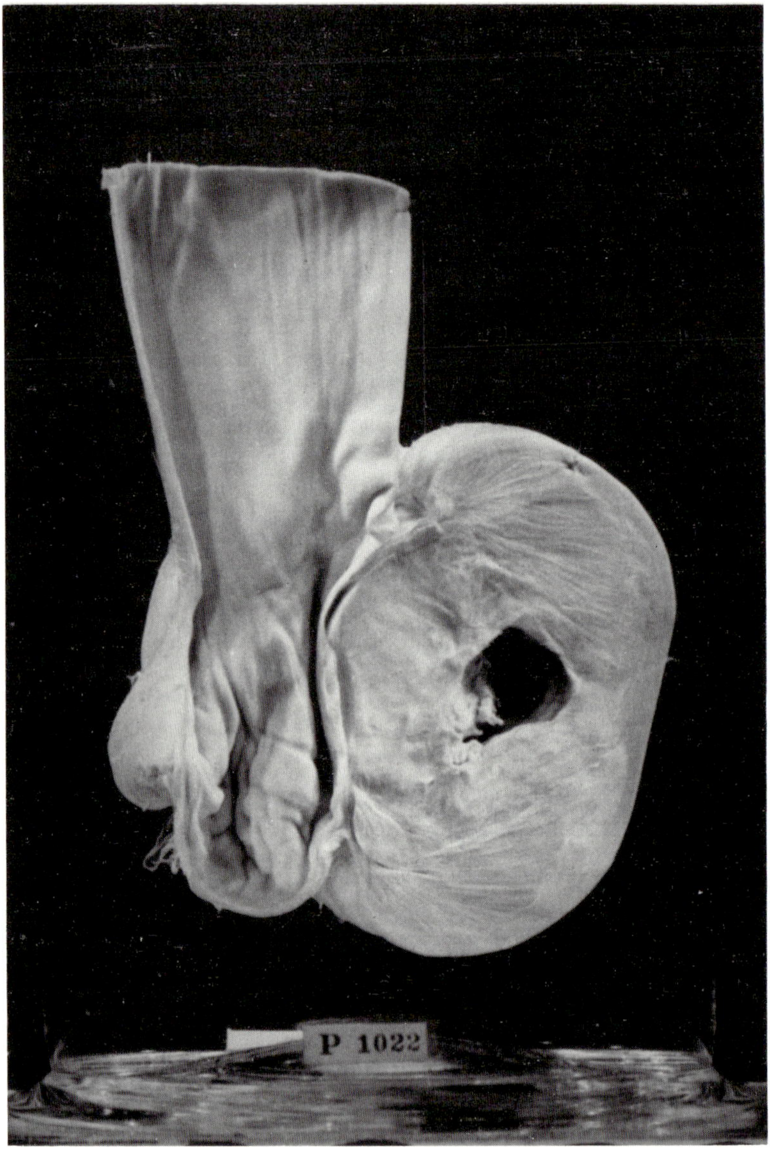

Fig. 8. Tumor of the stomach of a cod (*G. morhua*). Hunterian collection. Catalogue No. P 1022. Specimen is greatly magnified by containing vessel. (By kind permission of Miss Jessie Dobson, Curator of the Hunterian Museum, Royal College of Surgeons of England, London.)

future study had not been established. In the Hunterian collection, established by the great John Hunter (1728–1793) (Fig. 7), which contained about 13,465 specimens, only 4,829 were moist preparations, the remainder being dried. The use of spirit or wine as a preservative in the biological field was an event of great historical significance. In the Hunterian collection there exists a single fish tumor, a tumor of the stomach of a cod (*Gadus morhua*) (Fig. 8). The following description is appended.

> A longitudinal section of the stomach of a codfish, and of a large tumour attached to it. The tumour is of a somewhat oval form and measured about nine inches and five inches in its two chief diameters: it appears to have grown between the coats of the stomach, for the outer coat may be traced for a short distance over its surface. The greater part of it is composed of a very dense and compact semi-transparent substance, traversed by fine bundles of white shining fibres, which are variously arranged but chiefly radiate from the part at which the tumour is attached to the mucous membrane of the stomach. The exterior of the tumour is formed of a thick layer of pale fibrous tissue enveloping that just described; and in its centre is a large irregular cavity, formed apparently, by ulceration or softening of its substance. The mucous membrane and the other adjacent parts of the stomach appear healthy.

It remains a constant source of wonder that John Hunter had so wide a range of interests. There exists a paper presented by him (Hunter, 1782) to the Royal Society on "An Account of the Organ of Hearing in Fish" in which he wrote that we ought: "to consider whatever is uncommon in the structure of this organ in fishes as only a link in the chain of varieties displayed in its formation in different animals descending from the most perfect to the most imperfect, in regular progression." Such statements are of the utmost significance as they pre-date much Darwinian philosophy. As in the case of anatomy, so it is with pathology which in the final analysis is but "an altered anatomy." In the year of Hunter's death, Bell (1793) presented a paper to the Royal Society describing a species of *Chaetodon,* called by the Malays "Ecan bonna," and recorded osteomata of the ribs and other bones (Fig. 9). It is unfortunate that these osteomata have become inappropriately known as "Tilley bones" (Konnerth, 1966). Buniva (1802) wrote a short report on the physiology and pathology of fish, while Rayer (1843) was the first to write a comprehensive treatise on diseases of fish, in which he quotes Professors Scheidsweiler and Gody of the Veterinary School of Brussels as describing epithelial tumors of trout. Whether these represented papillomata or epithelial hyperplasia is a matter for conjecture. Gervais (1875)

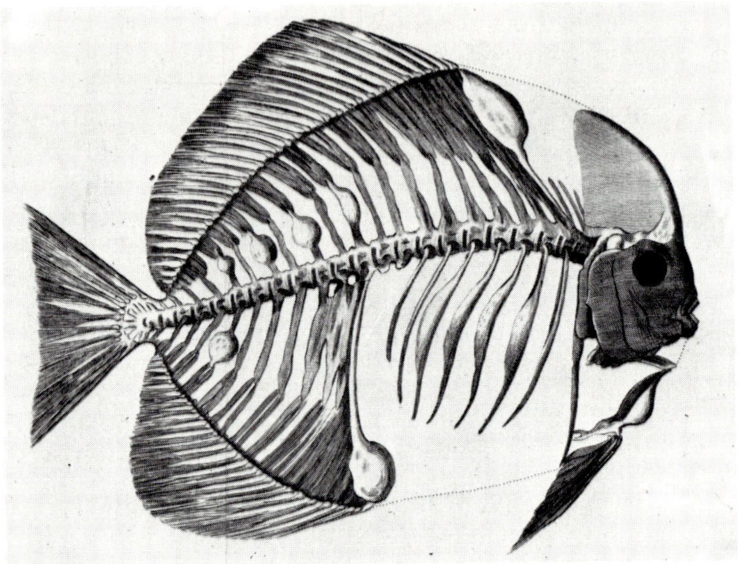

Fig. 9. Skeleton of a species of *Chaetodon* showing various exostoses described by Bell (1793).

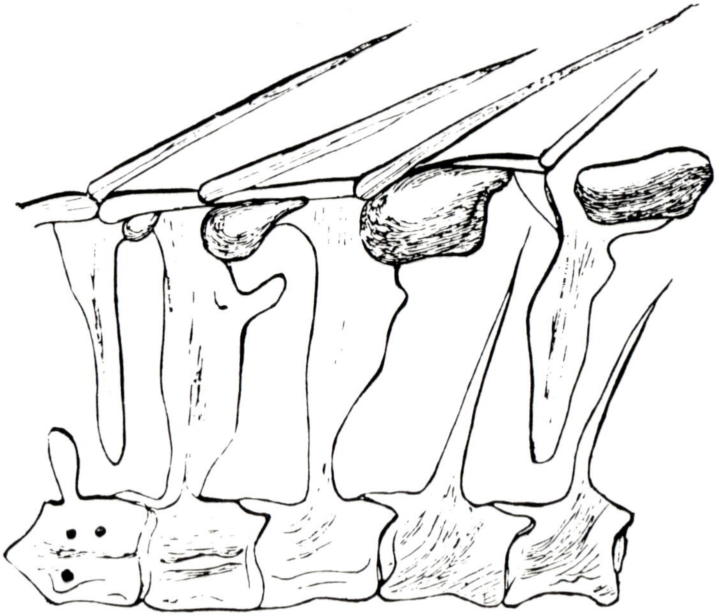

Fig. 10. Exostoses associated with the vertebral column (Gervais, 1875).

reported exostoses associated with the vertebrae of *Lepidopus* (Fig. 10). Finally, in this brief historical survey, mention must be made of Bland-Sutton (1885) who, as a Fellow of the Royal College of Surgeons of England, held the position of Lecturer on Comparative Anatomy at the Middlesex Hospital Medical College, London. He recorded many tumors of animals previously in the collection of the Royal College of Surgeons of England, the majority of which were destroyed in the bombing during the Second World War, thus providing an invaluable link with the past. Bland-Sutton described a fibrous tumor of the stomach of a cod similar to that reported by Hunter (Fig. 11), together with many examples of exostoses (Figs. 12 and 13) in a pike (*Esox lucius*) and a cod (*G. morhua*), and a spindle cell sarcoma in a goldfish (*Carassius auratus*). Bland-Sutton defined a tumor as "a new growth, characterized by histological diversity from the matrix in which it grows; it is distinguished from inflammatory new-formations by the variety of its form, mode of origin and the frequent inherent tendency it has to increase."

III. Classification of Tumors

The classification of tumors presents many problems as there must inevitably be exceptions and inadequacies. A useful classification considers the anatomical and histological type from which the tumors arise. The following classification of tumors has been modified after Willis.

(1) Tumors of epithelial tissues—consisting of papillomata, adenomata, or carcinomata

(2) Tumors of nonhemopoietic mesenchymal tissues—consisting of tumors of muscle, connective, skeletal, and vascular tissues

(3) Tumors of hemopoietic tissues—consisting of tumors of lymphatic tissue and other hemopoietic tissues

(4) Special classes of tumors—consisting of melanomata, teratomata, and tumors associated with the peripheral nervous system

It is worth emphasizing that the terms "benign" and "malignant" are used in reference to man to indicate a clinical significance in relation to prognosis and to this alone. As prognosis is not an established art in lower animals, to designate a tumor benign or malignant on a purely histological basis is to relegate pathology to the descriptive desert of the nineteenth century. Interspecies prognosis, if it exists at all, cannot be extrapolated without a most careful examination in the light of much experience. The hallmark of a malignant tumor, in man, is its invasiveness, whether local or distant; it is the behavior of the tumor that is significant

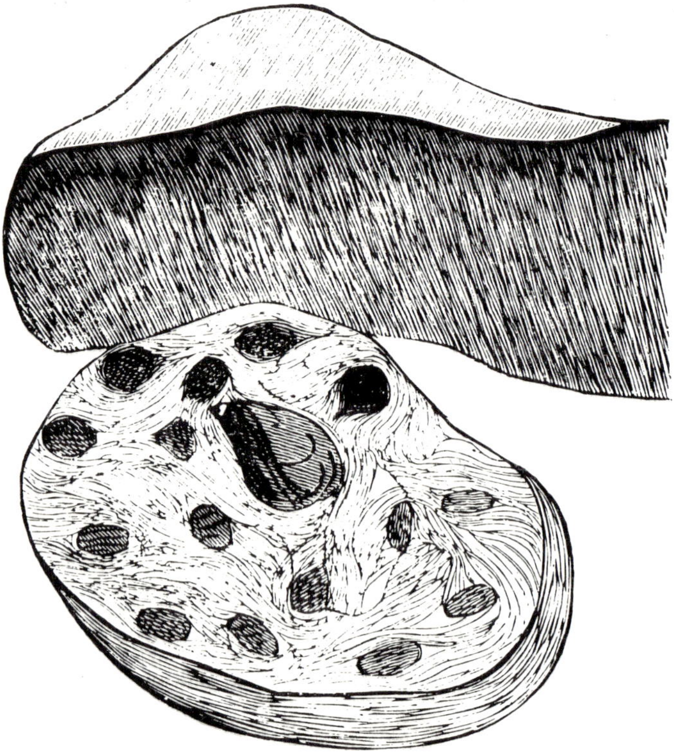

Fig. 11. A fibroma attached to the stomach of a cod (*G. morhua*). (Bland-Sutton, 1885.)

and not primarily its morphology. If the term malignant must be applied, it should not be used until the invasiveness of a tumor has been established beyond reasonable doubt.

In lower vertebrates, until more knowledge accumulates, tumors should not be designated solely on a basis of their morphology. We feel that animal tumors should be reviewed and reclassified in their own right, but no attempt has been made in this review to alter the status quo.

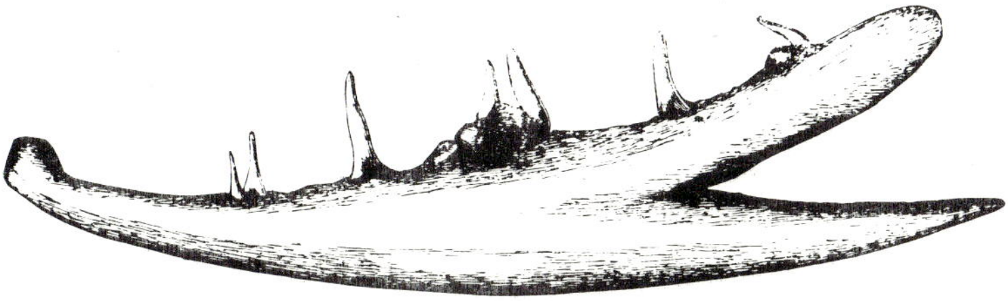

Fig. 12. Exostosis on the dentary bone of a pike (*E. lucius*). (Bland-Sutton, 1885.)

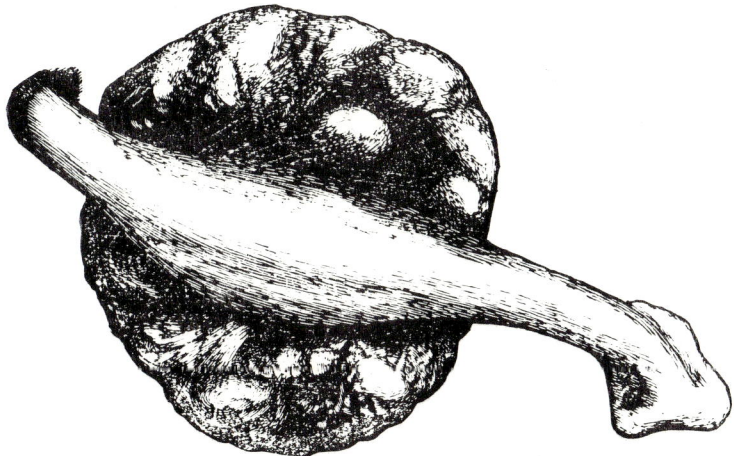

Fig. 13. Exostosis on the superior maxilla of a cod (*G. morhua*). (Bland-Sutton, 1885.)

IV. Epithelial Tumors

A. Skin

Tumors of the skin are the commonest types of tumors occurring in fish, probably because of their relative ease of recognition. Epidermal papillomata have been frequently reported together with epidermal carcinomata (Schlumberger and Lucké, 1948).

1. Papilloma

Papillomata present many difficulties and highlight two major problems: the relationship of hyperplasia to neoplasia, and the distribution of "species-specific" tumors (Schlumberger, 1957; Stolk, 1958g). Both problems are of interest to the comparative pathologist as they shed some light on the broader problems of environmental stress and neoplasia. Papillomata have been reported in many species (McIntosh, 1884–1885, 1885a,b; Sandeman, 1892a,b; Oxner, 1905; Keysselitz, 1908; Schroeders, 1908; Fiebiger, 1909a; Johnstone, 1911, 1924b; Breslauer, 1915; Anitschkow and Pawlowsky, 1923; Sagawa, 1925; Takahashi, 1929; Thomas, 1930, 1932e; Pacis, 1932; Coates *et al.*, 1938; Lucké, 1937; Good, 1940; Nigrelli and Smith, 1940; Finkelstein, 1944; Schlumberger and Lucké, 1948; Tavolga, 1951; Oota, 1952; Ketchen, 1953; Schlumberger, 1953; Ichikawa, 1954; Nishikawa, 1954; Stolk, 1954; Iwashita, 1955; Russell and Kotin, 1957; Nigrelli *et al.*, 1965; Reichenbach-Klinke, 1966; Kimura *et al.*, 1967a; Radulescu, 1967; Honma and Kon, 1968; Ljungberg and Lange, 1968; Winqvist *et al.*, 1968; Steeves, 1969). Those papillomata that have been reported in various species of flatfish are listed in Table I.

TABLE I
PAPILLOMATA IN FLATFISH

Species	Incidence	Reference
Butter sole (*Isopsetta isolepis*)	0.7% (3 per 430)	McArn *et al.* (1968)
Dover sole (*Microstomus pacificus*)	Epizootic	Young (1964)
English sole (*Parophyrs vetulus*)	3–28% (572–4507 per 15,739)	Cooper and Keller (1969)
	4.5%	Pacis (1932)
	4.8%	Good (1940)
	5.2% (93 per 1792)	McArn *et al.* (1968)
Flathead sole (*Hippoglossoides elassodon*)	6.4% (281 per 4,364)	Wellings *et al.* (1964)
	6.4% (336 per 5,250)	Wellings *et al.* (1965)
Sand sole (*Psettichthys melanosticus*)	3.3% (3 per 90)	McArn *et al.* (1968)
	31.7% (231 per 726)	Nigrelli *et al.* (1965)
Starry flounder (*Platichthys stellata*)	5.4% (57 per 1063)	McArn *et al.* (1968)

In many of the older references, uncertainties of diagnosis exist. Various specific etiologies have had to be considered when these tumors have occurred in larger numbers of fish in a specific geographical location. Keysselitz, as early as 1908, inferred the essential similarity between intracytoplasmic inclusions seen in some of these papillomata and those associated with vaccinia and other viral diseases. Harold and Innes

(1922) also noted the similarity of these tumors to the common wart and suggested a viral etiology. Further work on the etiology of this condition had to wait many years until Wellings, Nigrelli, and their colleagues commenced their studies with flatfish from the Pacific coast of North America (Wellings *et al.*, 1963, 1964, 1965, 1966, 1967; Chuinard, *et al.*, 1964, 1966; Wellings and Chuinard, 1964; Nigrelli *et al.*, 1965; McArn *et al.*, 1968; Cooper and Keller, 1969).

One of the interesting facts arising from these studies was that the highest incidence of tumors was found in the first year of life—no tumors were seen in fish over 4 years of age. While skin tumors were often multiple and showed a preference for the eye side, they were not associated with tumor formation elsewhere in the body and did not regress on subsequent laboratory observations. Histologically, these papillomata have been adequately described, and three main patterns have emerged—the angioepithelial nodule, the epidermal papilloma, and the angioepithelial polyp. Viruslike particles have been described and discussed by several workers (Oota, 1952; Nishikawa, 1954; Iwashita, 1955; Walker, 1958; Imai and Fujiwara, 1959; Nigrelli *et al.*, 1965; Wolf, 1966; Kimura *et al.*, 1967b; Wellings *et al.*, 1967), but their exact relationship to neoplasia has yet to be established. To pursue the argument as to whether these conditions represent a hyperplasia or a neoplasia is fruitless until all the facts become known. In other conditions associated with epidermal hyperplasia (Nigrelli, 1948), such as fish pox, epithelial proliferation is more controlled and the lesion often appears to be seasonally "self-limiting." These lesions have also been associated on occasions with cytoplasmic and intranuclear inclusions (Schubert, 1964). It is now thought that this condition, known since the sixteenth century, is attributable to a Herpes-type virus (Wolf, 1966; Mawdesley-Thomas and Bucke, 1967a). It has been commented that these papillomata are not transplantable. As so little is presently known about fish immunology however, any comment on the success or failure of tumor transplantation is premature (Bashford *et al.*, 1905).

Papillomata have been recorded in the eel (*Anguilla anguilla*) (Wolff, 1912; Thomas and Oxner, 1930; Ladreyt, 1935; Christiansen and Jensen, 1947; Schäperclaus, 1953; Lümann and Mann, 1956; Amlacher, 1961; Mann, 1962; Deys, 1969). These papillomata, often referred to as "cauliflower disease," have been reported most frequently from the Baltic Sea and along the northwestern coast of Europe. Available information suggests that this condition was extremely rare, or even unknown, before 1944, but since then it has occurred occasionally in epizootic proportions, causing much damage to local fishing industries. Deys (1969) noted a "remarkable annual and seasonal fluctuation" in Holland. In the spring tumors were seldom seen, but their incidence rose to about 5% in the autumn. As with papillomata in flatfish, a geographical locality was defined, suggestive of some external etiological agent. These tumors varied in size and were found anywhere on the body but had a predilection for the snout (Fig. 14). The tumors appeared as simple squamous papil-

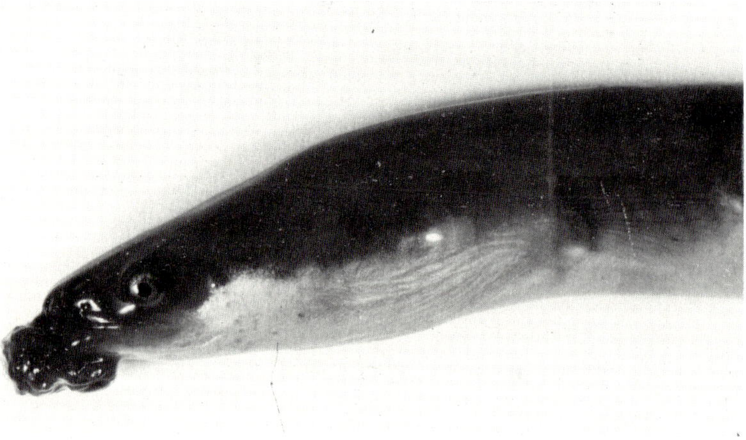

Fig. 14. "Cauliflower disease" affecting the snout of an eel (*A. anguilla*). (By kind permission of Dr. D. F. Deys.)

lomata, consisting of squamous epithelium in which mucous cells surrounded a central core of connective tissue (Fig. 15). Deys (1969), in further experimental work with the electron microscope, using virus-like particles seen in these tumors, showed a cytopathogenic effect of the particles on tissue culture (HeLa cells and eel gonad cells), but further work must be undertaken to ascertain their relation to the papillomata.

2. Squamous Cell Carcinoma (Epidermoid Carcinoma)

The first reported case (McFarland, 1901) of a malignant tumor of the skin epidermis in a fish was in the mouth of a white catfish (*Ameirus catus*). Since then, many other cases have been documented (Marsh, 1903; Dauwe and Pennemann, 1904; Bashford *et al.*, 1905; Loewenthal, 1907; Murray, 1908; Fiebiger, 1909a; Clunet, 1910; Drew, 1910; Schmey, 1911; Beatti, 1916; Johnstone, 1924b; Williams, 1929; Puente-Duany, 1930; Thomas, 1931a; Lucké and Schlumberger, 1941, 1942; Aronowitz

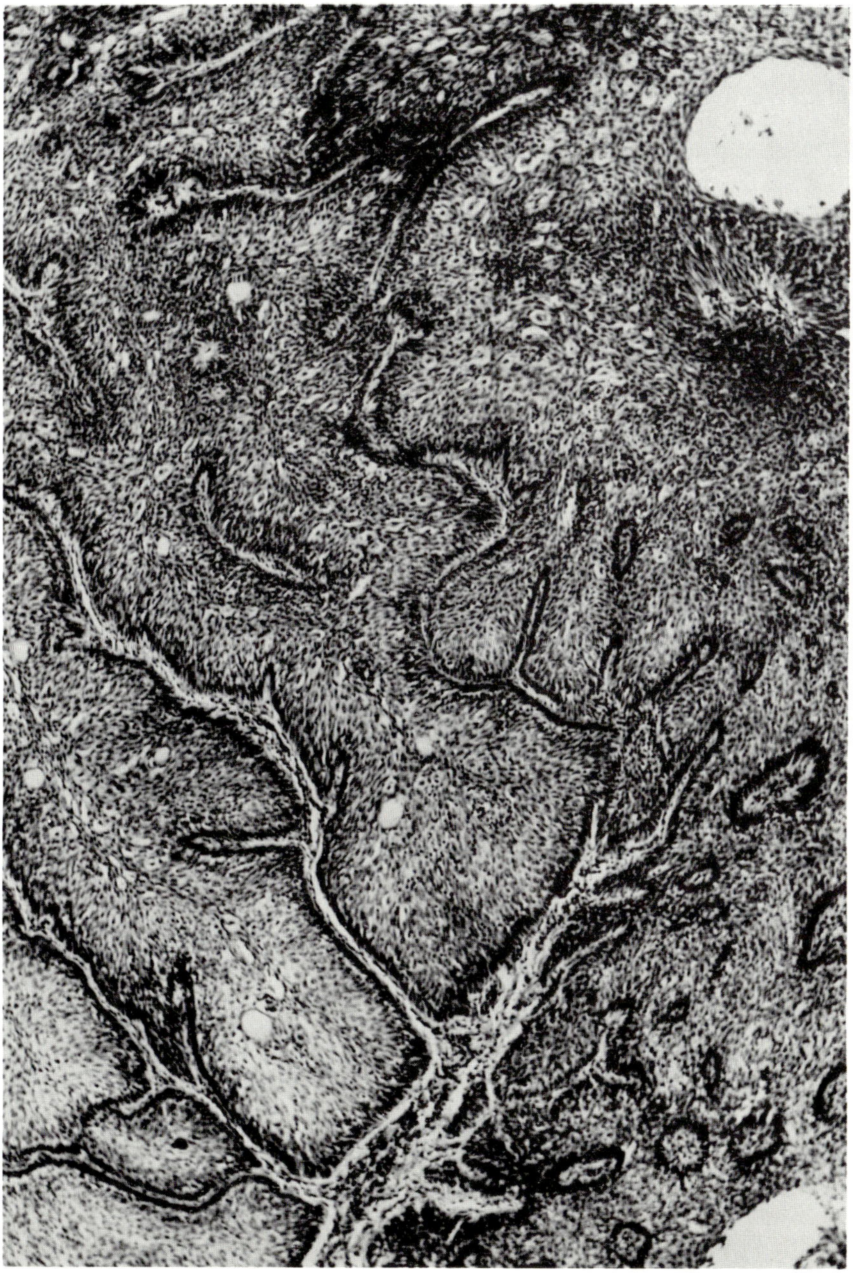

Fig. 15. Epithelial hyperplasia associated with "cauliflower disease" in eels, showing epithelial cells surrounding a fibrous core. Hematoxylin–eosin. 375×

et al., 1951; Nigrelli, 1951, 1952a, 1954; Sarkar and Dutta-Chaudhuri, 1953; Schlumberger, 1953; Stolk, 1953c, 1956d,h, 1958c, 1960b; Ermin, 1954; Reichenbach-Klinke, 1966; Mawdesley-Thomas and Bucke, 1967b; Harshbarger, 1968). The histological picture is well established in these tumors. The epithelial hyperplasia may be associated with "pegging" of the basement membrane before actual invasion occurs. Squamous cell tumors are usually slow growing and are often associated with a marked fibroblastic reaction in which epithelial cell nests are seen (Fig. 16). These cell nests (Fig. 17) are similar to those in tumors of mam-

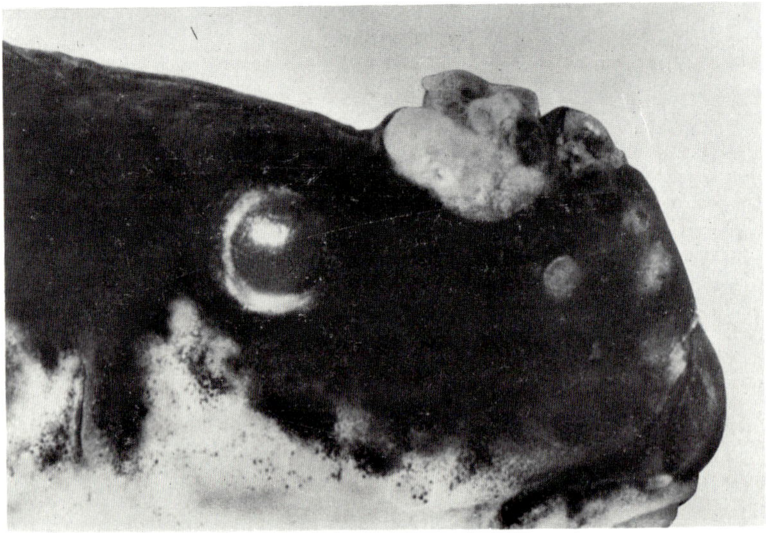

Fig. 16. Squamous cell carcinoma on the head of a gudgeon (*Gobio gobio*). (By courtesy of Dr. C. N. Barron).

mals, but the keratin is replaced by mucous cells. Metastatic deposits have never been reported. Recent work carried out off the European continental shelf has shown that several species of deep sea fish, especially *Parabassogigas crassus*, have epithelial tumors around the mouth. The macroscopic picture presented is one of a carcinoma rather than a papilloma (Fig. 18), but their histology has yet to be evaluated.

Finally, mention must be made of two skin conditions that are not truly neoplastic: one concerns an observation by Schmey (1911), who reported an interesting case of a keloid scar in a trout following possible trauma; the other concerns papillomata which appear on the fins and opercula of male goldfish during breeding season (Sagawa, 1925; Ghadially and Whiteley, 1952). These changes have been shown to

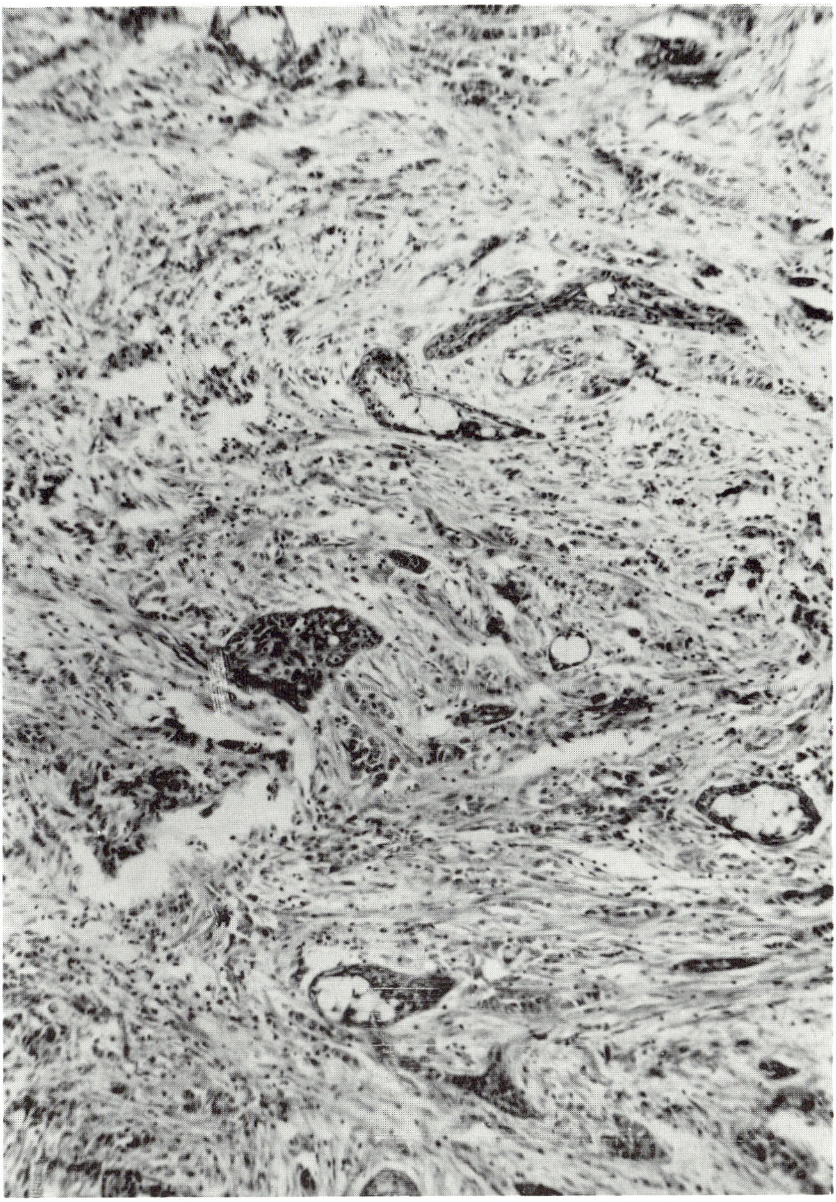

Fig. 17. Squamous cell carcinoma invading surrounding tissue. Epithelial cell nests are prominent. Hematoxylin–eosin. 100×.

be attributable to an androgenic-type response and one wonders if the "gibbosities" described by Aldrovandi (1613) might also have had a similar androgenic etiology (Pellegrin, 1901).

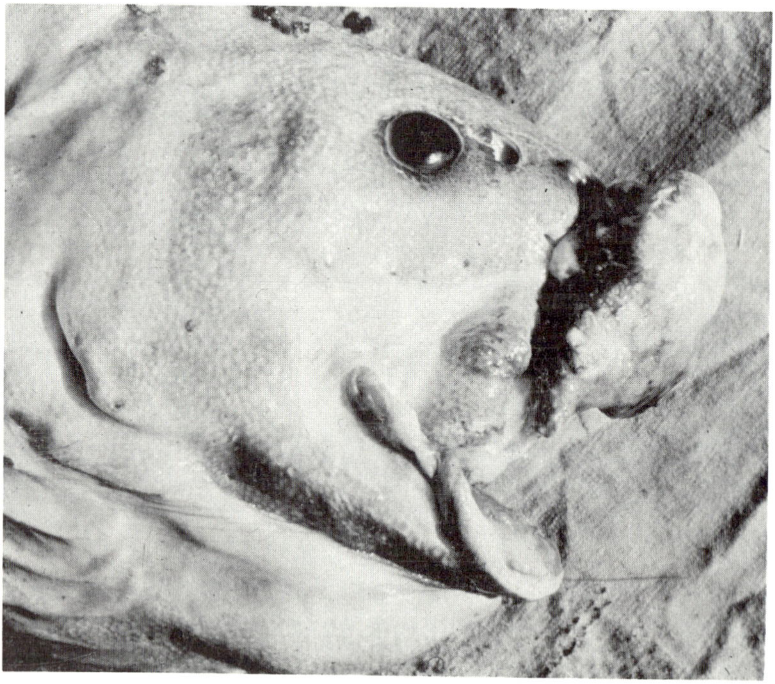

Fig. 18. Tumor of the snout in *P. crassus.*

3. Etiologies

Following the review of some instances of skin tumors in fish, a brief comment must be made on possible etiologies.

a. Genetic Factors. Evidence accumulated from a large number of animal species suggests that the genetic basis of disease is of much greater significance than previously supposed. The many elegant papers by Gordon and other workers (see Section VII,A) attest to this fact. Not only must the geographic distribution of skin tumors in some flatfish and eels be considered, but also the possible genetic factors must be more fully investigated. Genetic etiologies may also be involved in the nerve sheath tumors of goldfish (Schlumberger, 1952) and snapper fish (Lucké, 1942).

b. Trauma. It has been noted on several occasions (Deys, 1969) that many fish in which skin tumors are seen are bottom feeders. The implication that trauma may play a part in neoplasia must be considered, especially since many of these tumors are found in and around the mouth (Lucké and Schlumberger, 1941; Nigrelli, 1951; Russell and Kotin, 1957). Some tench (*Tinca tinca*) seen in our laboratory have shown evidence of bruising, hemorrhage, and even ulceration around the mouth, lower

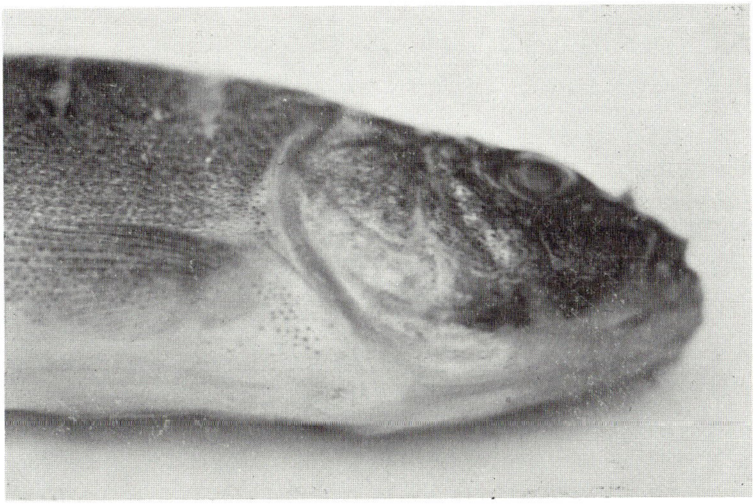

Fig. 19. Hemorrhage over the lower part of the operculum in a tench (*T. tinca*).

jaw, and operculum (Fig. 19), although no tumor formation has ever been observed.

c. Water Pollution. Water pollution is a worldwide problem and skin tumors have occurred in fish found in heavily polluted water (Lucké and Schlumberger, 1941; Russell and Kotin, 1957; Cooper and Keller, 1969). In any etiological discussion the effects of water pollution, with its potential carcinogenic action, must be considered. Hueper (1942) and Hueper and Ruchhoft (1954) anticipated many of these problems and showed that there was some ground for concern. In this context much more attention should be paid to the effects of pollution on the life in our seas and rivers (Mawdesley-Thomas, 1968).

d. Oncogenic Viruses. From the preceding comments it appears that a viral etiology is suspected in many tumors (Wessing, 1959; Wessing and Von Bargen, 1959), and it can only be a matter of time before this is established, at least in some instances. It is interesting to note where the various etiologies may overlap; the localized trauma in bottom-feeding fish may place the fish at greater risk to viral infections and the effects of water pollution. Oncogenic viruses may be carried in the water, or by other fish, or by the many parasites known to infest fish (Wellings *et al.*, 1964).

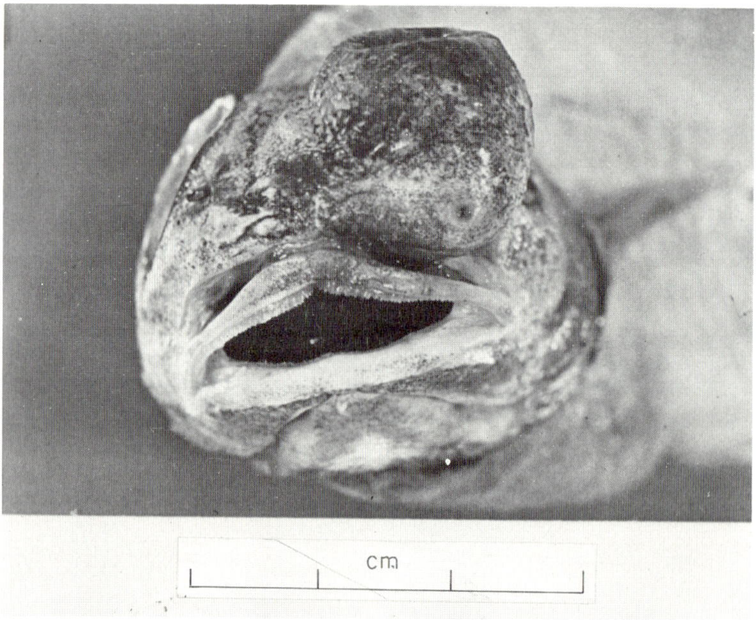

Fig. 20. Parasitic cyst on snout of a sea morid mimicking a neoplasm.

Many skin lesions that may appear as tumors may not be true tumors in the strict sense of the word. Many "tumors" of the skin and subcutaneous tissue have a non-neoplastic etiology. Many cystic conditions (Fig. 20), often associated with a parasitic infestation, are known (Smith, 1935). A definite diagnosis of neoplasia can be made only on microscopical examination.

B. *Thyroid*

The problem of hyperplasia and neoplasia, already seen to be of paramount importance in skin tumors, is even more acute where tumors of the thyroid are concerned. The majority of the earlier reported tumors (Bonnet, 1883; Scott, 1891; Gilruth, 1902; Plehn, 1902; Pick, 1905,

Jaboulay, 1908a,b; Gaylord, 1909, 1910, 1916; Gaylord and Marsh, 1912, 1914; Smith, 1909, Marsh, 1911; Schmey, 1911; Southwell, 1915; Southwell and Prashad, 1918; Schreitmüller, 1924; Klemm, 1927) have subsequently been assessed as representing a hyperplastic rather than a neoplastic condition. The designation of these tumors as malignant was the result of a failure to appreciate the normal anatomical distribution of the piscine thyroid, which does not possess the definite capsule seen in the majority of vertebrate species. The necessity for an appreciation of the normal anatomy (Chavin, 1956a,b) and histology is essential if meaningful comment is to be made on possible pathological change (Gardner and Wachowski, 1951). Aberrant thyroid tissue is extremely common in fish, and while found primarily between the first and second gill arches (Gudernatsch, 1910, 1911a,b; Gardner and Wachowski, 1951), it may also be found in surrounding muscle bundles and bone lamellae, in the heart, eye, kidney, ovary, spleen, gut, and ear but never in the liver, brain, or blood vessels (Baker *et al.*, 1954, 1955; Vivien and Ruhland-Gaiser, 1954; Chavin, 1956c; Baker, 1958; Sathyanesan, 1963).

While the majority of these tumors are now more correctly designated hyperplasias, true neoplasias have been reported (Dinulesco and Vasilescu, 1939). Gaylord and Marsh (1914), in a beautifully illustrated monograph, described among many examples of hyperplasia a metastasis in the wall of the rectum and a nodule on the tip of the mandible (Fig. 21). As comparative pathologists now realize (Schlumberger, 1954;

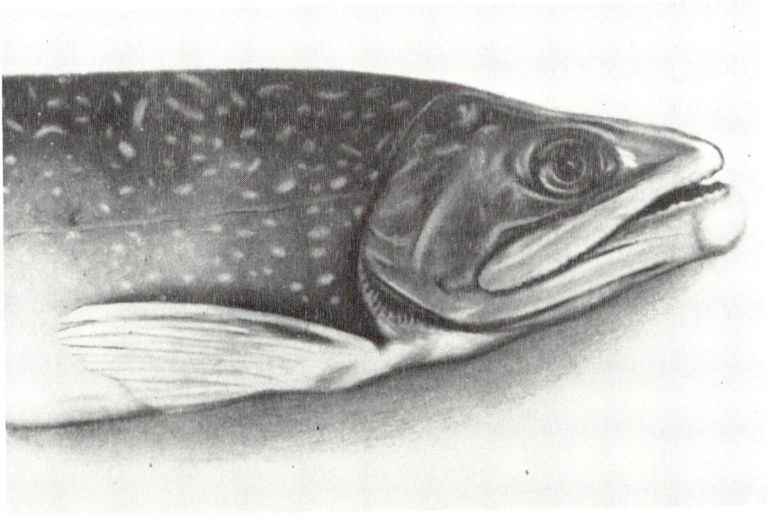

Fig. 21. Nodule on mandible of a trout. Metastasis (?) from thyroid tumor.

Wellings, 1969), it is often impossible in man to distinguish between thyroid hyperplasia and neoplasia. This is even more so the case with fish. It is often forgotten that much of the early work on thyroid pathology was associated with fish (Berg *et al.*, 1953; Gorbman, 1964), and the rationale of prescribing iodine for goitrous conditions was established from observations on fish. The major share of the credit for establishing the true etiology of thyroid tumors goes to Marine and Lenhart (1910a,b, 1911) and Marine (1914), who worked with brook trout (*Salvelinus fontinalis*), for it was they who showed that thyroid hyperplasia occurred as a result of an iodine deficiency in the water. Hyperplastic thyroid condition has since been shown to occur in laboratory and natural populations if the water iodine content is allowed to become depleted (Schlumberger and Lucké, 1948; Gorbman and Gordon, 1951; Nigrelli, 1952b,c; Robertson and Chaney, 1953; Berg and Gorbman, 1954; Vivien and Ruhland-Gaiser, 1954). The prevalence of thyroid hyperplasia in the Salmonidae may be associated with their high oxygen requirement (Duerst, 1941). While an iodine deficiency can be appreciated in freshwater or laboratory fish, it is difficult to find a physiological explanation for the thyroid tumors described in marine fish (Cameron and Vincent, 1915; Marsh and Vonwiller, 1916; Johnstone, 1924a; Burwash, 1929; Schlumberger and Lucké, 1948). The presence of thyroid hyperplasia in small tropical fish has been reported by several workers (Schreitmüller, 1924; Müller, 1926; Smith *et al.*, 1936; Smith and Coates, 1937; Berg *et al.*, 1953; Berg *et al.*, 1954). As a result of the investigations, it has been suggested that a genetic factor might also be involved. In some of these species, exceptionally high iodine requirements have been noted. Many cases of thyroid hyperplasia have subsequently been reported, in one instance associated with exophthalmia (Hamre and Nichols, 1926; Klemm, 1927; Peyron and Thomas, 1930; Thomas, 1931c; Dinulesco and Vasilescu, 1939; Nigrelli, 1943; Aronowitz *et al.*, 1951; Schlumberger, 1955; Stolk, 1955b, 1956a,b,e; MacIntyre, 1960; MacIntyre and Baker-Cohen, 1961; Woodhead and Ellett, 1967; Conroy, 1967; Ghittino *et al.*, 1967a,b; Radulescu *et al.*, 1968).

Thyroid adenomata can also be induced experimentally with thiouracil (Stolk, 1955b), and drug therapy can control the growth of goiters (Berg and Gordon, 1953).

C. *Kidney*

Renal tumors of fish have not been reported with the same frequency as those of amphibia (Schlumberger and Lucké, 1948). Ectopic thyroid in the teleostean kidney is not an infrequent finding (see Section IV,B), and several instances of functioning thyroid tumors of the kidney have been reported (Baker *et al.*, 1954, 1955; Baker, 1958; MacIntyre and Baker-Cohen, 1961; Sathyanesan, 1963). Primary tumors of the kidney have been described (Schmey, 1911, Plehn, 1924; Jahnel, 1939; Peyron, 1939; Nigrelli, 1943; Schlumberger and Lucké, 1948; Baker and Gordon, 1953; Stolk, 1957a,d; Conroy, 1965). Ashley (1967) reported renal neoplasia in rainbow trout fed experimental diets containing dimethylnitrosamine; histologically, these tumors resembled nephroblastomata and have characteristics similar to adenocarcinomata of man. The term "hypernephroma" is no longer considered valid for this type of tumor and should be avoided.

Stolk (1960c) described several dehydrogenase systems in renal tumors occurring in a cyprinodont (*Aplocheilus lineatus lineatus*) and noted the highest activity in DPN-linked diaphorase and lactate dehydrogenase. Polycystic kidneys have been reported in several species of fish, and this condition should always be considered a differential diagnosis in renal enlargement (Grafflin, 1937; Schlumberger, 1950; Stolk, 1955b, 1956b,c,g; Besse *et al.*, 1959; Sathyanesan, 1966; Mawdesley-Thomas and Jolly, 1967).

D. Urinary Bladder

Only one possible case of an adenocarcinoma of the urinary bladder has been reported (Plehn, 1909); it occurred in a goldfish (*C. auratus*).

E. Testis

Few primary tumors of the testis (seminomata) have been reported (Nigrelli and Jakowska, 1953; Dunbar, personal communication; Budd and Schroder, 1969). Interstitial cell tumors have been induced experimentally with sesame oil (Li and Baldwin, 1944). Other tumors reported are of the sarcomatous type (Thomas, 1931a; Johnstone, 1924a).

F. Ovary

Ovarian tumors also appear to be uncommon in fish. Johnstone (1914b) noted a papillary cystadenoma in a ling (*Molva molva*). Freudenthal (1928) described a possible fibroma in a goldfish (*Carassius vulgaris*), Haddow and Blake (1933) reported an ovarian adenocarcinoma in a pike (*E. lucius*), and Honma (1966) a lymphosarcoma in a *Plecoglossus altivelis.* Erdman (personal communication) reported ovarian tumors in *Coryhaena hippusus* and Sc*omberomorus regalis* but, unfortunately, no histological material was available. Ceretto (1968) reported an interesting ovarian tumor in a goldfish with cerebral metastasis. This tumor was considered to be a "psammomatous carcinoma." Stolk described several ovarian teratomata (see Section IX).

G. Liver

Tumors of the liver in fish, especially in the Salmonidae, are of particular significance not only to the fish pathologist but to the experimentalist in general. The outbreak of hepatomata in rainbow trout (*Salmo gairdneri*) in American hatcheries in 1960 focused the attention of many pathologists on this problem. Much of the credit for appreciating the nutritional etiology (Anonymous, 1964) must go to Ashley and Halver, who were able to show that the toxic agent was produced by a mold, *Aspergillus flavus,* that contaminates foodstuffs. This fungus is responsible for the production of aflatoxin (Ashley and Halver, 1961, 1963; Ghittino and Ceretto, 1961, 1962; Hueper and Payne, 1961; Nigrelli and Jakowska, 1961; Rucker *et al.*, 1961; Snieszko, 1961; Wood and Larson, 1961; Ashley *et al.*, 1962, 1964, 1965; Halver *et al.*, 1962, 1968; LaRoche *et al.*, 1962; Levaditi *et al.*, 1963a,b; Scarpelli *et al.*, 1963; Wolf and Jackson, 1963; Kraybill and Shimkin, 1964; Ashley, 1965; Halver, 1965a,b; Sinnhuber *et al.*, 1965, 1966, 1968a,b; Solomon *et al.*, 1965; Wales and Sinnhuber, 1966; Ghittino *et al.*, 1967a,b; Halver and Mitchell, 1967; Lee *et al.*, 1967; Jackson *et al.*, 1968). Credit must also be given to these workers for tackling and solving such a pressing problem, with its many overtones involving man, so quickly. This is an example of a problem being supported by government agencies with a degree of urgency, adequate funds, and skilled workers. The "art of the soluble" (Medowar, 1967) played a significant part. One could only wish that this was more typical of the approach to more mundane problems that are nevertheless equally as pressing. The association of liver tumor formation and aflatoxin in relation to various aflatoxin components has been reviewed and discussed by Halver and Mitchell (1967). (See Coates *et al.*, 1967; Dollar *et al.*, 1967; Falk, 1967; Halver, 1967, 1968, 1969; Halver *et al.*, 1967, 1969; Novelli, 1967; Phelps, 1967; Scarpelli, 1967; Simon *et al.*, 1967; Sims, 1967; Sinnhuber, 1967; Wales, 1967; Wogan, 1967; Wolf and Jackson, 1967; Yasutake and Rucker, 1967; Mawdesley-Thomas, 1970).

More recently, several workers (Rodricks *et al.*, 1968) isolated a new toxin from *A. flavus* called aspertoxin. Further experiments must be made with this substance to determine its effect on fish liver. Tumors of the liver had of course been described before 1960 under various histological headings. A critical review of the histopathogenesis of experimental liver tumors in the rat (Stewart and Snell, 1957) sheds much light on liver tumors in general. In fish the main histological types include hepatoma, or hepatocellular adenoma; adenocarcinoma, a tumor of the hepatic cell; and cholangioma or cholangiosarcoma, a tumor of the bile duct epithelium. Various workers have also reported cystadenomata. The majority of tumors have been reported in the Salmonidae (Plehn, 1909; Loeb, 1910; Schmey, 1911; Haddow and Blake, 1933; Scolari, 1953; Nigrelli, 1954; Cudkowicz and Scolari, 1955; Kubota, 1955a; Nigrelli and Jakowska, 1955; Honma and Shirai, 1959; Besse *et al.*, 1960, 1966; Levaditi et *al.*, 1960; Dollar *et al.*, 1963; Ghittino, 1963; Halver *et al.*, 1964; Scarpelli *et al.*, 1963; Snieszko and Miller, 1966; Codegone *et al.*, 1968; Ellis, personal communication). Occasional papers concerning liver neoplasm in other species of fish also exist. Dawe *et al.* (1964) reported liver neoplasia in the bottom-feeding fish *Catostomus commersoni* and *Ictalurus nebulosus*. These neoplasms consisted of cholangiomata and a single minimal deviation hepatoma. Stanton (1966) described liver tumors in fish attributable to *Cycas-circinalis*. Various environmental hazards were considered, and the suggestion was made that fish might prove useful indicators of environmental carcinogens. Recent work with carcinogens (Stanton, 1965, Ashley and Halver, 1968), using dimethylnitrosamine fed to *Brachydanio rerio* and *S. gairdneri*, resulted in liver tumor formation. Several investigators have studied the carcinogen 2-acetylaminofluorene (Lotlikar *et al.*, 1967). The significant point made by Stanton (1965) is that "*the high sensitivity of small fish to a known carcinogen, their poikilothermic physiology and the ease with which their aquatic environment can be controlled are particular advantages in studies on carcinogenesis.*" This sentence may well be the most important statement in this chapter.

H. Gastrointestinal Tract

While some reports of mesenchymal tumors associated with the gastrointestinal tract have been documented (see Section V), few descriptions of epithelial tumors are available. Takahashi (1929) noted an adenocarcinoma of the rectal gland. Labbé (1930) reported a tumorlike condition in the gut of a whiting (*Merlangus merlangus*), which in all probability represented a congenital anomaly rather than a true neoplasm. Thomas (1931a,b) described an adenoma and adenocarcinoma of the small intestine; Raabe (1939) a possible adenocarcinoma; and Nigrelli (1946a,b) a "fibro-carcinoma-like growth" in the stomach of a *Borophyrne apogon.*

I. Pancreas

As in the case of the gastrointestinal tract, tumors of the pancreas have been rarely reported. Nigrelli and Gordon, as recently as 1951, were the first to describe a pancreatic tumor occurring in a hybrid platyfish (Nigrelli and Gordon, 1951), although Drew (1910) suggested the possibility of such a tumor in *Pleuronectes platessa.* Otte (1964) reported an adenocarcinoma occurring in a goldfish.

J. Swim Bladder

The earliest report of a tumor in piscian swim bladder is by Bashford and Murray (1904) of a spindle cell sarcoma in a cod. Johnstone (1924b) reported an angiosarcoma in a cod (*G. morhua*). Stolk (1957j) also noted an adenoma in a guppy (*Lebistes reticulatus*).

K. Dental Tumors

Relatively few examples of dental tumors have been reported in fish (Plehn, 1915; Roffo, 1925; Thomas, 1926; Ladreyt, 1929; Schlumberger, 1953; Schlumberger and Katz, 1956; Stolk, 1957k). The tumors were described as odontomata or ameloblastomata, although Willis (1967) has advised caution in regard to the latter term, "carcinoma of the tooth-germ residue" being a more precise term. Schlumberger and Katz (1956) have suggested that a genetic etiology may be involved in the dental tumors occurring in the Salmonidae, thus again stressing the importance of the genetic basis of disease.

L. Tumors of Parabranchial Bodies and Allied Structures

The parabranchial bodies are two small organs which lie in front of the true gills and have no counterpart in man. It is only fair to state however, that there is some doubt as to their function or even presence (Wellings, 1969). Several workers have described tumors of these structures (Peyron and Thomas, 1929; Takahashi, 1929; Wellings, 1969). Tumors of the pharynx and gills have also been reported (Takahashi, 1934; Stolk, 1953d, 1957h,i, 1962; Sarkar and Dutta-Chaudhuri, 1964).

V. Mesenchymal Tumors

The connective tissue cells of the animal body and their response to various stimuli are possibly of greater importance to the pathologist than any other class of tissue. The histogenesis of mesenchymal tumors is debatable, that is, whether they arise from differentiated or embryonic mesenchymal cell is of little more than academic interest. The difficulty associated with their histogenesis is illustrated by the use of a polysyllabic nomenclature—"myxoendotheliosarcoma." As in the case of epithelial tumors, the terms benign and malignant are only of prognostic significance. In many of the cases reported, it is impossible to establish a definitive diagnosis. Mesenchymal tumors have been grouped according to their most likely cell type.

A. Tumors of Muscle

1. Rhabdomyoma

Rhabdomyoma is a tumor of skeletal muscle. Relatively few of these tumors have been reported in the animal kingdom, and even fewer among the lower vertebrates (Adami, 1908; Bergman, 1921; Young, 1923; Kolmer, 1928; Ladreyt, 1930; Williams, 1931; Thomas, 1932a; Hoshina, 1952; Blaehser, 1961; Finkelstein and Danchenko-Ryzchkova, 1965). All occurred in the trunk musculature. Fiebiger (1909c) reported a visceral rhabdomyoma. Two further tumors have been seen in our laboratory, both arising from the trunk musculature: one occurred in an adult trout (*S. gairdneri*), arising from the dorsal musculature lateral to the dorsal fin and was approximately 5 cm in diameter; the other was in a herring (*Clupea harengus*). Both tumors consisted of striated muscle fibers running in various directions (Fig. 22). A false capsule was noted in one of the trout, but no evidence of local invasion was observed.

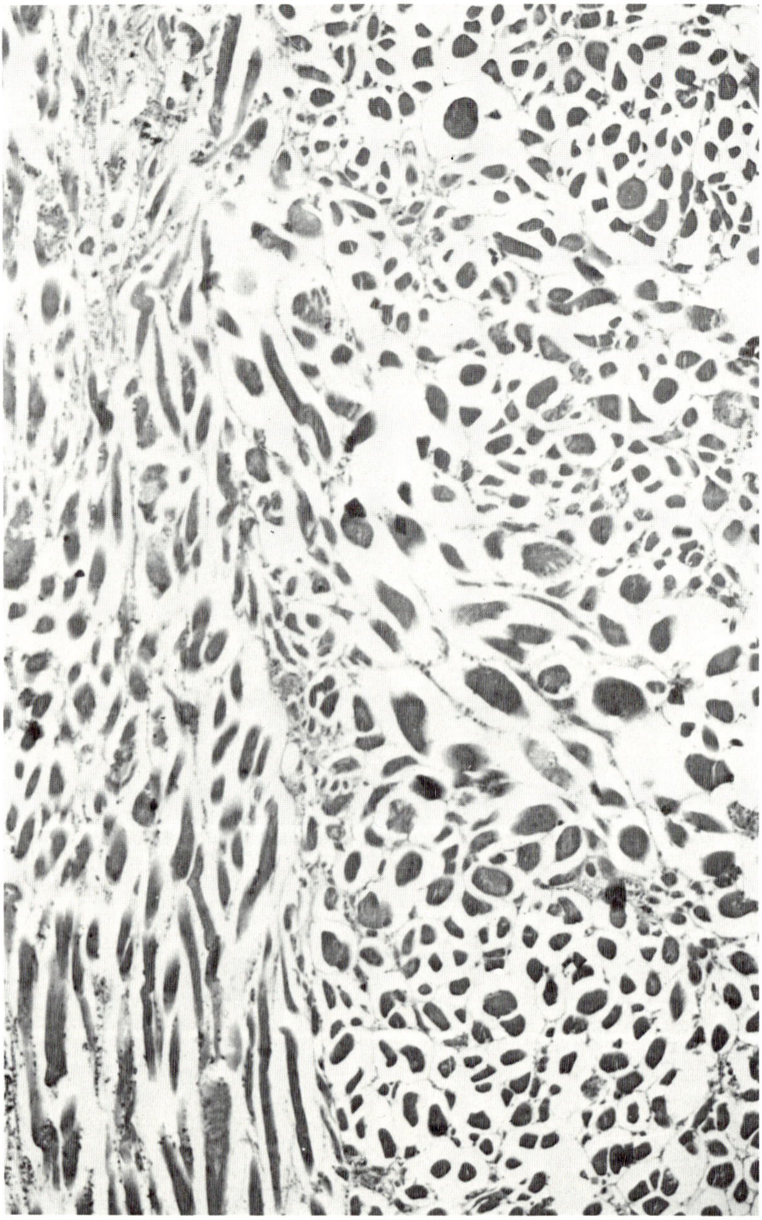

Fig. 22. Rhabdomyoma seen in the lateral musculature of a herring (*C. harengus*). Hematoxylin–eosin. 113×.

2. Leiomyoma

Leiomyoma is a tumor of smooth muscle and has been reported most frequently in association with the upper gastrointestinal tract (Plehn, 1906; Pesce, 1907; Thomas, 1933a,c; Andre, 1939; Kubota, 1955b; Sarkar *et al.*, 1955), although the possibility of some type of granulomatous lesion must be considered as a differential diagnosis (Woodhead, 1884–1885). This anatomical distribution is interestingly paralleled in

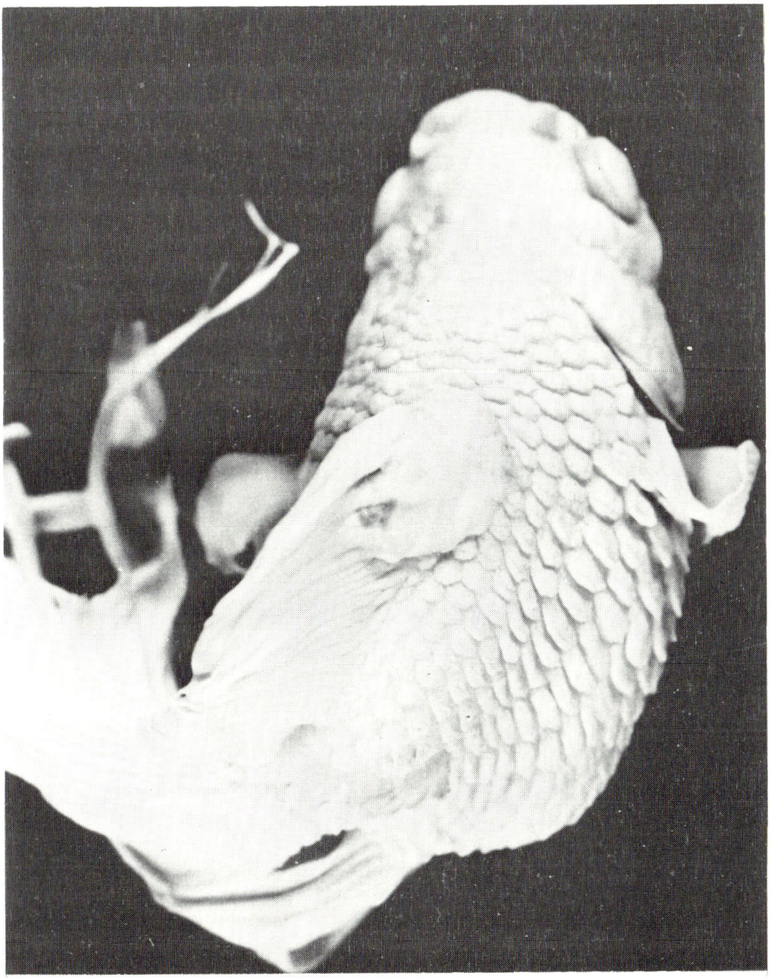

Fig. 23. Leiomyoma arising from the dorsal musculature of a goldfish (*C. auratus*).

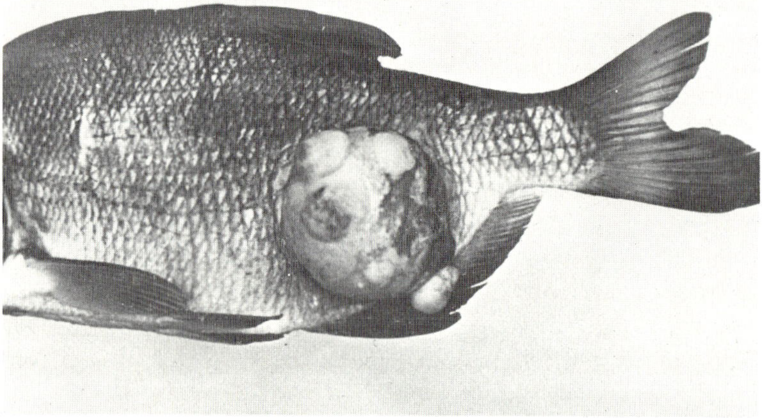

Fig. 24. Lipoma in a bream (*A. brama*) suggestive of a multifocal origin.

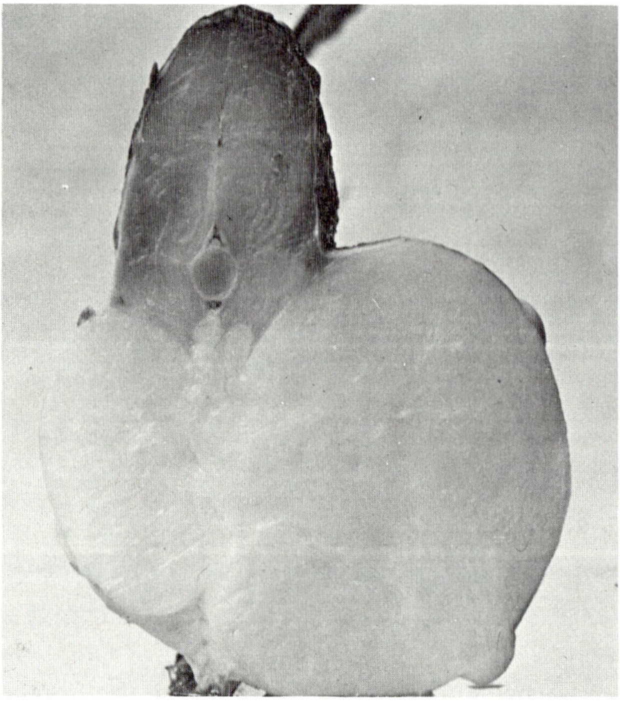

Fig. 25. Lipoma in a bream (*A. brama*) showing a capsule separating the tumor from the musculature.

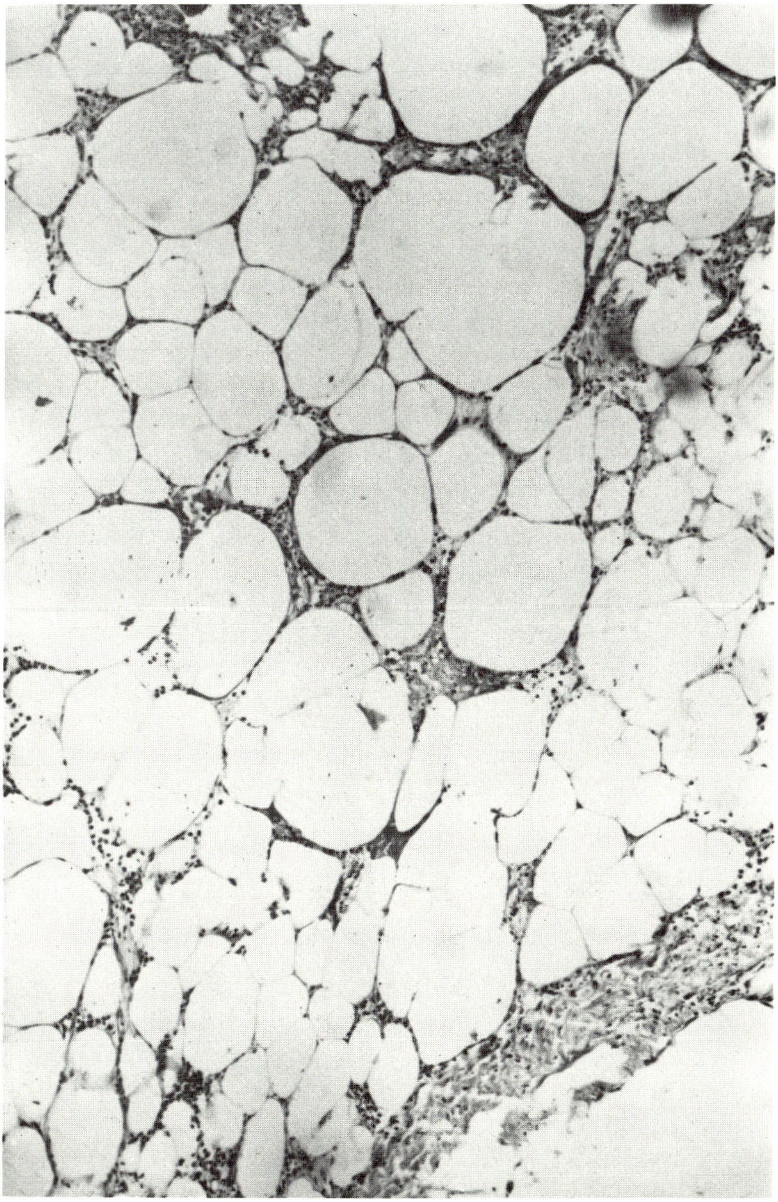

Fig. 26. Transverse section through surface of lipoma showing chronic inflammatory cells and fibroblasts interspersed between the adipose cells. Hematoxylin–eosin. 113×.

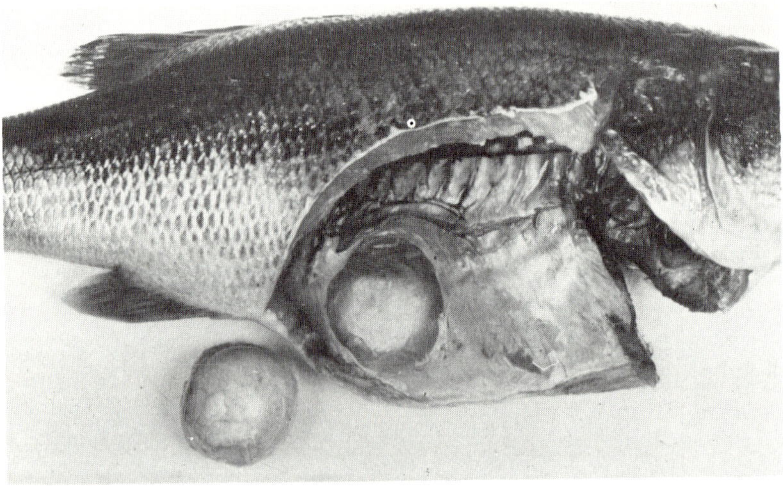

27

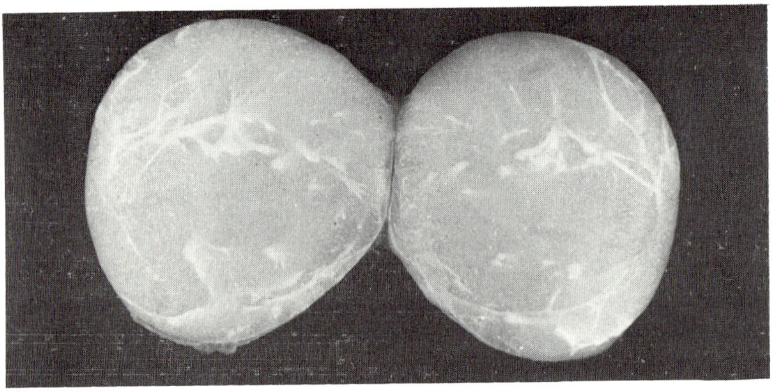

28

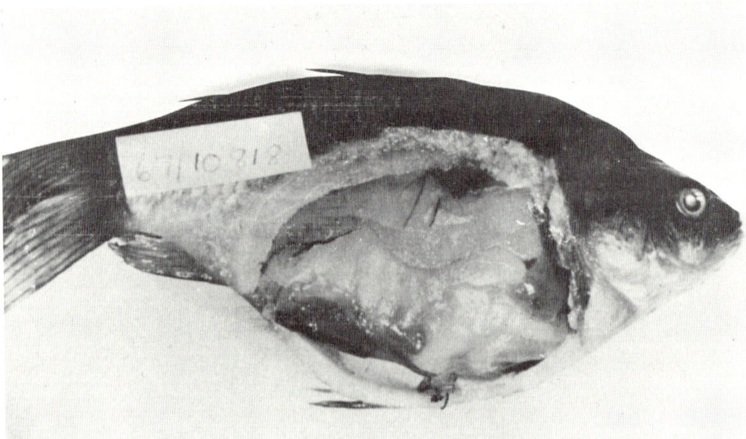

29

man (Golden and Stout, 1941). The histological picture of these tumors is one of bundles of smooth muscle fibers arranged as trabeculae coarsing throughout the tumor. Often there is definite regimentation of the nuclei, which may cause the tumor to be confused with a neurilemmoma. Such difficulty has already been encountered in the case of the goldfish (Schlumberger, 1949, 1952, 1957). Dunbar (personal communication) recently found a leiomyoma arising in the trunk musculature of a goldfish (Fig. 23).

B. Lipoma

Although lipoma is a relatively common type of tumor in mammals, including man, only a few cases have been reported in fish (Bergman, 1921; Kazama, 1924; Takahashi, 1929; Williams, 1929; Thomas, 1933d; Anadon, 1956; Bertullo and Bellagamba, 1964; Mawdesley-Thomas and Bucke, 1968; Harshbarger and Bane, 1969; Wellings, 1969). The lipoma reported from our laboratory was in a bream (*Abramis brama*). The tumor (Fig. 24) measured 8.2×9.0 cm, and the fish weighed 4.8 kg. On histological examination it was found to be surrounded by a false capsule (Fig. 25) and consisted mainly of mature fat cells. Blood vessels were seen throughout the tumor associated with a fibroblastic response (Fig. 26). If the fibroblastic elements predominate, then the term fibrolipoma can be used. The tumors examined to date have not shown any invasive tendencies. A lipoma in a largemouth bass (*Micropterus salmoides*) has been sent to our laboratory (Figs. 27 and 28). Occasionally, an increase of fat in the fat depots is seen, which is not associated with any definite tumor formation. The exact etiology is still unknown. We have observed it on several occasions in goldfish (*C. auratus* (Fig. 29).

C. Fibroma and Fibrosarcoma

Fibromata and fibrosarcomata are tumors in which collagen-forming fibroblasts predominate. If other cellular elements are present, their

---

Fig. 27. Lipoma arising in the lateral musculature of a largemouth bass (*M. salmoides*). (By kind permission of Dr. N. Fijan.)

Fig. 28. Enucleated lipoma from a largemouth bass (*M. salmoides*). (By kind permission of Dr. N. Fijan.)

Fig. 29. Goldfish (*C. auratus*) showing massive deposition of adipose tissue, presenting as an abdominal swelling. Etiology as yet unknown.

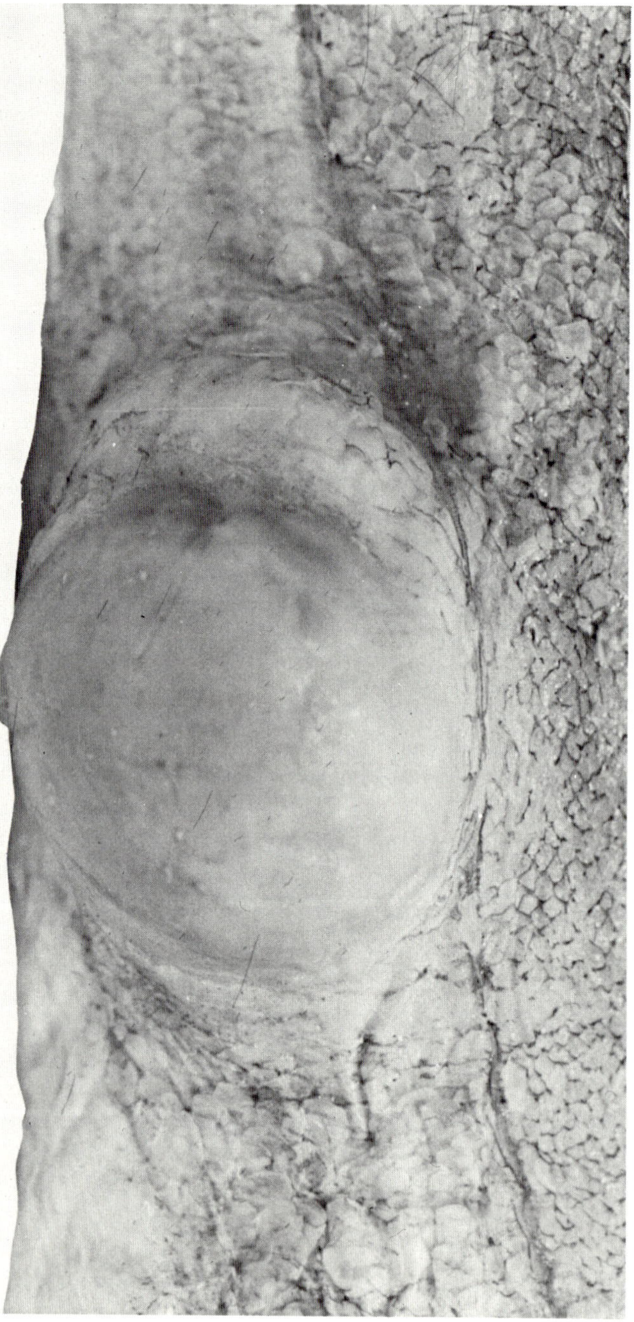

Fig. 30. Fibroma arising from the dorsal musculature of a whiting (*M. merlangus*).

presence may be indicated by such terminology as "chondrofibroma." This type of terminology is still a matter of personal preference (Bertullo and Bellagamba, 1964). Fibromata may be associated with a range of clinical and histological features, their varying degrees of cellularity and collagen content accounting for their color and consistency. Some of the earliest tumors to be reported were fibromata (Hunter, 1782; Bland-Sutton, 1885: see Section II). This is in contradistinction to man (Willis, 1967). Of all the mesenchymal tumors, fibromata are the most frequently described. This incidence is attributable in part to their predilection for subcutaneous tissues. It is interesting to note that the earlier references date back to the late nineteenth century (Crisp, 1854; Bugnion, 1875; Gervais, 1876; Eberth, 1878; Bland-Sutton, 1885; Semer, 1888; Lawrence, 1895), although in some instances the exact diagnosis is in doubt. Other cases were reported by Sandeman (1892a,b), Plehn (1906), Fiebiger (1909a, 1912), Drew (1910), Guglianetti (1910), Johnstone (1910, 1911, 1913, 1914a,b, 1920, 1922a,b, 1923a,b, 1924a,b, 1926b), Williamson (1911), Ronca (1914), Beatti (1916), Kazama (1922), Schamberg and Lucké (1922), Wago (1922), Plehn (1924), Roffo (1924, 1926), Leger (1925), Eguchi and Oota (1926), Thomas (1927a, 1933a), Dominguez (1928), Freudenthal (1928), Takahashi (1929), Williams (1931), Montpellier and Dieuzeide (1932), Smith *et al.* (1936), Kreyberg (1937), Jahnel (1939), Nigrelli (1946a,b), Walker (1947), Lucké *et al.* (1948), Hoshina (1950, 1952), Stolk (1954, 1957b,c,g), Nishikawa (1955a,b), Wadsworth (1961), Mattheis (1964), Biavati and Mancini, 1967; Mawdesley-Thomas (1967), and Wellings (1969). In our laboratory a fibroma in the dorsal musculature of a whiting (*M. merlangus*) and the lateral muscle of a haddock (*Melanogrammus aeglefinus*) have been recorded (Figs. 30–32). These tumors were well defined and consisted of whorls of fibroblasts. A fibrosarcoma has also been noted in a trout (*S. gairdneri*). This tumor was seen in the lateral musculature (Fig. 33) and measured about 4.5 cm in diameter. Invasion of the musculature was suspected on macroscopic examination. The tumor was whitish in appearance and of rubbery consistency. When examined histologically, much infiltration of the surrounding musculature by cells of the fibrosarcomatous type was seen (Figs. 34 and 35).

D. Myxoma and Myxosarcoma

It should be remembered that this type of tumor is but a variant of a fibroma or a fibrosarcoma in which mucin is found. There is no such cell as a "myxoblast," and myxomata and myxosarcoma are composed essentially of fibroblasts. They are relatively rare tumors in the majority of fish species and should not be confused with edematous fibromata. A diagnosis should only be made after mucin has been demon-

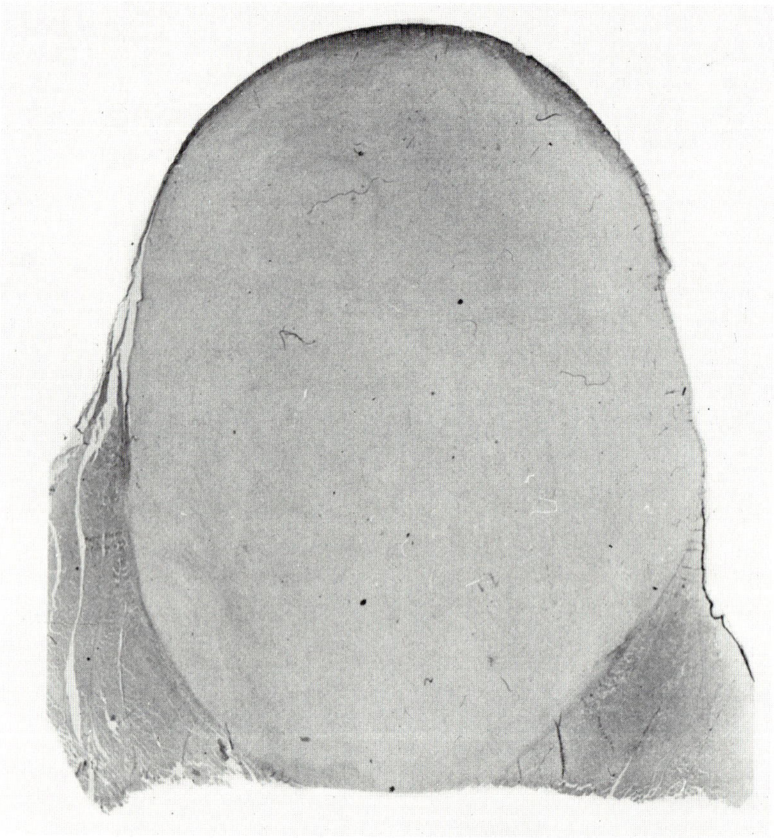

Fig. 31. Transverse section of fibroma showing clear differentiation between the tumor and the surrounding musculature. Hematoxylin–eosin. 4×.

strated. The following investigators have reported myxomata in fish: Plehn (1906), McIntosh (1908), Schroeders (1908), Wago (1922), Johnstone (1926a), Williams (1929), Stolk (1958a), Honma (1965), and Ashley and Halver (1968).

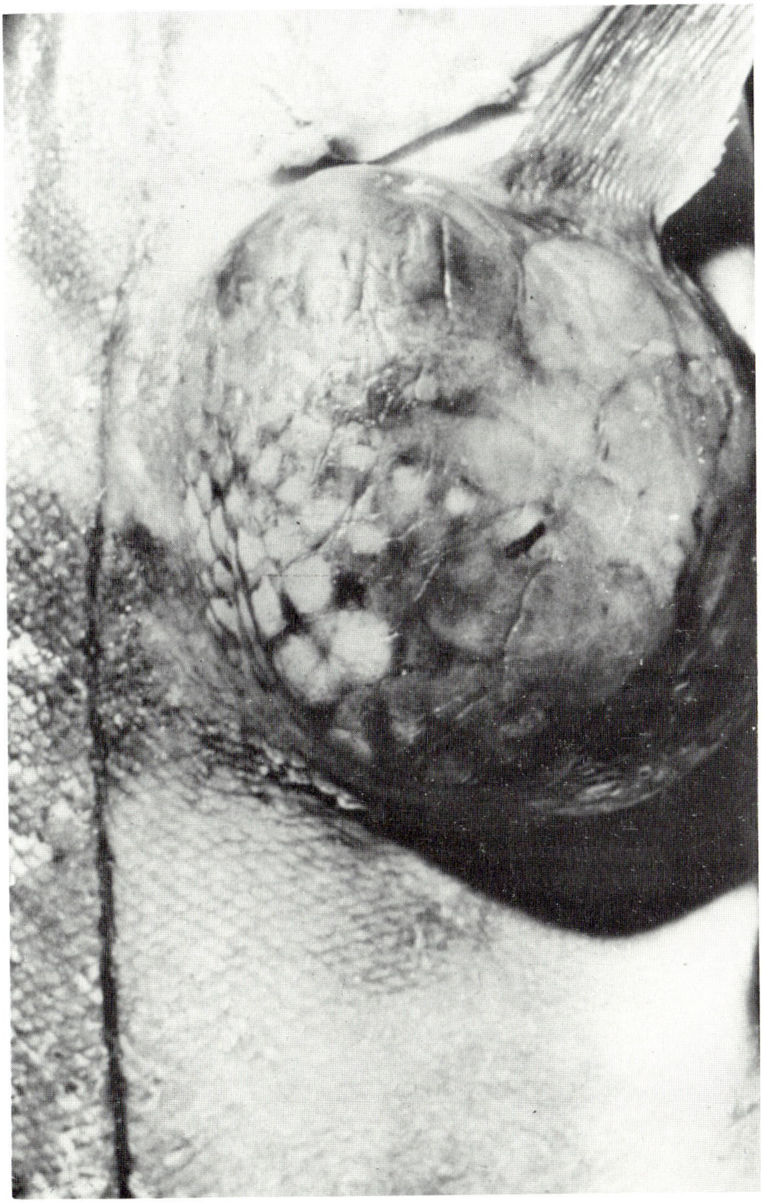

Fig. 32. Fibroma in a haddock (*M. aeglifinus*) arising caudally to the right operculum. Note the hypertrophy of overlying scales.

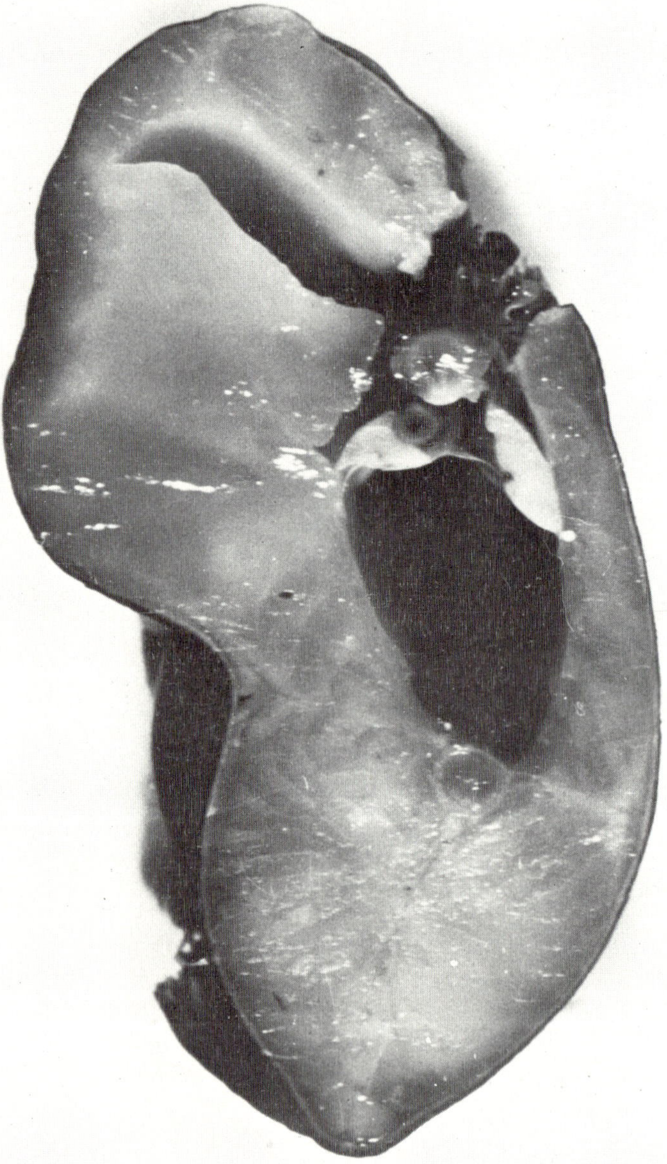

Fig. 33. Section through trout showing a fibrosarcoma.

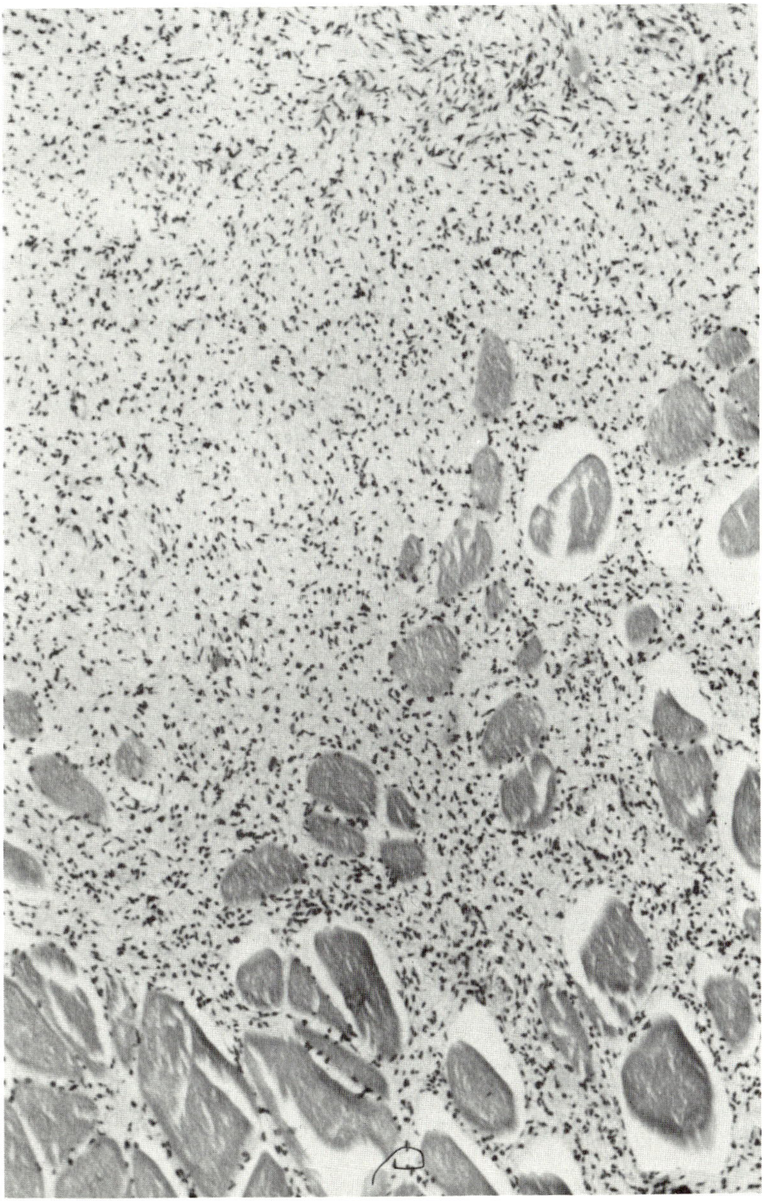

Fig. 34. Transverse section of fibrosarcoma showing invasion by skeletal muscle. Hematoxylin–eosin. 113×.

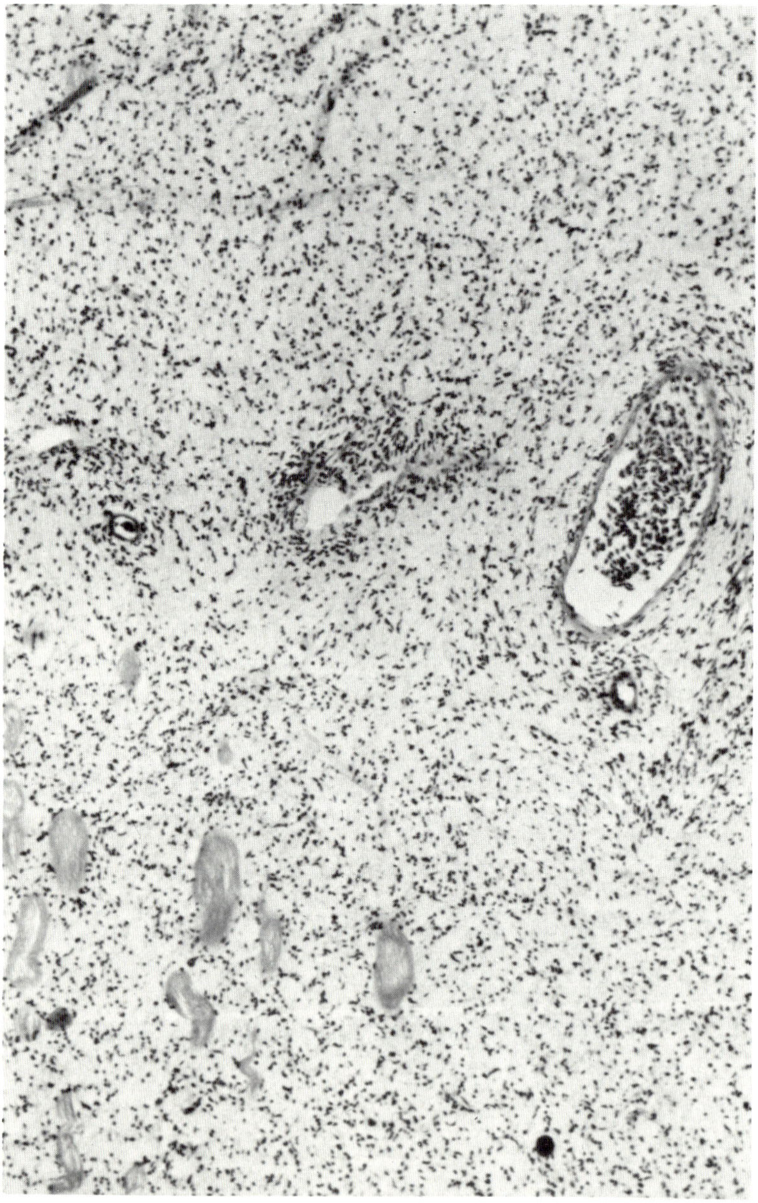

Fig. 35. Transverse section of fibrosarcoma showing a cellular tumor containing blood vessels and an occasional muscle fiber. Hematoxylin–eosin. 113×.

E. Osteoma and Osteosarcoma

Osteomata were among the first piscine neoplasms to be reported (Worm, 1655; Olearius, 1674; Bell, 1793; Cuvier and Valenciennes, 1831; Rayer, 1843). Bland-Sutton (1885) mentioned an exostosis in connection with the vertebrae of a cod, the dentary bone of a pike (*E. lucius*), and the superior maxillary of a cod. In another fish (*Pagrus unicolor*), an exostosis of the occipital crest was seen which histologically resembled vasodentine (Fig. 36). A tumor in the mouth of a striped marlin (*Makaira audax*), which may be of bony origin (Fig. 37), has been noted by Wares (personal communication). Other reports of osteoma and osteosarcoma include those of Wahlgren (1876), Plehn (1906), Murray (1908), Schroeders (1908), Fiebiger (1909b), Starks (1911), Williamson (1911), Beatti (1916), Kazama (1924), Sagawa (1925), Takahashi (1929, 1934), Williams (1929), Thomas (1932b, 1933b), Nigrelli (1938), Schlumberger and Lucké (1948), Bertullo and Traibel (1955), Sarkar and Dutta-Chaudhuri (1958), Barcellos (1962), and Wellings (1969). Many tumors of this type were reported by Takahashi (1929) and Chabanaud (1926) in *Pagrosomes major.* A traumatic etiology was considered most likely, as fine fracture lines were seen in the specimens. The subsequent "callus" formation was considered a true tumor formation. This etiology, however, is no longer considered valid.

F. Chondroma

Despite the fact that the elasmobranchs form a major group of fish, tumors of cartilage are uncommon. No report exists of the occurrence of a chondrosarcoma. Only eight reports of chondroma formation have been noted to date (Surbeck, 1917; André, 1927; Takahashi, 1929; Thomas, 1932b,d, 1933b; Nigrelli and Gordon, 1946).

G. Hemangioma

In the strict sense of the word, many benign angiomata are not true neoplasms but rather malformations (Willis, 1967), and a detailed examination is not particularly relevant to this chapter. As in the case of many other types of tumors, an exact diagnosis is not always possible. Several workers have reported hemangiomata in fish (Plehn, 1906; Murray, 1908; Drew, 1912; Johnstone, 1915, 1924a,b, 1926a; Stolk, 1958b; Honma, 1966). The inclusion of these cases in a discussion on neoplasia must remain in doubt however.

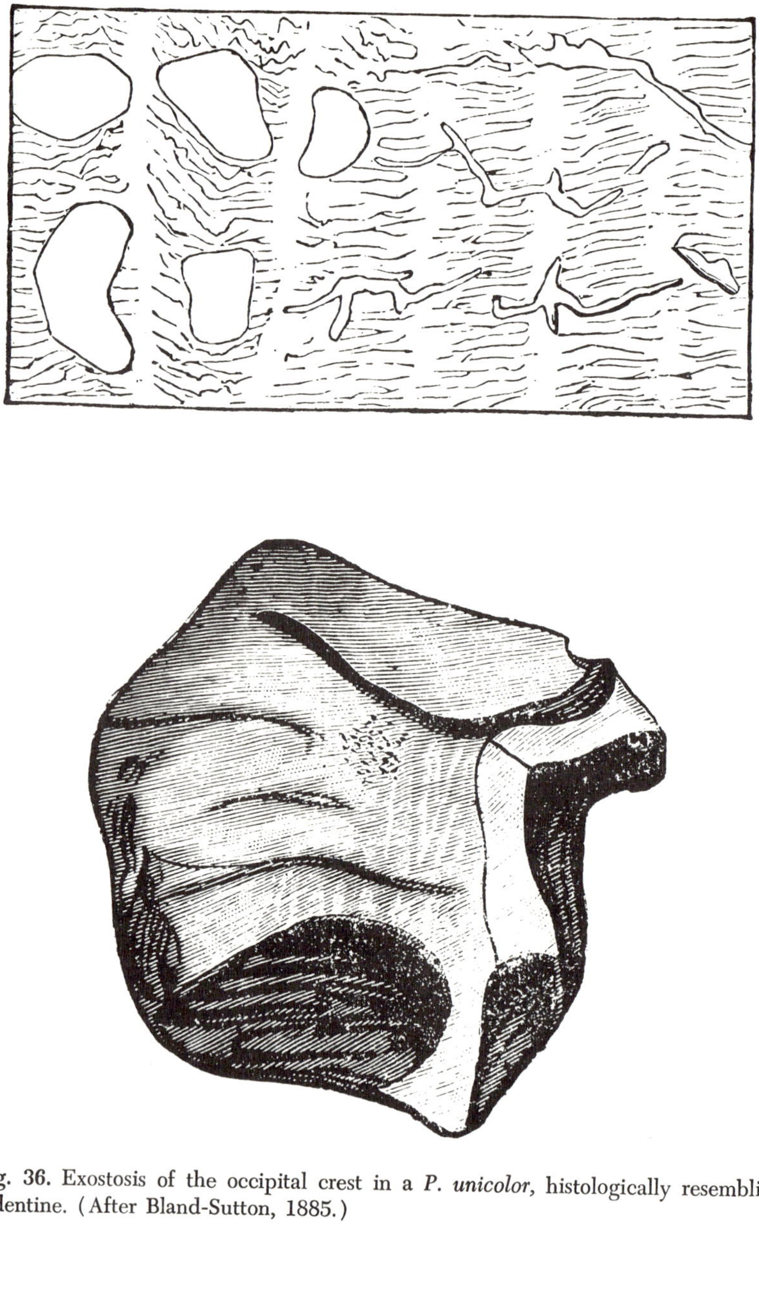

Fig. 36. Exostosis of the occipital crest in a *P. unicolor,* histologically resembling vasodentine. (After Bland-Sutton, 1885.)

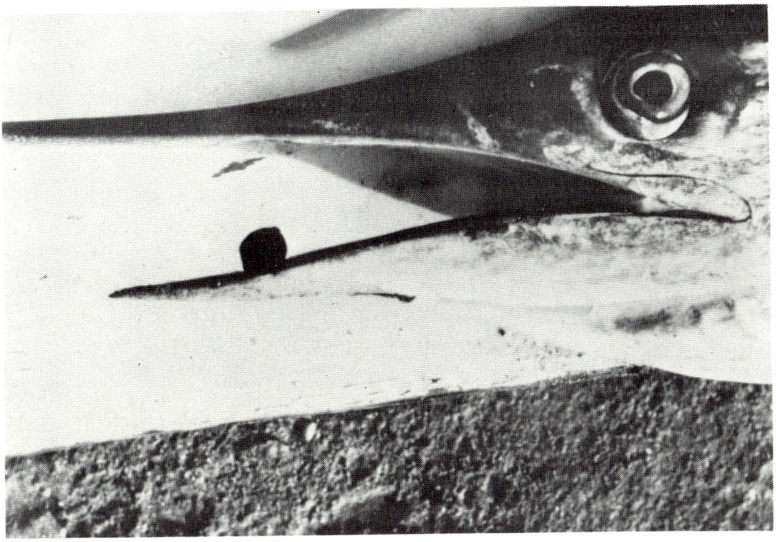

Fig. 37. Tumor arising from the mandible in a striped marlin (*M. audax*). (By kind permission of Dr. Paul C. Wares.)

VI. Tumors of Hemopoietic Tissues

In teleostean fish hematopoiesis occurs primarily in parts of the kidney (mesonephros), spleen, thymus, and submucosa of the gut. These anatomical and physiological facts often explain the distribution of some of the tumors of this system. This subject has recently been reviewed in some detail by Dawe (1969).

While the occurrence of lymphosarcomata has been reported over the past 50 years, the diagnosis is dubious in many instances since detailed histological examinations were lacking. In the earlier references no clear division exists between the various types of sarcomata, the group being treated as a single entity. The following workers have reported lymphosarcomata in fish: Ohlmacher (1898), Johnstone (1911), Plehn (1924), Johnstone (1926a), Williams (1931), Haddow and Blake (1933), Smith *et al.* (1936), Nigrelli (1947), Rasquin and Hafter (1951), Rasquin and Rosenbloom (1954), Wessing and Von Bargen (1959), Ehlinger (1963), Mulcahy (1963), Mulcahy and O'Rourke (1964a,b), Honma and Hirosaki (1966), Dunbar (1969), and Wolke and Wyard (1969).

The problems of classification of these tumors are many, as there is relatively little available information on fish blood. Until more is known about fish blood cell types and counts together with the erythroblastic and lymphoblastic maturation of cells, a more precise classification is not advisable. As Dawe (1969) has pointed out, the relatively high incidence of lymphosarcomata in pike (*E. lucius*) in Ireland provides a useful source of material for further investigation. As in the case of lymphosarcomata in other animal species, epizootic outbreaks occur from time to time (Nigrelli, 1947; Schlumberger, 1957; Mulcahy and O'Rourke, 1964a,b), and the possibility of a viral etiology must be considered, together in some instances with a genetic factor. Mulcahy (1970) is now actively following up her earlier work on lymphosarcomata in Irish pike.

VII. Tumors of Pigment Cells

Tumors of pigment cells in fish are well documented. This is not surprising, since pigment cells are frequently found in the epidermis and subcutaneous tissues as well as in the meninges, peritoneum, mesentery, and abdominal viscera. The hypothesis suggested by Schlumberger and Lucké (1948) that all pigment cell tumors are derived from a common undifferentiated mesenchymal cell cannot be supported. To suggest that all have a similar origin whether it be mesodermal, epithelial, or neuroectodermal (Borcca, 1909; Becher, 1929) is inaccurate, and a more logical classification is demanded (Willis, 1967).

There are several types of pigment cell tumors in fish: those containing melanin, the melanomata; those containing a red pigment (erythropterin), the erythrophoromata (Goodrich *et al.*, 1941); those containing a yellow pigment (composed of lutein and zeaxanthin), the xanthophoromata; and those containing guanine crystals, the guanophoromata. While these pigments may exist in relatively pure states, various complex color combinations occur (Gordon, 1948; Gordon and Nigrelli, 1950), such as is seen in xanthoerythrophoromata (Gordon, 1950). It is worth noting that the iridescence frequently associated with many fish species is attributable to the presence of iridiocytes which contain crystals of various inorganic salts that reflect light.

A. *Melanoma*

Melanoma is the commonest of all pigment cell tumors. Melanomata of the fish skin are known (Prince, 1892; Prince and Steven, 1892; Hofer,

1904; Schmey, 1911; Johnstone, 1911, 1912, 1913, 1915, 1924b; Bergman, 1921; Osburn, 1925; Haüssler, 1928, 1934; Ingleby, 1929; Kosswig, 1929a,b, 1931; Takahashi, 1929, 1934; Reed and Gordon, 1931; Haddow and Blake, 1933; Montpellier and Dieuzeide, 1934; Gordon, 1937, 1951; Gordon and Smith, 1938a,b; Breider, 1938, 1939, 1956; Dollfus *et al.*, 1938; Gordon and Lansing, 1943; Nigrelli and Gordon, 1944; Breider and Schmidt, 1951; Nigrelli *et al.*, 1951; Ermin, 1953; Stolk, 1953e, 1958e,f,g, 1960a; Proewig, 1954; Greenberg *et al.*, 1956; Elwin, 1957; Ghadially and Gordon, 1957; Dupont and Vandaele, 1959; Greenberg

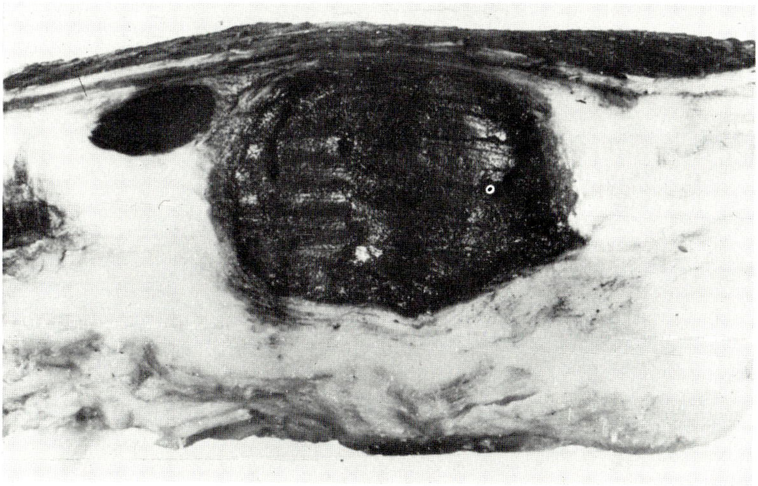

Fig. 38. Section through dorsal musculature of cod (*G. morhua*) showing several melanosarcomata. (By kind permission of Dr. Calvert Appleby, Royal Veterinary College, London.)

and Kopac, 1960, 1963; MacIntyre and Baker-Cohen, 1961; Anders and Klinke, 1965; Anders, 1967; Erdman, personal communication). Melanomata have seldom been reported in trunk musculature (Stolk, 1953e). In our laboratory a melanosarcoma of the trunk musculature was observed in a cod (*G. morhua*) (Fig. 38). In fact, several such tumors have been seen (Fig. 39); however, whether they represent true metastasis rather than multifocal tumors is uncertain. Melanomata have also been reported in the eyes of fish (Gordon, 1946; Levine and Gordon, 1946; Stolk, 1958e; Cohen, 1965). Recently, a melanoma of the eye was seen in an angelfish (*Pterophyllum eimekei*) (Fig. 40).

A renal melanoma has been reported in the African lungfish (*Protopterus annectens*) (Nigrelli and Jakowska, 1953). Melanosis or

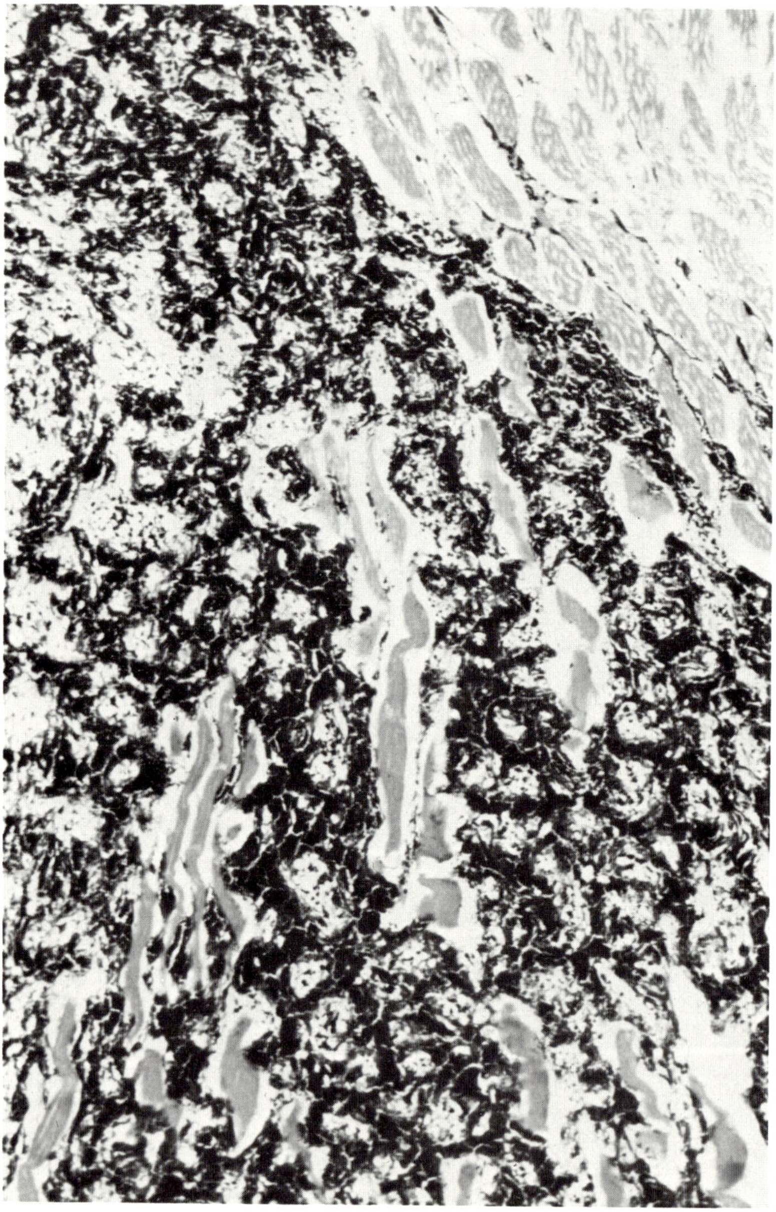

Fig. 39. Transverse section showing infiltration of skeletal muscle by pigment cells. 88×.

melanoma formation is often associated with physical, chemical, or parasitic insult (Hsiao, 1941; Mawdesley-Thomas and Young, 1967). Ghadially (1966), however, showed that repeated trauma to *Xiphophorus maculatus* × *Xiphophorus helleri* hybrids did not produce tumors

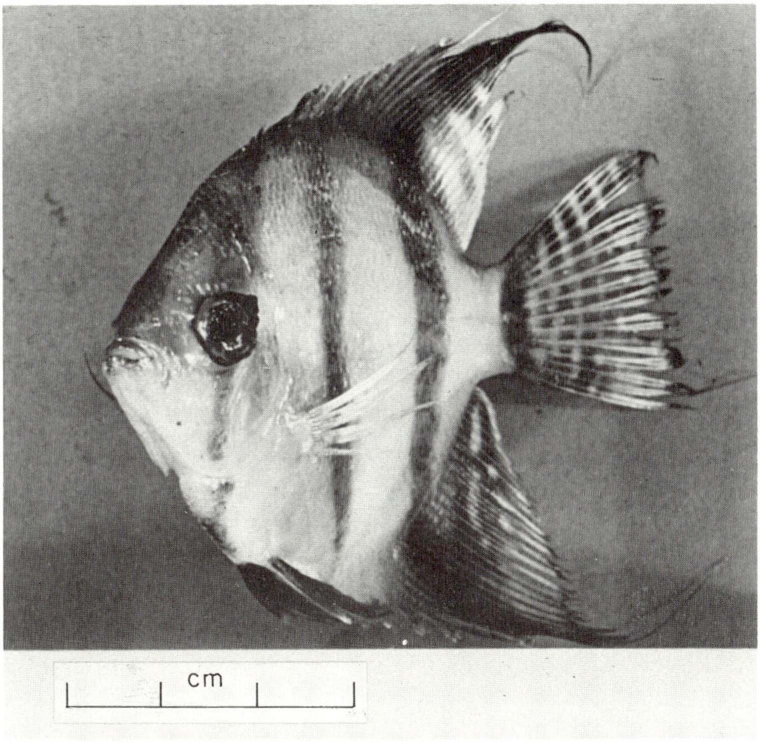

Fig. 40. Melanoma of the left eye in an angelfish (*P. eimekei*).

although these hybrids are genetically prediposed to melanoma formation.

B. Erythrophoroma

Erythrophoromata have been reported from only a few species of fish (Kosswig, 1929a, 1931; Takahashi, 1929; Thomas, 1931a; Smith, 1934; Smith *et al.*, 1936; Gordon and Nigrelli, 1950; Nigrelli *et al.*, 1950; Ghadially and Whiteley, 1951; Ermin, 1953; Stolk, 1959b).

C. *Xanthoerythrophoroma*

Mixed-pigment xanthoerythrophoromata have occasionally been observed in fish (Nigrelli *et al.*, 1951; Ermin, 1953).

D. *Guanophoroma*

Only two cases of guanophoromata have been recorded. These occurred in a specimen of *Hexagrammos atakii* (Takahashi, 1929) and in a specimen of *Ctenobrycon spilurus* (Stolk, 1959c).

E. *Xanthophoroma*

Schroeders (1908) reported a xanthophoromata in a specimen of blenny and, subsequently, another was seen in a *Rivulus xanthonotus* (Stolk, 1959d).

VIII. Tumors of Nervous Tissue

No tumor of the brain or spinal cord has been recorded in fish apart from a pineal tumor reported by Charlton (1929). Present evidence suggests their relative rarity, but not until many more systems have been examined can any valid assessment be made. Parasitic infestation of the central nervous system has been described, and cerebral cysts have also been reported in *Cichlasoma facetum* and *L. reticulatus* (Stolk, 1957e,f) and should not be confused with true neoplasms (Hoffman and Hoyme, 1958).

Tumors of the Pituitary

The first tumor recorded from a fish pituitary occurred in a guppy (*L. reticulatus*) (Stolk, 1953b). Subsequent cases have been recorded (Stolk, 1958d; Sathyanesan, 1962). The majority of these tumors were seen in smaller, warm-water fishes and were of the chromophobe adenoma type. Several of the tumorous fish represented intersexes, hence some endocrine dysfunction is suggested (Stolk, 1956f). The anatomy of the base of the brain in these fish is such that the optic chiasm may be displaced without causing any optic atrophy as a result of pressure. The embryology of the pituitary gland predisposes it to developmental anomalies.

Pituitary cysts resulting from craniopharyngeal remnants are relatively common in many animal species. In some breeds of dogs a 90% incidence has been noted.

Hypophysial cysts have been described in teleostean fish (Schreibman and Charipper, 1962; Schreibman, 1966). These cysts must be considered in any differential diagnosis of a pituitary tumor. While no tumor of the spinal cord or central nervous system has been reported, cerebral parasitic infection of the cerebrum may give the appearance of a tumor.

Neoplasms of spinal ganglia and peripheral nerves have been reported (Thomas, 1927b, 1932c; Takahashi, 1929, 1933; Haddow and Blake, 1933; Picchi, 1933; Lucké, 1942; Schlumberger, 1951, 1952; Finkelstein and Danchenko-Ryzchkova, 1965; McArn and Wellings, 1967; Fajen, personal communication; Wellings, 1969). An understanding of the histogenesis of this group of tumors presents many difficulties. Recent electron microscope studies (Duncan and Harkin, 1968) have shown that neurilemmoma in the goldfish is dissimilar to that in man, thus emphasizing the difficulty in diagnosing many neural tumors. Willis (1967) has commented on the distinct regimentation of nuclei in certain leiomyomata, which can be confused with neurilemmomata (Stewart, 1931; Golden and Stout, 1941; Willis, 1962). Several neurilemmomata have been seen in goldfish (Figs. 41 and 42). The interest in some of the pituitary tumors reported lies in their possible value as experimental models for further studies. Lucké (1942) showed that species-specific nerve sheath tumors in the family Lutianidae, known locally as "cancer fish," occurred in up to 1.0% of certain species. Schlumberger (1951) suggested a relationship between the limbus tumors in the eye of the goldfish (*C. auratus*) and Von Recklinghausen's neurofibromatosis. Young and Olafson (1944) described neurilemmomata in a family of brook trout (*S. fontinalis*), but it has been subsequently suggested (Schlumberger and Lucké, 1948; Snieszko, 1961) that these tumors represent a non-neoplastic condition and Snieszko suggested "visceral granuloma" as a more realistic description. Parasitic infestation should always be considered in a differential diagnosis (Petrushevski, 1957). More recently, Ashley *et al.* (1969) have reported several visceral tumors in trout (*S. gairdneri*) and salmon (*Oncorhynchus tshawytscha*) which were considered reticulocytomata.

IX. Miscellaneous Conditions

Evidence of cataract formation in the rainbow trout has been reported following the dietary administration of thioacetamide (von Sallmann *et al.*, 1966). The proliferation of the lens epithelium has been likened to a "tumorous growth pattern." While proliferation of the lens epithelium was well shown, it does not appear to be a property peculiar to a thioacetamide diet. Many similar cataracts have been seen in rainbow trout (Figs. 43 and 44) to which thioacetamide has not been supplied (Mawdesley-Thomas and Jolly, 1968). The etiology of the latter cataracts is uncertain. Hess (1937) suggested that some cataracts may have a nutritional etiology, and similar proliferations have been seen associated with parasitic infections of the lens (Fig. 45). It is thought that this hyperplasia of the lens epithelium is not a true neoplastic condition but rather a nonspecific cellular response to a noxious influence. Tumorlike lesions of the notochord of fish have been produced experimentally in several species of fish by immersing embryos in a solution of β-aminoproprionitrile (Levy, 1962). It is, however, doubtful that these lesions represent a truly neoplastic condition.

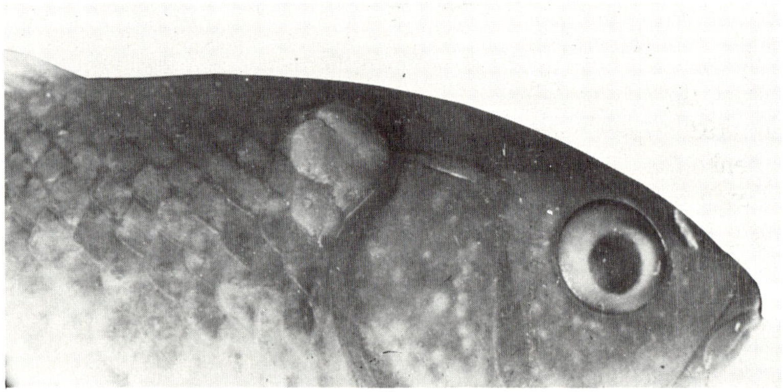

Fig. 41. Neurilemmoma in a goldfish (*C. auratus*).

Teratoma

In the majority of definitions applied to types of tumors, it is usually Willis (1962) who has the last word. According to him, "A teratoma is

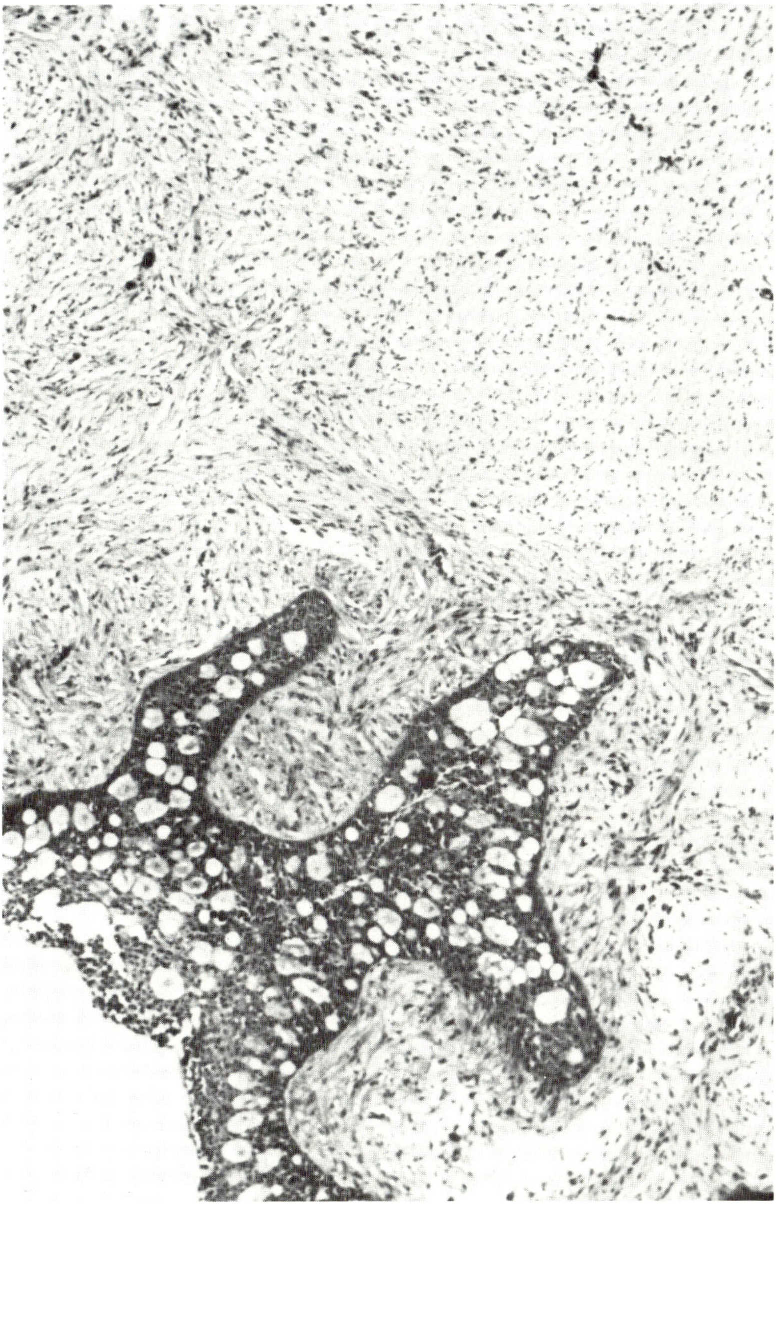

Fig. 42. Transverse section of skin showing underlying neurilemmoma. Hematoxylin–eosin. 113×.

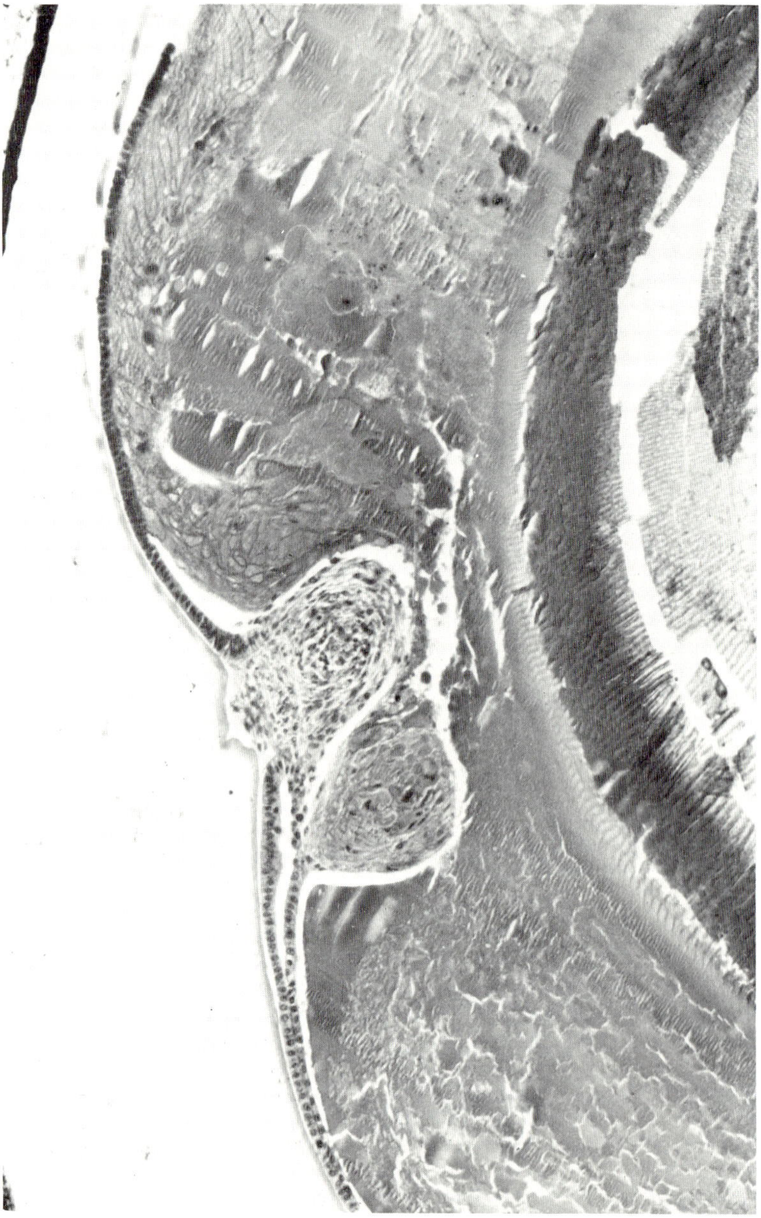

Fig. 43. Transverse section of trout lens showing proliferation of the lens epithelium. Hematoxylin–eosin. 113×.

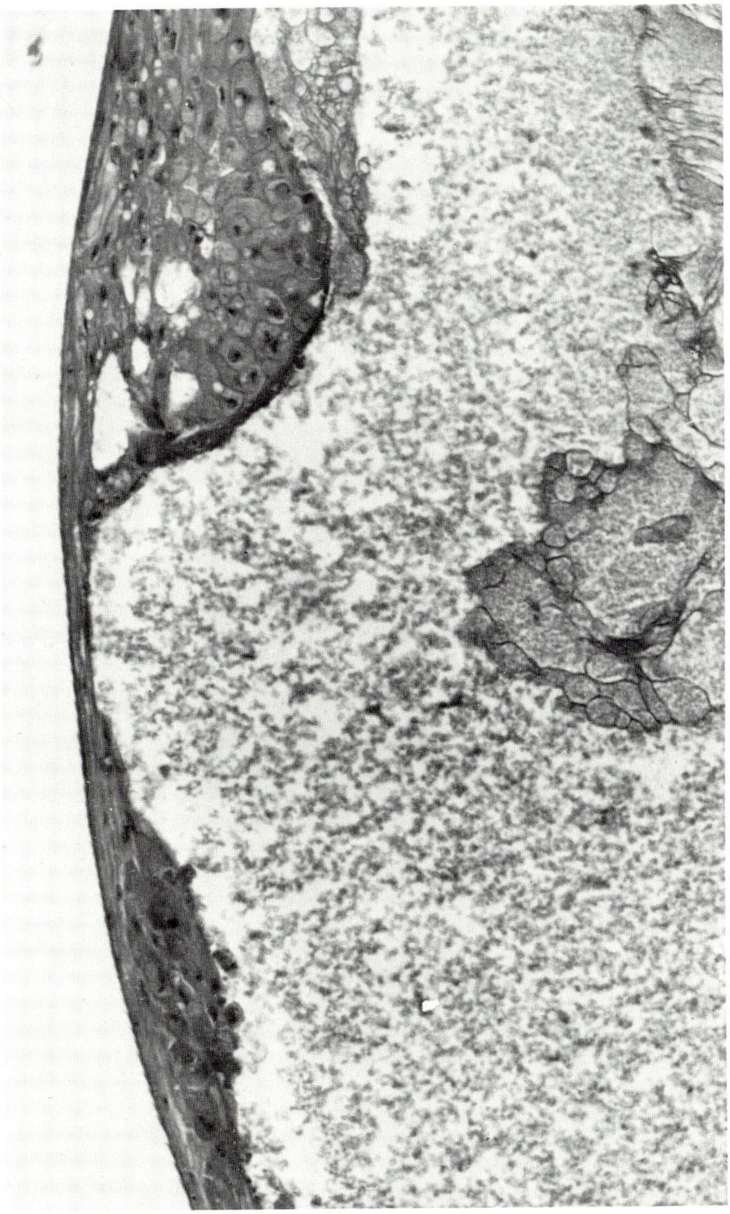

Fig. 44. Transverse section of trout lens showing proliferation of lens epithelium and underlying fiber degeneration. Hematoxylin–eosin. 215×.

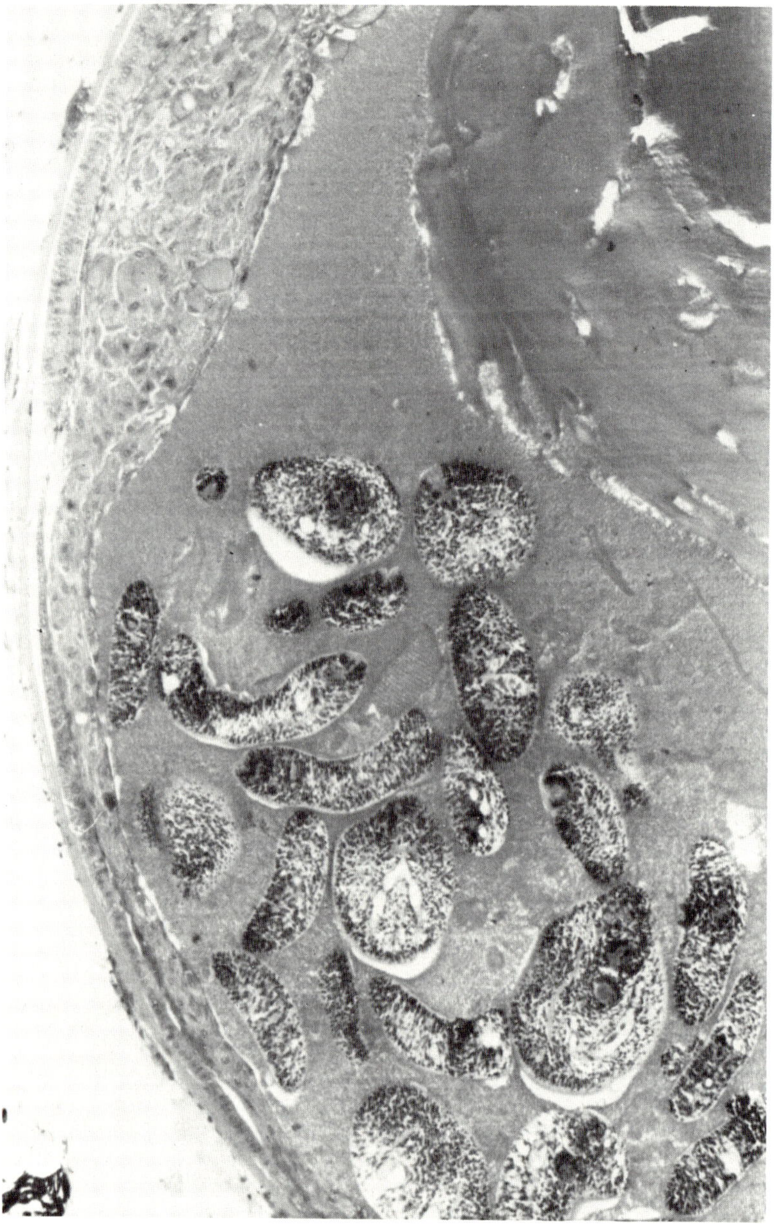

Fig. 45. Transverse section of trout lens showing proliferation of lens epithelium associated with a parasitic infestation. Hematoxylin–eosin. 113×.

a true tumour or neoplasm composed of multiple tissues of kinds foreign to the part in which it arises."

Until 1953 teratomata has not been reported in fish, giving some indication of the rarity of this tumor (Stolk, 1953a, 1955a; Hisaoka, 1961). The majority of recorded cases occurred in the guppy or million fish (*L. reticulatus*), although Stolk (1959a) also reported teratomata in viviparous toothcarps.

X. Summary and Conclusions

Neoplastic transformation might be considered a direct consequence of life, such is its frequency and range throughout the animal kingdom and the Vertebrata in particular (Bashford, 1904; Dean, 1923; Cramer, 1932). The universality of neoplasia, although not completely established at this time, is in all probability a fact (Finkelstein, 1962). The absence of reported cases of neoplasia of the brain and spinal cord in fish does not preclude their existence. Documentation of neoplasia of the nervous system generally has lagged behind that of other systems in many species.

Neoplasia of all cell types has been seen in fish. Tumors have been recorded in mesenchymal, epithelial, hemopoietic, and nervous tissues. Pigment cell tumors appear to be more frequent in fish than in other categories of animals. This may be accounted for by the widespread distribution of the various pigment cell types in fish.

In general, it is considered unwise to assess animal tumors as anything more than analogous to tumors in man. They should certainly not be considered homologous. One of the main problems of comparative pathology is the tendency to relate all tumors to those of man. This is a natural tendency, as human pathology has been studied in greater detail than any of the comparative branches. Close analogy should be resisted for, as any experimentalist appreciates, "only man is like man" and animal tumors should be treated, not in relation to those of man but on their own individual and particular merits (Pick and Poll, 1903). A great disservice has been rendered to comparative pathology over the years, particularly by medical pathologists, by forcing a "man-made" discipline onto infrahuman branches of the animal kingdom. Nowhere is this more apparent than in the realms of the benign or malignant condition—a term of prognostic significance only in man and a point repeatedly stressed by Willis (1967), one of the greatest tumor pathologists of our time. Much objective thinking has been brought to bear recently by Daniel and Prichard (1967) on this topic in relation to mammary tumors in the rat.

While many etiologies have been considered in the preceding discussion, many might well be investigated as experimental models for further basic research into neoplasia. The species-specific tumors of poikilothermic vertebrates (Lucké and Schlumberger, 1949; Schlumberger, 1957; Stolk, 1958g) offer ideal models for epidemiological investigations. The extreme sensitivity of the fish liver to tumor formation, for example, the effects of aflatoxin, could be of great significance (Bonser, 1967). Researchers interested in hepatomagenesis should consider further research using the trout as a laboratory animal. Fish are easily kept and maintained under laboratory conditions, much background information is already available, and intercurrent infection and disease are not serious problems. The use of fish and fish tumor formation as a bioassay of natural pollution cannot be overstressed, particularly in regard to skin neoplasia. This type of investigation has significance in relation to man as well as to various fish species.

Finally, it is hoped that fish, the commonest occurring vertebrate, can be more fully exploited by investigators in the field of neoplasia, for within their particular biological systems may lie many clues to the basic mechanisms involved.

Acknowledgments

I would like to express my thanks to the Trustees of the British Museum; A. Wheeler and G. Bridson, British Museum (Natural History); Dr. D. W. Jones, Liverpool; M. Bulleid, Wales; Miss J. Dobson, Royal College of Surgeons of England; Mr. P. Wade, Royal Society of Medicine, London; Dr. C. Appleby, Royal College of Veterinary Surgeons, London; Mr. G. R. Foster, Plymouth; D. A. Conroy, Aberdeen, Scotland; Dr. P. Besse, Paris; Dr. O. Ljungberg, Sweden; J. P. Wise, Florida; Prof. O. V. Bauer, Leningrad; D. S. Erdman, Puerto Rico; The American Fisheries Society; Dr. J. C. Harshbarger, Smithsonian Institution, Washington, D. C.; Dr. B. F. Deys, Leiden; Dr. P. G. Wares, California; Dr. N. Fijan, Yugoslavia; Prof. S. R. Wellings, Davis, California; Prof. J. E. Deacon, Los Vegas, Nevada; Dr. M. Wiles, Halifax, Canada; Dr. J. W. Ellis, Hawaii; O. F. Fajen, Columbia, Missouri; Dr. L. M. Ashley, Cook, Washington; Prof. J. Seno, Tokyo; Prof. R. Walker, New York; and Dr. C. Dawe, Washington—many of whom have kindly sent photographs—but particularly to my chief librarian, Miss M. G. Shafto, and her assistant, Miss V. Orbell, for invaluable assistance with the bibliography; to Mr. A. Creed for proofreading the manuscript; to my secretary, Mrs. L. Williams, without whose help this manuscript would never have been produced; and finally to my director-general, Prof. A. Worden, for encouragement and helpful discussions of the manuscript.

References

Adami, J. G. (1908). On a giant-celled rhabdomyosarcoma from the trout. *Montreal Med. J.* **37**, 163–165.

Aldrovandi, U. (1613). "De Piscibus." Bologna.

Amlacher, E. (1961). Taschenbuch der Fischkrankheiten. *Jenaer Rundschau* **11**, 286.

Anadon, E. (1956). Nota sobre un tumor en *Trachurus trachurus* L. *Invest. Pesq.* **5**, 13–15.

Anders, F. (1967). Tumour formation in platyfish-swordtail hybrids as a problem of gene regulation. *Experientia* **23**, 1–10.

Anders, F., and Klinke, K. (1965). Untersuchungen über die erbbedingte Aminosäurenkonzentration, Farbenmanifestation und Tumorbildung bei lebendgebärenden Zahnkarpfen (Poeciliidae). *Z. Verebungslehre* **96**, 49–65.

André, E. (1927). Sur un chondrome du vairon. *Bull. Suisse Pêche Piscicult.* **28**, 177–178.

André, E. (1939). Myome chez un poisson. *Bull. Franç. Piscicult.* **118**, 173–174.

Anitschkow, N., and Pawlowsky, E. N. (1923). Über die Hautpapillome bei Gobius und ihre Beziehung zur normalen Struktur der Fischhaut. *Z. Krebsforsch.* **20**, 128–147.

Anonymous (1964). Hepatomas in trout. *Nutr. Rev.* **22**, 208–210.

Aronowitz, O., Nigrelli, R. F., and Gordon, M. (1951). A spontaneous epithelioma in the platyfish, *Xiphophorus* (*Platypoecilus*) *variatus*. *Zoologica* (*New York*) **36**, 239–241.

Ashley, L. M. (1965). Histopathology of rainbow trout aflatoxicosis. *In* "Trout Hepatoma Research Conference Papers" (J. E. Halver and I. A. Mitchell, eds.). *Fish Wildl. Serv.* (*U.S.*), *Res. Rep.* **70**, 103–120.

Ashley, L. M. (1967). Renal neoplasms of rainbow trout. *Bull. Wildl. Dis. Ass.* **3**, 86. (Abstr.)

Ashley, L. M., and Halver, J. E. (1961). Hepatomagenesis in rainbow trout. *Fed. Proc. Fed. Amer. Soc. Exp. Biol.* **20**, 290. (Abstr.)

Ashley, L. M., and Halver, J. E. (1963). Multiple metastasis of rainbow trout hepatoma. *Trans. Amer. Fish. Soc.* **92**, 365–371.

Ashley, L. M., and Halver, J. E. (1968). Dimethylnitrosamine-induced hepatic cell carcinoma in rainbow trout. *J. Nat. Cancer Inst.* **41**, 531–552.

Ashley, L. M., Halver, J. E., and Johnson, C. L. (1962). Histopathology of induced trout hepatoma. *Fed. Proc. Fed. Amer. Soc. Exp. Biol.* **21**, 304. (Abstr.)

Ashley, L. M., Halver, J. E., and Wogan, G. N. (1964). Hepatoma and aflatoxicosis in trout. *Fed. Proc. Fed. Amer. Soc. Exp. Biol.* **23**, 105. (Abstr.)

Ashley, L. M., Halver, J. E., Gardner, W. K., Jr., and Wogan, G. N. (1965). Crystalline aflatoxins cause trout hepatoma. *Fed. Proc. Fed. Amer. Soc. Exp. Biol.* **24**, 627. (Abstr.)

Ashley, L. M., Halver, J. E., and Wellings, S. R. (1969). Case reports of three teleost neoplasms. *In* "Neoplasms and Related Disorders of Invertebrate and Lower Vertebrate Animals" (C. J. Dawe and J. C. Harshbarger, eds.). *Nat. Cancer Inst. Monogr.* **31**, 157–166.

Baker, K. F. (1958). Heterotopic thyroid tissue in fish. *J. Morphol.* **103**, 91–129.

Baker, K. F., and Gordon, M. (1953). Preliminary studies of the differential susceptibility of various strains of the platyfish to a kidney tumor. *Genetics* **38**, 655. (Abstr.)

Baker, K. F., Berg, O., Nigrelli, R. F., Gorbman, A., and Gordon, M. (1954). Thyroid cell origin of spontaneous adenocarcinomas of the kidneys in fishes. *Proc. Amer. Ass. Cancer Res.* **1**, 3. (Abstr.)

Baker, K. F., Berg, O., Gorbman, A., Nigrelli, R. F., and Gordon, M. (1955). Functional thyroid tumors in the kidneys of platyfish. *Cancer Res.* **15**, 118–123.

Barcellos, B. N. (1962). Anomalias do esqueleto da corvina. *Cienc. Cult.* (*Maracaibo*) **14**, 111–113.

Bashford, E. F. (1904). The zoological distribution of cancer. *Sci. Rep. Invest. Imp. Cancer Res. Fund* **1**, 3–11.

Bashford, E. F., and Murray, J. A. (1904). Spindle cell sarcoma of the swim bladder in a cod (*Gadus morhua,* Linnaeus). *Sci. Rep. Invest. Imp. Cancer Res. Fund* **1**, 5–9.

Bashford, E. F., Murray, J. A., and Cramer, W. (1905). Transplantation of malignant new growths. *Sci. Rep. Invest. Imp. Cancer Res. Fund* **2**, 13–17.

Bean, T. H. (1907). *12th Annu. Rep. Forest Fish Game Comm., N.Y. State.* [Eng. Transl. of part of Hofer (1904).]

Beatti, M. (1916). Geschwülste bei Tieren. *Z. Krebsforsch.* **15**, 452–491.

Becher, H. (1929). Über die Entwicklung der Farbstoffzellen in der Haut der Knockenfische. *Verh. Anat. Ges.* **38**, 164–181.

Bell, W. (1793). Description of a species of *Chaetodon,* called by the Malays "Ecan bonna." *Phil. Trans. Roy. Soc. London* **83**, 7–9.

Berg, O., and Gorbman, A. (1954). Iodine utilization by tumorous thyroid tissue of the swordtail, *Xiphophorus montezumae. Cancer Res.* **14**, 232–236.

Berg, O., and Gordon, M. (1953). Thyroid drugs that control growth of goiters in xiphophorin fishes. *Proc. Amer. Ass. Cancer Res.* **1**, 5. (Abstr.)

Berg, O., Edgar, M., and Gordon, M. (1953). Progressive growth stages in the development of spontaneous thyroid tumors in inbred swordtails, *Xiphophorus montezumae. Cancer Res.* **13**, 1–8.

Berg, O., Gordon, M., and Gorbman, A. (1954). Comparative effects of thyroidal stimulants and inhibitors on normal and tumorous thyroids in Xiphophorin fishes. *Cancer Res.* **14**, 527–533.

Bergman, A. M. (1921). Einige Geschwülste bei Fischen: Rhabdomyom, Lipom und Melanom. *Z. Krebsforsch.* **18**, 292–302.

Bertullo, V. H., and Bellagamba, C. J. (1964). Neoplasmas en los peces de las costas uruguayas. II. Lipofibroma en corvina. *Rev. Inst. Invest. Pesq.* **1**, 261–264.

Bertullo, V. H., and Traibel, R. M. (1955). Neoplasma de los peces de las costas uruguayas. I. Osteoma de la costilla pleural de la corvina (*Micropogon opercularis*). *Anales de la Facultad de Veterinaria del Uruguay* **3**, 55–59.

Besse, P., Levaditi, J. C., Destombes, P., and Nazimoff, O. (1959). Reins polykystiques observés chez des Cyprinides d'un étarg de l'Eure. *Bull. Acad. Vet. Fr.* **32**, 421–426.

Besse, P., Levaditi, J., Vibert, R., and Nazimoff, O. (1960). Sur l'existence de tumeurs hepatiques primitives chez la truite arc-en-ciel (*Salmo irideus*). *C. R. Acad. Sci.* **251**, 482–483.

Besse, P., Levaditi, J. C., Doublet-Normand, A. M., and de Kinkelin, P. (1966). Incidence de l'hépatome dans les piscicultures françaises. *Bull. Off. Int. Epizoot.* **65**, 1071–1076.

Biavati, S. T., and Mancini, L. (1967). Un caso di fibroma in sardina *Pilchardus sardina*. *Nuova Vet.* **43**, 11–14.

Blaehser, S. (1961). Contribution à l'étude des tumeurs de la fibre musculaire striée chez les animaux. 74 pp. Thesis, Univ. de Paris.

Bland-Sutton, J. (1885). Tumors in animals. *J. Anat. Physiol.* **19**, 415–475.

Bonnet, R. (1883). Studien zur Physiologie und Pathologie der Fische. *Bayerische Fischerie Zeitschrift* **6**, 79.

Bonser, G. M. (1967). Factors concerned in the location of human and experimental tumours. *Brit. Med. J.* **2**, 655–660.

Borcca, M. I. (1909). Sur l'origine du coeur des cellules vasculaires migratices et des cellules pigmentaires chez les teleosteens. *C. R. Acad. Sci.* **149**, 688–689.

Breider, H. (1938). Die genetischen, histologischen und cytologischen Grundlagen der Geschwulstbildung nach Kreuzung verschiedener Rassen und Arten lebendgebärender Zahnkarpfen. *Z. Zellforsch. Mikrosk. Anat.* **28**, 784–828.

Breider, H. (1939). Über die Pigmentbildung in den Zellen von Sarkomen albinotischer und nichtalbinotischer Gattungsbastarde lebendgebärender Zahnkarpfen. *Z. Wiss. Zool., Abt. A* **152**, 107–128.

Breider, H. (1956). Farbgene und Melanosarkomhäufigkeit. *Zool. Anz.* **156**, 129–140.

Breider, H., and Schmidt, E. (1951). Melanosarkome durch Artkreuzung und Spontantumoren bei Fischen. *Strahlentherapie* **84**, 498–523.

Breslauer, T. (1915). Zur Kenntnis der Epidermoidalgeschwülste von Kaltblütern. *Arch. Mikrosk. Anat. Entwicklungsmech.* **87**, 200–262.

Budd, J., and Schroder, J. D. (1969). Testicular tumors of yellow perch. *Perca flavescens* (Mitchill). *Bull. Wildl. Dis. Ass.* **5**, 315–318.

Bugnion, E. (1875). Ein Fall von Sarkome beim Fische. *Deut. Z. Tiermed. Vergl. Pathol.* **1**, 132–134.

Buniva, M. F. (1802). Sur la physiologie et la pathologie des poissons. *Mem. Accad. Sci. Torin* **12**, 78–121.

Burwash, F. M. (1929). The iodine content of the thyroid of two species of elasmobranchs and one species of teleost. *Contrib. Can. Biol. Fish.* **4**, 117–120.

Cameron, A. T., and Vincent, S. (1915). Notes on an enlarged thyroid occurring in an elasmobranch fish (*Squalus suckleyi*). *J. Med. Res.* **27**, 251–256.

Ceretto, F. (1968). Carcinoma di tipo psammomatoso in *Carassius auratus*. *Riv. Ital. Piscic. Ittiopat.* A III, 37–40.

Chabanaud, P. (1926). Fréquence, symétrie et constance spécifique d'hyperostoses externes chez divers poissons de la famille des sciaenides. *C. R. Acad. Sci.* **182**, 1647–1649.

Charlton, H. H. (1929). A tumor of the pineal organ with cartilage formation in the mackerel, *Scomber scombrus*. *Anat. Rec.* **43**, 271–276.

Chavin, W. (1956a). Thyroid distribution and function in the goldfish, *Carassius auratus* L., as determined by the uptake of tracer doses of radio-iodine. *Anat. Rec.* **124**, 272. (Abstr.)

Chavin, W. (1956b). Thyroid distribution and function in the goldfish, *Carassius auratus* L. *J. Exp. Zool.* **133**, 259–279.

Chavin, W. (1956c). Thyroid follicles in the head kidney of the goldfish, *Carassius auratus* L. *Zoologica* (*New York*) **41**, 101–104.

Christiansen, M., and Jensen, A. J. C. (1947). On a recent and frequently occurring tumor disease in eel. *Rep. Dan. Biol. Sta. Bod. Agr.* **50**, 31–44.

Chuinard, R. G., Wellings, S. R., Bern, H. A., and Nishioka, R. (1964). Epidermal papillomas in pleuronectid fishes from the San Juan Islands, Washington. *Fed. Proc. Fed. Amer. Soc. Exp. Biol.* **23**, 337. (Abstr.)

Chuinard, R. G., Berkson, H., and Wellings, S. R. (1966). Surface tumors of starry flounder and English sole from Puget Sound, Washington. *Fed. Proc. Fed. Amer. Soc. Exp. Biol.* **25**, 661. (Abstr.)

Clunet, J. (1910). "Recherches Expérimentales sur les Tumeurs Malignes." Steinhell, Paris.

Coates, C. W., Cox, R. T., and Smith, G. M. (1938). Papilloma of the skin occurring in an electric eel, *Electrophorus electricus* L. *Zoologica (New York)* **23**, 247–251.

Coates, J. A., Potts, T. J., and Wilcke, H. L. (1967). Interim hepatoma research report. *In* "Trout Hepatoma Research Conference Papers" (J. E. Halver and I. A. Mitchell, eds.). *Fish Wildl. Serv. (U.S.), Res. Rep.* **70**, 34–38.

Codegone, M. L., Provana, A., and Ghittino, P. (1968). Evolution of the early hepatoma in rainbow trout. *Tumori* **54**, 419–426.

Cohen, S. (1965). Malignant melanoma of the eye of a catfish, *Corydoras julii. Copeia* **3**, 382–383.

Cole, F. J., and Eales, N. B. (1917). The history of comparative anatomy. A statistical analysis of the literature. *Sci. Progr. (London)* **11**, 578–590.

Conroy, D. A. (1965). Anormalidades patologicas en los peces marinos de la zona del Mar del Plata (Argentina). *Rev. Inst. Invest. Pesq.* **1**, 341–343.

Conroy, D. A. (1967). Thyroid tumour in Argentine pearl fish. *British Ichthyology Society Newsletter* Dec. 7–8.

Cooper, R. C., and Keller, C. A. (1969). Epizootiology of papillomas in English sole, *Parophyrs vetulus. In* "Neoplasms and Related Disorders of Invertebrate and Lower Vertebrate Animals" (C. J. Dawe and J. C. Harshbarger, eds.). *Nat. Cancer Inst. Monogr.* **31**, 173–186.

Cramer, W. (1932). The comparative study of cancer. *Cancer Rev.* **7**, 241–257.

Crisp, E. (1854). Large fungoid tumour in a carp. *Transactions of the Pathological Society of London* **5**, 347–348.

Cudkowicz, G., and Scolari, C. (1955). Un tumore primitive epatico a diffusione epizootica nella trota iridea di allevamento (*Salmo irideus*). *Tumori* **41**, 524–537.

Cuvier, Baron G. L. C. F. D., and Valenciennes, A. (1831). "Histoire Naturelle des Poissons," vol. 8, p. 249. Paris. (22 Vols., 1828–1849.)

Daniel, P. M., and Prichard, M. M. L. (1967). Further studies on mammary tumours induced in rats by 7,12-Dimethylbenz(α)anthracine (DMBA). *Int. J. Cancer* **2**, 163–177.

Dauwe, F., and Pennemann, G. (1904). Contributions à l'étude du cancer chez les poissons. *Ann. Soc. Med. Gand.* **84**, 41–52.

Dawe, C. J. (1969). Neoplasms of blood cell origin in poikilothermic animals. A review. *In* "Comparative Morphology of Hematopoietic Neoplasms" (C. H. Lingeman and F. M. Garner, eds.). *Nat. Cancer Inst. Monogr.* **32**, 7–28.

Dawe, C. J., and Harshbarger, eds. (1968). "Neoplasms and Related Disorders of Invertebrate and Lower Vertebrate Animals." *Nat. Cancer Inst. Monogr.* **31**.

Dawe, C. J., Stanton, M. F., and Schwartz, F. J. (1964). Hepatic neoplasms in native bottom-feeding fish of Deep Creek Lake, Maryland. *Cancer Res.* **24**, 1194–1201.

Dean, B. (assisted by Gudger, E. W., and Henn, A. W.) (1923). "A Bibliography of Fishes," Vol. 3, pp. 546–550. Amer. Mus. Natur. Hist. Press, New York.

Deys, B. F. (1969). Papillomas in the Atlantic eel, *Anguilla vulgaris*. *In* "Neoplasms and Related Disorders of Invertebrate and Lower Vertebrate Animals" (C. J. Dawe and J. C. Harshbarger, eds.). *Nat. Cancer Inst. Monogr.* **31**, 187–194.

Dinulesco, G., and Vasilescu, C. (1939). Thyroid cancer disease in two specimens of rainbow trout (*Salmo gairdneri irideus*). *Z. Fisch. Hilfswiss.* **37**, 689.

Dollar, A. M., Katz, M., Tripple, M. F., and Simon, R. C. (1963). Trout hepatoma. *Research in Fisheries* **139**, 23–25.

Dollar, A. M., Smuckler, E. A., and Simon, R. C. (1967). Etiology and epidemiology of trout hepatoma. *In* "Trout Hepatoma Research Conference Papers" (J. E. Halver and I. A. Mitchell, eds.). *Fish Wildl. Serv. (U.S.), Res. Rep.* **70**, 1–17.

Dollfus, R. P., Timon-David, J., and Mosinger, M. (1938). À propos des tumeurs mélaniques des poissons. *Bull. Ass. Fr. Etude Cancer* **27**, 37–50.

Dominguez, A. G. (1928). Fibroblastic sarcoma in a goldfish. *Clin. Med. Surg.* **35**, 256–257.

Drew, G. H. (1910). Some notes on parasitic and other diseases of fish. *Parasitology* **3**, 54–62.

Drew, G. H. (1912). Some cases of new growths in fish. *J. Mar. Biol. Ass. U.K.* **9**, 281–287.

Duerst, J. U. (1941). "Die Ursachen der Entstehung des Kropfes." Huber, Bern.

Dunbar, C. E. (1969). Lymphosarcoma of possible thymus origin in salmonid fishes. *In* "Neoplasms and Related Disorders of Invertebrate and Lower Vertebrate Animals" (C. J. Dawe and J. C. Harshbarger, eds.). *Nat. Cancer Inst. Monogr.* **31**, 167–172.

Duncan, T. E., and Harkin, J. C. (1968). Ultrastructure of spontaneous goldfish tumors previously classified as neurofibromas. *Amer. J. Pathol.* **52**, 33a.

Dupont, A., and Vandaele, R. (1959). Un cas de tumeur mélanique chez un poisson albinos, *Protopterus annecteus,* Owen du Congo. *Bull. Soc. Zool. Anvers* **8**, 252–253.

Eberth, C. J. (1878). Fibrosarcom der Kopfhaut einer Forelle. *Arch. Pathol. Anat. Physiol. Klin. Med.* **72**, 107–108.

Eguchi, S., and Oota, K. (1926). Of a tumour in a fish. *Aichi Igakkwai Zasshi* **33**, 24–26.

Ehlinger, N. F. (1963). Kidney disease in lake trout complicated by lymphosarcoma. *Progr. Fish Cult.* **25**, 3–7.

Elwin, M. C. (1957). Pathological melanosis in an intergenic hybrid. *Nature (London)* **179**, 1254–1255.

Ermin, R. (1953). *Platypoecilus maculutus* var. *fugilinosus* da Ksanto-eritroforoma Teşekkülü Hakkinda. *Istanbul Univ. Fen. Fak. Mecm., Seri B* **18**, 301–314.

Ermin, R. (1954). Bir Anatolichthys Melezinde Tesekkül Eden Göz Tümörü Hakkinda. *Istanbul Univ. Fen. Fak. Mecm., Seri B* **19**, 203–211.

Falk, H. L. (1967). Potential hepatocarcinogens for fish. *In* "Trout Hepatoma Research Conference Papers" (J. E. Halver and I. A. Mitchell, eds.). *Fish Wildl. Serv. (U.S.), Res. Rep.* **70**, 175–177, 182–192.

Fiebiger, J. (1909a). Ueber Hautgeschwülste bei Fischen nebst Bemerkungen über die Pockenfrankheit der Karpfen. *Z. Krebsforsch.* **7**, 165–179.

Fiebiger, J. (1909b). Ein Osteochondrom bei einem Karpfen. *Z. Krebsforsch.* **7**, 371–381.

Fiebiger, J. (1909c). Ein Rhabdomyom bei einem Kabljau. *Z. Krebsforsch.* **7**, 382–388.

Fiebiger, J. (1912). Bösartige Neubildung (Fibrosarkom) bei einem Seefisch. *Oestesreichische Fischerie Zeitung* **9**, 308.

Finkelstein, E. A. (1944). Development of tumours in invertebrates and lower vertebrates. *Usp. Sovrem. Biol.* **17**, 324–339.

Finkelstein, E. A. (1960). Tumours of fish. *Arkh. Patol.* **22**, 56–61.

Finkelstein, E. A. (1962). On some aspects of tumour distribution in the classes of fishes. *Usp. Sovrem. Biol.* **53**, 2.

Finkelstein, E. A., and Danchenko-Ryzchkova, L. K. (1965). Neurinoma in the perch *Perca fluviatilis*. *Arkh. Patol.* **27**, 81–84.

Freudenthal, P. (1928). Fibrom (Spindelzellensarkom) im Ovarium einer Karausche (*Carassius vulgaris*). *Z. Krebsforsch.* **26**, 414–417.

Gaillard, C. (1923). Recherches sur les poissons representés dans quelques tombeaux Egyptiens de l'ancien Empire. *Mémoires publiées par les Membres de l'Institut Français d'Archéologie Orientale du Caire* p. 51.

Gardner, L. W., and Wachowski, H. E. (1951). The thyroid gland and its function in cold-blooded vertebrates. *Quart. Rev. Biol.* **26**, 123–128.

Gaylord, H. R. (1909). An epidemic of cancer of the thyroid in brook trout in a fish hatchery. *J. Amer. Med. Ass.* **52**, 411.

Gaylord, H. R. (1910). An epidemic of carcinoma of the thyroid gland among fish. *J. Amer. Med. Ass.* **54**, 227.

Gaylord, H. R. (1916). Further observations on so-called carcinoma of the thyroid in fish. *J. Cancer Res.* **1**, 197–204.

Gaylord, H. R., and Marsh, M. C. (1912). Relation of feeding to thyroid hyperplasia in Salmonidae. *Z. Krebsforsch.* **12**, 436–438.

Gaylord, H. R., and Marsh, M. C. (1914). Carcinoma of the thyroid in the Salmonoid fishes. *Bull. U.S. Fish. Bur.* **32**, 363–524.

Gervais, P. (1875). De l'hyperostose chez l'homme et chez les animaux. *J. Zool.* **4**, 272–284, 445–465.

Gervais, P. (1876). Carpe atteinte d'une énorme tumeur fibreuse de l'abdomen. *J. Zool.* **5**, 466.

Gessner, C. (1558). "Historiae Animalium Liber IIII, qui est de Piscium et Aquatilium Animantium Natura." Tiguri, Zurich.

Ghadially, F. N. (1966). Trauma and melanoma production. *Nature (London)* **211**, 1199.

Ghadially, F. N., and Gordon, M. D. (1957). A localized melanoma in a hybrid fish *Lebistes X Mollienesia*. *Cancer Res.* **17**, 597–599.

Ghadially, F. N., and Whiteley, H. J. (1951). An invasive red-pigmented tumour (erythrophoroma) in a red male platyfish (*Platypoecilus maculatus* var. *rubra*). *Brit. J. Cancer* **5**, 405–408.

Ghadially, F. N., and Whiteley, H. J. (1952). Hormonally induced epithelial hyperplasia in the goldfish (*Carassius auratus*). *Brit. J. Cancer* **6**, 246–248.

Ghittino, P. (1963). Caso di epatoma nel salmerino di allevamento (*Salvelinus fontinalis*). *Atti Soc. Ital. Sci. Vet.* **17**, 574–579.

Ghittino, P., and Ceretto, F. (1961). Studio istologico ed ezio-patogenetico dell'epatoma della trota iridea di allevamento (*Salmo gairdneri*). *Atti Soc. Ital. Sci. Vet.* **15**, 579–585.

Ghittino, P., and Ceretto, F. (1962). Studio sulla eziopatogenesi dell'epatoma della trota iridea di allevamento. *Tumori* **48**, 393–409.

Ghittino, P., Dalforna, S., Provana, A., and Codegone, M. L. (1967a). Aspetti istologici di tumore tiroideo in una trota iridea di laboratorio. *Riv. Ital. Piscic. Ittiopat. A II,* 30–31.

Ghittino, P., Provana, A., and Codegone, M. L. (1967b). Experimental dietary hepatoma in rainbow trout. The role of cottonseed meals and other diets. *Cancro* **20,** 3–24.

Gilruth, J. A. (1902). Epithelioma affecting the branchial arches of salmon and trout. *New Zealand Department of Agriculture, Veterinary Division, Report* **1901/1902,** 312–315.

Golden, T., and Stout, A. P. (1941). Smooth muscle tumors of the gastro-intestinal tract and retro-peritoneal tissues. *Surg. Gynecol. Obstet.* **73,** 784–810.

Good, H. V. (1940). A study of an epithelial tumor of *Parophyrus vetulus.* M.S. Thesis, Univ. of Washington, Seattle, Washington.

Goodrich, H. B., Hill, G. A., and Arrick, M. S. (1941). The chemical identification of gene-controlled pigments in platypoecilus and Xiphophorus and comparisons with other tropical fish. *Genetics* **26,** 573–586.

Gorbman, A. (1964). Comparative pathology of the thyroid. *In* "The Thyroid," Int. Acad. of Pathol. Monogr. (J. Beach Hazard and D. E. Smith, eds.), pp. 32–48. Williams & Wilkins, Baltimore, Maryland.

Gorbman, A., and Gordon, M. (1951). Spontaneous thyroidal tumors in the swordtail, *Xiphophorus montezumae. Cancer Res.* **11,** 184–187.

Gordon, M. (1937). The production of spontaneous melanotic neoplasms in fishes by selective matings. II. Neoplasms with macromelanophores only. III. Neoplasms in day old fish. *Amer. J. Cancer* **30,** 362–375.

Gordon, M. (1946). Genetics of ocular-tumor development in fishes (preliminary report). *J. Nat. Cancer Inst.* **7,** 87–92.

Gordon, M. (1948). Effects of five primary genes on the site of melanomas in fishes and the influence of two color genes on their pigmentation. *In* "The Biology of Melanomas." *N.Y. Acad. Sci. Spec. Publ.* **4,** 216–268.

Gordon, M. (1950). Heredity of pigmented tumours in fish. *Endeavour* **9,** 26–34.

Gordon, M. (1951). The variable expressivity of a pigment cell gene from zero effect to melanotic tumor induction. *Cancer Res.* **11,** 676–686.

Gordon, M., and Lansing, W. (1943). Cutaneous melanophore eruptions in young fish during stages preceding melanotic tumor formation. *J. Morphol.* **73,** 231–245.

Gordon, M., and Nigrelli, R. F. (1950). The effect of two linked color genes upon the atypical growth of erythrophores and macromelanophores to form erythromelanomas in four generations of hybrid fishes. *Cancer Res.* **10,** 220. (Abstr.)

Gordon, M., and Smith, G. M. (1938a). Progressive growth stages of a heritable melanotic neoplastic disease in fishes from the day of birth. *Amer. J. Cancer* **34,** 255–272.

Gordon, M., and Smith, G. M. (1938b). The production of a melanotic neoplastic disease in fishes by selective matings. *Amer J. Cancer* **34,** 543–565.

Grafflin, A. L. (1937). Cyst formation in the glomerular tufts of certain fish kidneys. *Biol. Bull.* **72,** 247–257.

Greenberg, S. S., and Kopac, M. J. (1960). The amino acids of Xiphophorin fishes and their tumorous hybrids. *Anat. Rec.* **137,** 360. (Abstr.)

Greenberg, S. S., and Kopac, M. J. (1963). Studies of gene action and melanogenic enzyme activity in melanomatous fishes. *Ann. N.Y. Acad. Sci.* **100,** 887–923.

Greenberg, S. S., Kopac, M. J., and Gordon, M. (1956). Tissue culture studies of fish melanomas. *Anat. Rec.* **124**, 488–489.

Gudernatsch, J. F. (1910). The structure, distribution and variation of the thyroid gland in fish. *J. Amer. Med. Ass.* **54**, 227.

Gudernatsch, J. F. (1911a). The thyroid gland of teleosts. *J. Morphol.* **21**, 709–782.

Gudernatsch, J. F. (1911b). The relationship between the normal and pathological thyroid gland of fish. *Johns Hopkins Hosp. Bull.* **22**, 152–155.

Gudger, E. W. (1934). The five great naturalists of the sixteenth century: Belon, Rondelet, Salviani, Gessner and Aldrovandi. A chapter in the history of ichthyology. *Isis* **22**, 21–40.

Gudger, E. W. (1936). The beginnings of fish teratology, 1555–1642. *Sci. Mon.* **43**, 252–261.

Guglianetti, L. (1910). Fibroma dell'orbita in un ciprino. *Arch. Ottalmol.* **17**, 289–297.

Gusseva, V. V. (1963). Data on the investigation of fish tumours. Tumours of the pike-perch. Papers of the Leningrad Veterinary High School, p. 25. (In Russ.)

Haddow, A., and Blake, I. (1933). Neoplasms in fish: A report of six cases with a summary of the literature. *J. Pathol. Bacteriol.* **36**, 41–47.

Halver, J. E. (1965a). Aflatoxicosis and rainbow trout hepatoma. *In* "Mycotoxins in Foodstuffs" (G. N. Wogan, ed.), pp. 209–234. M.I.T. Press, Cambridge, Massachusetts.

Halver, J. E. (1965b). Hepatomas in fish. *In* "Primary Hepatomas" (W. J. Burdette, ed.), pp. 103–112. Univ. of Utah Press, Salt Lake City, Utah.

Halver, J. E. (1967). Crystalline aflatoxin and other vectors for trout hepatoma. *In* "Trout Hepatoma Research Conference Papers" (J. E. Halver and I. A. Mitchell, eds.). *Fish Wildl. Serv. (U.S.), Res. Rep.* **70**, 78–102.

Halver, J. E. (1968). Aflatoxicosis and trout hepatoma. *Bull. Off. Intl. Epizoot.* **69**, 1249–1278.

Halver, J. E. (1969). Aflatoxicosis and trout hepatoma. *In* "Aflatoxin, Scientific Background, Control and Implications" (L. A. Goldblatt, ed.), pp. 265–306. Academic Press, New York.

Halver, J. E., and Mitchell, I. A., eds. (1967). "Trout Hepatoma Research Conference Papers." *Fish Wildl. Serv. (U.S.), Res. Rep.* **70**, 1–199.

Halver, J. E., Johnson, C. L., and Ashley, L. M. (1962). Dietary carcinogens induce fish hepatoma. *Fed. Proc. Fed. Amer. Soc. Exp. Biol.* **21**, 390. (Abstr.)

Halver, J. E., LaRoche, G., and Ashley, L. M. (1963). Experimental hepatocellular carcinoma in rainbow trout. *Proc. 6th Int. Cong. Nutr. Edinburgh, 1963* p. 603.

Halver, J. E., Ashley, L. M., Smith, C. E., and Wogan, G. N. (1967). Early acute aflatoxicosis stimulates rainbow trout hepatomagenesis. *Toxicol. Appl. Pharmacol.* **10**, 398. (Abstr.)

Halver, J. E., Ashley, L. M., Smith, R. R., and Wogan, G. N. (1968). Age and sensitivity of trout to aflatoxin B_1. *Fed. Proc. Fed. Amer. Soc. Exp. Biol.* **27**, 552. (Abstr.)

Halver, J. E., Ashley, L. M., and Smith, R. R. (1969). Aflatoxins and neoplasia in Coho salmon. *In* "Neoplasms and Related Disorders of Invertebrate and Lower Vertebrate Animals" (C. J. Dawe and J. C. Harshbarger, eds.). *Nat. Cancer Inst. Monogr.* **31**, 141–149.

Hamre, C., and Nichols, M. S. (1926). Exophthalmia in trout fry. *Proc. Soc. Exp. Biol. Med.* **26**, 63–65.

Harold, E. S., and Innes, K. F. (1922). "The Shrimp and Associated Organisms of San Francisco Bay." Steinhart Aquarium, Calif. Acad. of Sci., Golden Gate Park, San Francisco.

Harshbarger, J. C. (1968). "Activities Report. Registry of Tumors in Lower Animals, April 1967–March 1968." Smithson. Inst., Washington, D.C.

Harshbarger, J. C., and Bane, C. W. (1969). Case report of fibrolipoma in a rockfish, *Sebastodes diploproa*. *In* "Neoplasms and Related Disorders of Invertebrate and Lower Vertebrate Animals" (C. J. Dawe and J. C. Harshbarger, eds.). *Nat. Cancer Inst. Monogr.* **31**, 219–222.

Haüssler, G. (1928). Über Melanombildungen bei Bastarden von *Xiphophorus hellerii* und *Platypoecilus maculatus* var. rubra. *Klin. Wochenschr.* **7**, 1561–1562.

Haüssler, G. (1934). Über die Melanome der *Xiphophorus platypoecilus Bastarde*. *Z. Krebsforsch.* **40**, 280–292.

Hess, W. N. (1937). Production of nutritional cataract in trout. *Proc. Soc. Exp. Biol. Med.* **37**, 306–309.

Hisaoka, K. K. (1961). Congenital teratomata in the guppy, *Lebistes reticulatus*. *J. Morphol.* **109**, 93–100.

Hofer, B. (1904). "Handbuch der Fischkrankheiten." Verlag der Allg. Fischerei, Munich.

Hoffman, G. L., and Hoyme, J. B. (1958). The experimental histopathology of the "tumour" on the brain of the stickleback caused by *Diplostomum baeri eucaliae* Hoffman and Hundley, 1957 (Trematoda-Strigeoidea). *J. Parasitol.* **44**, 374–378.

Honma, Y. (1965). A case of the myxoma developed in the head of the salmonoid fish, the Ayu, *Plecoglossus altivelis* Temminck et Schlegel. *Nippon Suisan Gakkaishi*, **31**, 192–197.

Honma, Y. (1966). Studies on the endocrine glands of the salmonoid fish, the Ayu, *Plecoglossus altivelis* Temminck and Schlegel. VI. Effect of artificially controlled light on the endocrines of the pond-cultured fish. *Nippon Suisan Gakkaishi* **32**, 32–40.

Honma, Y., and Hirosaki, Y. (1966). Histopathology on the tumors and endocrine glands of the immature chum salmon, *Oncorhynchus keta* reared in the Enoshima aquarium. *Gyoruigaku Zasshi* **14**, 74–83.

Honma, Y., and Kon, T. (1968). A case of the epidermal papilloma in the witch flounder from the Sea of Japan. *Nippon Suisan Gakkaishi* **34**, 1–5.

Honma, Y., and Shirai, K. (1959). Cystoma found in the liver of rainbow trout (*Salmo gairdneri irideus* Gibbons). *Nippon Suisan Gakkaishi* **24**, 966–970.

Hoshina, T. (1950). A case of fibroblastic sarcoma developed in *Hypomesus olidus* (Pallas). *Gyoruigaku Zasshi* **1**, 53–56.

Hoshina, T. (1952). Four cases of tumorous growths in fish. *Gyoruigaku Zasshi* **2**, 81–88.

Hsiao, S. C. T. (1941). Melanosis in the common cod, *Gadus callarias* L., associated with trematode infection. *Biol. Bull.* **80**, 37–44.

Hueper, W. C. (1942). "Occupational Tumors and Allied Diseases," pp. 5 and 33. Thomas, Springfield, Illinois.

Hueper, W. C., and Payne, W. W. (1961). Observations on the occurrence of hepatomas in rainbow trout. *J. Nat. Cancer Inst.* **27**, 1123–1143.

Hueper, W. C., and Ruchhoft, C. C. (1954). Carcinogenic studies on adsorbates of industrially polluted raw and finished water supplies. *AMA Arch. Ind. Hyg. Occup. Med.* **9**, 488–495.

Hunter, J. (1782). An account of the organ of hearing in fish. *Phil. Trans. Roy. Soc. London* **72**, 379–383.

Ichikawa, R. (1954). Studies on the abnormalities of scales in the tumour appearing on the skin of Japanese common goby. *Gyoruigaku Zasshi* **3**, 188–192.

Imai, T., and Fujiwara, N. (1959). An electron microscopic study of a papilloma-like hyperplastic growth in a goby, *Acanthogobius flavimanus*. *Kyushu J. Med. Sci.* **10**, 135–147.

Ingleby, H. (1929). Melanotic tumor in *Lophius piscatorius*. *Arch. Pathol.* **8**, 1016–1021.

Iwashita, M. (1955). On the tumour of gobies. *Collecting and Breeding, Tokyo* **17**, 50.

Jaboulay, M. (1908a). Poissons atteints de goitres malins héréditaires et contagieux. *J. Méd. Chir. Prat.* **79**, 239–240.

Jaboulay, M. (1908b). Poissons atteints de goitres malins héréditaires et contagieux. *Lyon Med.* **110**, 335–336.

Jackson, E. W., Wolf, H., and Sinnhuber, R. O. (1968). The relationship of hepatoma in rainbow trout to aflatoxin contamination and cottonseed meal. *Cancer Res.* **28**, 987–991.

Jahnel, J. (1939). Über einige Geschwülste bei Fischen, ein Beitrag zur Erblichkeitsfrage von Tumoren. *Wein Tieraerztl. Monatsschr.* **26**, 325–333.

Johnstone, J. (1910). Internal parasites and diseased conditions of fishes. *Proceedings and Transactions of the Liverpool Biological Society* **25**, 88–122.

Johnstone, J. (1911). Internal parasites and diseased conditions of fishes. *Proceedings and Transactions of the Liverpool Biological Society* **26**, 103–144.

Johnstone, J. (1912). Internal parasites and diseased conditions of fishes. *Proceedings and Transactions of the Liverpool Biological Society* **26**, 103–104.

Johnstone, J. (1913). Diseased conditions in fishes. *Proceedings and Transactions of the Liverpool Biological Society* **27**, 196–218.

Johnstone, J. (1914a). Internal parasites and diseased conditions in fishes. *Proceedings and Transactions of the Liverpool Biological Society* **28**, 127–142.

Johnstone, J. (1914b). Diseased and abnormal conditions of marine fishes. *Rep. Lancashire Sea-Fish. Lab.* **23**, 18–56.

Johnstone, J. (1915). Diseased and abnormal conditions of marine fishes. *Proceedings and Transactions of the Liverpool Biological Society* **29**, 80–113.

Johnstone, J. (1920). On certain parasites, diseased and abnormal conditions in fishes. *Proceedings and Transactions of the Liverpool Biological Society* **34**, 120–129.

Johnstone, J. (1922a). Diseases and parasites of fishes. *Proceedings and Transactions of the Liverpool Biological Society* **36**, 286–301.

Johnstone, J. (1922b). On some malignant tumours in fishes. *Rep. Lancashire Sea-Fish. Lab.* **31**, 87–99.

Johnstone, J. (1923a). On some malignant tumours in fishes. *Proceedings and Transactions of the Liverpool Biological Society* **37**, 145–157.

Johnstone, J. (1923b). Malignant tumours in fishes. *J. Mar. Biol. Ass. U.K.* **13**, 447–471.

Johnstone, J. (1924a). Diseased conditions in fishes. *Proceedings and Transactions of the Liverpool Biological Society* **38**, 183–213.

Johnstone, J. (1924b). Malignant tumours in fishes. *Proceedings and Transactions of the Liverpool Biological Society* 39, 169–200.

Johnstone, J. (1926a). Malignant and other tumours in marine fishes. *Proceedings and Transactions of the Liverpool Biological Society* **40**, 75–98.

Johnstone, J. (1926b). Diseased conditions in fishes. *Proceedings and Transactions of the Liverpool Biological Society* **41**, 162–167.

Kazama, Y. (1922). On a spindle cell sarcoma in a salmon. *Gann* **16**, 12–13.

Kazama, Y. (1924). Einige Geschwülste bei Fischen (*Pagrus major* et *Paralichthys olivaceus*). *Gann* **18**, 35–37.

Ketchen, K. S. (1953). Tumorous Infection in Sand Soles of Northern Hecate Strait (British Columbia). Report on the Survey of Hecate Strait in July, 1953. Manuscript, 3 pp.

Keysselitz, G. (1908). Über ein Epitheliom der Barben. *Arch. Protistenk.* **11**, 326–333.

Kimura, I., Miyake, T., and Ito, Y. (1967a). Studies on tumours in fishes. II. Papillomatous growths of skin in the goby, *Acanthogobius flavimanus*. *Proc. Jap. Cancer Ass. 26th Annu. Meet.* p. 154. (In Jap.)

Kimura, I., Sugiyama, T., and Ito, Y. (1967b). Papillomatous growth in sole from Wakasa Bay area. *Proc. Soc. Exp. Biol. Med.* **125**, 175–177.

Klemm, E. (1927). Über die Schilddrüsengeschwülste bei Aquarienfischen. *Mikrokosmos* **20**, 184–187.

Kolmer, W. (1928). Partieller Riesenwuchs in Verbindung mit grossem Rhabdomyom bei einer Schleie, *Tina tinca*. *Virchows Arch. Pathol. Anat. Physiol.* **268**, 574–575.

Konnerth, A. (1966). Tilly bones. *Oceanus* **12**, 6–9.

Kosswig, C. (1929a). Melanotische Geschwülstbildungen bei Fischbastarden. *Munchen. Med. Wochenschr.* **76**, 1070.

Kosswig. C. (1929b). Zur Frage der Geschwülstbindungen bei Gattunsbastarden der Zahnkarpfen, *Xiphophorus* und *Platypoecilus*. *Z. Indukt. Abstamm.-Verebungslehre* **52**, 114–120.

Kosswig, C. (1931). Über Geschwülstbindungen bei Fischbastarden. *Z. Indukt. Abstamm.-Verebungslehre* **59**, 61–76.

Kraybill, H. F., and Shimkin, M. B. (1964). Carcinogenesis related to foods contaminated by processing and fungal metabolics. *Advan. Cancer Res.* **8**, 191–248.

Kreyberg, L. (1937). An intra-abdominal fibroma in a brown trout. *Amer. J. Cancer.* **30**, 112–114.

Kubota, S. S. (1955a). Notes on liver cell carcinoma found on the rainbow trout, *Salmo irideus* Gibbons. *Mie Kenritsu Daigaku Suisangakubu Kiyo* **2**, 27–32.

Kubota, S. S. (1955b). A case of leiomyoma found in rainbow trout *Salmo irideus* Gibbons. *Nippon Suisan Gakkaishi* **20**, 1060–1062.

Labbé, A. (1930). Une tumeur complexe chez un merlan. *Bull. Ass. Fr. Etude Cancer* **19**, 138–158.

Ladreyt, F. (1929). Sur une odontome cutane chez un *Scyllium catulus*. *Bull. Inst. Oceanogr.* **539**, 1–4.

Ladreyt, F. (1930). Sur un rhabdomyosarcome chez un *Labrus mixtus*. *Bull. Inst. Oceanogr.* **550**, 1–4.

Ladreyt, F. (1935). Sur un epitheliome de la muqueuse palatine chez une murène (*Muraena helena*). *Bull. Inst. Oceanogr.* **677**, 1–16.

LaRoche, G., Halver, J. E., Johnson, C. L., and Ashley, L. M. (1962). Hepatomainducing agents in trout diets. *Fed. Proc. Fed. Amer. Soc. Exp. Biol.* **21**, 300. (Abstr.)

Lawrence, G. (1895). Note on a tumour found attached to the stomach of a Saithe. *Report of the Fishery Board of Scotland* **13**, 236.

Lee, D. J., Wales, J. H., Sinnhuber, R. O., Ayres, J. L., and Roehm, J. N. (1967). A comparison of cyclopropenes and other possible promoting agents for aflatoxin-induced hepatoma in rainbow trout. *Fed. Proc. Fed. Amer. Soc. Exp. Biol.* **26**, 322. (Abstr.)

Leger, L. (1925). Tumeurs observés chez les salmonides d'élevage. *C. R. Ass. Fr. Avan. Sci.* **49**, 395–396.

Levaditi, J. C., Besse, P., Vibert, R., and Nazimoff, O. (1960). Sur les critères histopathologiques et biologiques de malignité propres aux tumeurs épithéliales hépatiques des salmonides. *C. R. Acad. Sci.* **251**, 608–610.

Levaditi, J. C., Besse, P., Vibert, R., Destombes, P., Guillon, J.-C., Nazimoff, O., and Normand, A. M. (1963a). Apparition d'hépatomes malins dans les élevages de truites arc-en-ciel (*Salmo gairdneri*). Aspects géographiques et histologiques; facteurs génétiques et nutritionnels. *Press. Med.* **71**, 2743–2746.

Levaditi, J. C., Besse, P., Vibert R., Guillon, J.-C., and Nazimoff, O. (1963b). Particularités actuelles de l'hépatome de la truite arc-en-ciel d'élevage (*Salmo irideus*). *C. R. Acad. Sci.* **257**, 1739–1741.

Levine, M., and Gordon, M. (1946). Ocular tumours with exophthalmia in Xiphophorin fishes. *Cancer Res.* **6**, 197–204.

Levy, B. M. (1962). Experimental induction of tumour-like lesions of the notochord of fish. *Cancer Res.* **22**, 441–442.

Li, M. H., and Baldwin, F. M. (1944). Testicular tumors in the teleost (*Xiphophorus helleri*) receiving sesame oil. *Proc. Soc. Exp. Biol. Med.* **57**, 165–167.

Ljungberg, O., and Lange, J. (1968). Skin tumors of northern pike (*Esox lucius* L.). I. Sarcoma in a baltic pike population. *Bull. Off. Int. Epizoot.* **69**, 1007–1022.

Loeb, L. (1910). Demonstration of tumors of fish. *J. Amer. Med. Ass.* **54**, 228.

Loewenthal, W. (1907). Einschlüssartige Zell- und Kernveranderungen in der Karpfenpocke. *Z. Krebsforsch.* **5**, 197–204.

Lombard, C. (1962). *Cancérologie Comparée* **25**, 49–52, 144–147.

Lotlikar, P. D., Miller, E. C., Miller, J. A., and Halver, J. E. (1967). Metabolism of the carcinogen 2-acetylaminofluorene by rainbow trout. *Proc. Soc. Exp. Biol. Med.* **124**, 160–163.

Lucké, B. (1937). "Studies on Tumors in Cold-Blooded Vertebrates," pp. 92–94. Annu. Rept. Tortugas Lab., Carnegie Inst., Washington, D.C.

Lucké, B. (1942). Tumors of the nerve sheaths in fish of the snapper family (Lutianidae). *Arch. Pathol.* **34**, 133–150.

Lucké, B., and Schlumberger, H. G. (1941). Transplantable epithelioma of the lip and mouth of catfish. I. Pathology. Transplantation to anterior chamber of eye and into cornea. *J. Exp. Med.* **74**, 397–408.

Lucké, B., and Schlumberger, H. G. (1942). Common neoplasms in fish, amphibians and reptiles. *J. Tech. Meth. Bull. Int. Ass. Med. Mus.* **22**, 4–9.

Lucké, B., and Schlumberger, H. G. (1949). Neoplasia in cold-blooded vertebrates. *Physiol. Rev.* **29**, 91–126.

Lucké, B., Schlumberger, H. G., and Breedis, C. (1948). A common mesenchymal tumor of the corium of goldfish, *Carassius auratus*. *Cancer Res.* **8**, 473–493.

Lümann, M., and Mann, H. (1956). Beobachtungen über die Blumenkohl Krankheit der Aale. *Arch. Fischereiwiss.* **3**, 229–239.

McArn, G., and Wellings, S. R. (1967). Neurofibroma in a teleost fish, *Lumpenus sagitta. J. Fish. Res. Bd. Can.* **24**, 2007–2009.

McArn, G., Chuinard, R. G., Miller, B. S., Brooks, R. E., and Wellings, S. R. (1968). Pathology of skin tumors found on English sole and starry flounder from Puget Sound, Washington. *J. Natl. Cancer Inst.* **41**, 229–242.

McFarland, J. (1901). Epithelioma of the mouth and skin of a catfish. *Proceedings of the Pathology Society Philadelphia* **4**, 79–81.

McGregor, E. A. (1963). Publications on fish parasites and diseases, 330 B.C.–A.D. 1923. *U.S. Fish. Wildl. Serv., Spec. Sci. Rep.* **474**, 84.

McIntosh, W. C. (1884–1885). Multiple tumours in plaice and common flounders. *3rd and 4th Reports of the Fishery Board of Scotland* pp. 66–67.

McIntosh, W. C. (1885a). Further remarks on the multiple tumours of common flounders, etc. *Report of the Fishery Board of Scotland* **4**, 214–215.

McIntosh, W. C. (1885b). On the spawning of certain marine fishes. *Annual Magazine of Natural History (Series 5)* **15**, 429–437.

McIntosh, W. C. (1908). On a tumour in a plaice. *Annual Magazine of Natural History (Series 8)* **1**, 373–387.

MacIntyre, P. A. (1960). Tumors of the thyroid gland in teleost fishes. *Zoologica (New York)* **45**, 161–170.

MacIntyre, P. A., and Baker-Cohen, K. F. (1961). Melanoma, renal thyroid tumor and reticulo-endothelial hyperplasia in a non-hybrid platyfish. *Zoologica (New York)* **46**, 125–131.

Mann, H. (1962). Beobachtungen uber Krankheiten und Parasiten an Elbfischen. *Fischwirt* **10**, 300–308.

Marine, D. (1914). Further observations and experiments on goitre in brook trout. *J. Exp. Med.* **19**, 70–88.

Marine, D., and Lenhart, C. H. (1910a). On the occurrence of goitre (active thyroid hyperplasia) in fish. *Johns Hopkins Hosp., Bull.* **21**, 95–98.

Marine, D., and Lenhart, C. H. (1910b). Observations and experiments on the so-called thyroid carcinoma of brook trout (*Salvelinus fontinalis*) and its relation to ordinary goitre. *J. Exp. Med.* **12**, 311–327.

Marine, D., and Lenhart, C. H. (1911). Further observations and experiments on the so-called thyroid carcinoma of the brook trout (*Salvelinus fontinalis*) and its relation to endemic goitre. *J. Exp. Med.* **13**, 455–475.

Marsh, M. C. (1903). Epithelioma in trout. *Wash. Med. Ann.* **2**, 59.

Marsh, M. C. (1911). Thyroid tumor in salmonoids. *Trans. Amer. Fish. Soc.* **40**, 377–392.

Marsh, M. C., and Vonwiller, P. (1916) Thyroid tumour in the sea bass (*Serranus*). *J. Cancer Res.* **1**, 183–196.

Mattheis, T. (1964). Fälle von Zystenbildung und Geschwulsten bei Aalen (*Anguilla vulgaris*). *Z. Fisch. Hilfswiss.* **12**, 709–715.

Mawdesley-Thomas, L. E. (1967). Fish pathology. *Proceedings of the Third British Coarse Fish Conference, Univ. of Liverpool* pp. 27–29.

Mawdesley-Thomas, L. E. (1968). Fish and their environment. *J. Inst. Pub. Health Eng.* **67**, 96–105.

Mawdesley-Thomas, L. E. (1969). Neoplasia in fish—A bibliography. *J. Fish. Biol.* **1**, 187–207.

Mawdesley-Thomas, L. E. (1970). Significance of liver tumour induction in animals. *In* "Metabolic Aspects of Food Safety" (F. J. C. Roe, ed.), pp. 481–531. Blackwell, Oxford.

Mawdesley-Thomas, L. E., and Bucke, D. (1967a). Fish pox in the roach (*Rutilus rutilus* L.). *Vet. Rec.* **81**, 56.

Mawdesley-Thomas, L. E., and Bucke, D. (1967b). Squamous cell carcinoma in a gudgeon (*Gobio gobio* L.). *Pathol. Vet.* **4**, 484–489.

Mawdesley-Thomas, L. E., and Bucke, D. (1968). A lipoma in a bream (*Abramis brama* L.). *Vet. Rec.* **82**, 673–674.

Mawdesley-Thomas, L. E., and Jolly, D. W. (1967). Diseases of fish. II. The goldfish (*Carassius auratus*). *J. small Anim. Pract.* **8**, 33–54.

Mawdesley-Thomas, L. E., and Jolly, D. W. (1968). Diseases of fish. III. The trout. *J. small Anim. Pract.* **9**, 167–188.

Mawdesley-Thomas, L. E., and Young, P. C. (1967). Cutaneous melanosis in a flounder (*Platichthys flesus*). *Vet. Rec.* **81**, 384.

Medowar, P. B. (1967). "The Art of the Soluble," 160 pp. Methuen, London.

Montpellier, J., and Dieuzeide, R. (1932). Sur une production de tumeurs cutanées du cyprin (*Carassius auratus*). *Bull. Ass. Fr. Etude Cancer* **21**, 295–306.

Montpellier, J., and Dieuzeide, R. (1934). Tumeurs melaniques de le peau du cyprin. *Bull. Stat. Agr. Peche Castiglione* pp. 97–103.

Mulcahy, M. F. (1963). Lymphosarcoma in the pike, *Esox lucius* L., (Pisces; Esocidae) in Ireland. *Proc. Roy. Irish Acad., Sect. B* **63**, 103–129.

Mulcahy, M. F. (1970). The thymus glands and lymphosarcoma in the pike, *Esox lucius* L., in Ireland. "Proceedings of the Fourth International Symposium of Comparative Leukaemia Research. Bibliotheca Haematologica," pp. 600–609. S. Carter, Basel.

Mulcahy, M. F., and O'Rourke, F. J. (1964a). Lymphosarcoma in the pike (*Esox lucius* L.) in Ireland. *Life Sci.* **3**, 719–720.

Mulcahy, M. F., and O'Rourke, F. J. (1964b). Cancerous pike in Ireland. *Irish Natur. J.* **14**, 312–315.

Müller, F. W. (1926). Über Schilddrüsendewächse bei Kaltblütern. *Virchows Arch. Pathol. Anat. Physiol.* **260**, 405–427.

Murray, J. A. (1908). The zoological distribution of cancer. *Sci. Rep. Invest. Imp. Cancer Res. Fund.* **3**, 52–60.

Nicholson, G. W. (1926). "The Nature of Tumour Formation," Erasmus Wilson Lectures, 1925. Heller, Cambridge.

Nigrelli, R. F. (1938). Fish parasites and fish diseases. I. Tumors. *Trans. N.Y. Acad. Sci. Ser.* 2 **1**, 4–7.

Nigrelli, R. F. (1943). Causes of diseases and death of fishes in captivity. *Zoologica (New York)* **28**, 203–216.

Nigrelli, R. F. (1946a). Studies on the marine resources of southern New England. V. Parasites and diseases of the ocean pout, Macrozoarces americanus.—(IV) On a fibro-epithelial growth on the snout. *Bull. Bingham Oceanogr. Coll.* **9**, 218–221.

Nigrelli, R. F. (1946b). Spontaneous neoplasms in fishes. II. Fibro-carcinoma-like growth in the stomach of *Borophryne apogon* Regan, a deep-sea ceratioid fish. *Zoologica (New York)* **31**, 183–184.

Nigrelli, R. F. (1947). Spontaneous neoplasms in fishes. III. Lymphosarcoma in *Astyanax* and *Esox. Zoologica (New York)* **32**, 101–108.

Nigrelli, R. F. (1948). Hyperplastic epidermal disease in the bluegill sunfish, *Lepomis macrochirus* Rafinesque. *Zoologica (New York)* **33**, 133–137.

Nigrelli, R. F. (1951). Lip tumors in fishes kept in captivity. *Cancer Res.* **2**, 272. (Abstr.)

Nigrelli, R. F. (1952a). Virus and tumors in fishes. *Ann. N.Y. Acad. Sci.* **54**, 1076–1092.

Nigrelli, R. F. (1952b). Spontaneous neoplasms in fishes. VI. Thyroid tumors in marine fishes. *Cancer Res.* **12**, 286.

Nigrelli, R. F. (1952c). Spontaneous neoplasms in fishes. VI. Thyroid tumors in marine fishes. *Zoologica (New York)* **37**, 185–189.

Nigrelli, R. F. (1954). Tumors and other atypical cell growths in temperate fresh-water fishes of North America. *Trans. Amer. Fish Soc.* **83**, 262–296.

Nigrelli, R. F., and Gordon, M. (1944). A melanotic tumor in the silverside, *Menidia beryllina peninsulae* (Good and Bean). *Zoologica (New York)* **29**, 45–47.

Nigrelli, R. F., and Gordon, M. (1946). Spontaneous neoplasms in fishes. I. Osteochondroma in the jewelfish, *Hemichromis bimaculatus*. *Zoologica (New York)* **31**, 89–92.

Nigrelli, R. F., and Gordon, M. (1951). Spontaneous neoplasms in fishes. V. Acinar adenocarcinoma of the pancreas in a hybrid platyfish. *Zoologica (New York)* **36**, 121–125.

Nigrelli, R. F., and Jakowska, S. (1953). Spontaneous neoplasms in fish. VII. A spermatocytoma and renal melanoma in an African lungfish, *Protopterus annectens* (Owen). *Zoologica (New York)* **38**, 109–112.

Nigrelli, R. F., and Jakowska, S. (1955). Spontaneous neoplasms in fish. IX. Hepatomas in rainbow trout, *Salmo gairdneri*. *Proc. Amer. Ass. Cancer Res.* **2**, 38. (Abstr.)

Nigrelli, R. F., and Jakowska, S. (1961). Fatty degeneration, regenerative hyperplasia and neoplasia in the livers of rainbow trout, *Salmo gairdneri*. *Zoologica (New York)* **46**, 49–55.

Nigrelli, R. F., and Smith, G. M. (1940). A papillary cystic disease affecting the barbels of *Ameiurus nebulosus* (LeSueur), caused by the myxosporidian *Henneguya ameiurensis* sp. *Zoologica (New York)* **25**, 89–96.

Nigrelli, R. F., Jakowska, S., and Gordon, M. (1950). Histological and cytological observations on hereditary erythromelanomas in platyfish-swordtail hybrids. *Cancer Res.* **10**, 234. (Abstr.)

Nigrelli, R. F., Jakowska, S., and Gordon, M. (1951). The invasion and cell replacement of one pigmented neoplastic growth by a second and more malignant type in experimental fishes. *Brit. J. Cancer* **5**, 54–68.

Nigrelli, R. F., Ketchen, K. S., and Ruggieri, G. D. (1965). Studies on virus diseases of fishes. Epizootiology of epithelial tumors in the skin of flatfishes of the Pacific coast, with special reference to the sand sole (*Psettichthys melanostictus*) from Northern Hecate Strait, British Columbia, Canada. *Zoologica (New York)* **50**, 115–122.

Nishikawa, S. (1954). On the tumorous growth observed in two fishes. *Collecting and Breeding, Tokyo* **16**, 236.

Nishikawa, S. (1955a). A case of spindle cell sarcoma developed in the Japanese common goby (*Acanthogobius flavimanus*). *Norinsho Suisan Koshusho Kenkyu Hokoku* **5**, 171–174.

Nishikawa, S. (1955b.) A case of fibroblastic sarcoma developed in *Theragra chalcogramma* (Pallas). *Norinsho Suisan Koshusho Kenkyu Hokoku* **4**, 666–669.

Novelli, G. D. (1967). Amino acid incorporation in rat and trout liver. *In* "Trout Hepatoma Research Conference Papers" (J. E. Halver and I. A. Mitchell, eds.). *Fish Wildl. Serv.* (*U.S.*), *Res. Rep.* **70**, 72–77.

Ohlmacher, N. (1898). Several examples illustrating the comparative pathology of tumors. *Bull. Ohio Hosp. Epilep.* **1**, 223–226.

Olearius, A. (1674). "Gottorf Museum of Arts in Which Are All Sorts of Extraordinary Things/Partly Natural History/Partly of Artificial Origins Have Been Brought and Prepared. Out of All Four Corners of the World This Has Been Carried Before One Year Has Been Described." 2nd Ed.

Oota, K. (1952). An epidemic occurrence of tumor-like hyperplasia of epidermis in a species of fish, *Acanthogobius flavimanus. Gann* **43**, 264–265.

Osburn, R. C. (1925). Black tumor of the catfish. *Bulletin of the Bureau of Fisheries Wash.* **91**, 9–13.

Otte, E. (1964). Eine bösartige Neubildung in der Bauchhöhle eines Goldfisches (*Carassius auratus* L.). *Wien. Tieraerztl. Monatsschr.* **51**, 485–488.

Oxner, M. (1905). Über die Kolbenzellen in der Epidermis der Fische; ihre Form, Verteilung, Entstehung und Bedeutung. *Jena. Z. Naturwiss.* **40**, 589–646.

Pacis, M. R. (1932). An epithelial tumor of *Parophyrs vetulus.* M.S. Thesis, Univ. of Washington, Seattle, Washington.

Pellegrin, J. (1901). Les poissons à gibbosité frontale. *Bull. Soc. Philomath. Paris* **3**, 81–91.

Pesce, P. (1907). Contributo alla conoscenza dei tumori nei pesci. *Riv. Mens. Pesca* **9**, 223–225.

Petrushevski, G. K. (1937). The diseases of White Lake—"Belogo Ozera" fish. *In* "Parasites and Diseases of Fish" (G. K. Petrushevski, ed.), pp. 274–277. Fish Ind. Dep. of the State Planning Comm. of the P.S.F.S.R., Leningrad.

Peyron, A., and Thomas, L. (1929). Contribution à l'étude des tumeurs du revêtement branchial chez les poissons. *Bull. Ass. Fr. Etude Cancer* **18**, 825–837.

Peyron, A., and Thomas, L. (1930). Les tumeurs thyroidiennes des salmonides. *Bull. Ass. Fr. Etude Cancer* **19**, 795–819.

Peyron, A. (1939). Sur la fréquence des tumeurs dans les divers ordres de vertebres a sang froid et leur rareté dans les espèces venimeuses. *C. R. Acad. Sci.* **209**, 261–263.

Phelps, R. A. (1967). Aflatoxins in feeds—A review. *In* "Trout Hepatoma Research Conference Papers" (J. E. Halver and I. A. Mitchell, eds.). *Fish Wildl. Serv.* (*U.S.*), *Res. Rep.* **70**, 145–159.

Picchi, L. (1933). Di un non commune tumore di un pesce (neurinoma). *Sperimentale* **86**, 128–130.

Pick, L. (1905). Der Schilddrüsenkrebs der Salmoniden (Edelfische). *Berlin. Klin. Wochenschr.* **42**, 1435, 1477, 1498, 1532.

Pick, L., and Poll, H. (1903). Über einige bemerkenswerte Tumorbildungen bei Kaltblütern. *Berlin Klin. Wochenschr.* **40**, 23–25.

Plehn, M. (1902). Bösartiger Kropf (Adenocarcinoma der Thyroidea) bei Salmoniden. *Allg. Fischwirtschaftsztg.* **27**, 117–118.

Plehn, M. (1906). Über Geschwülste bei Kaltblütern. *Z. Krebsforsch.* **4**, 525–564.

Plehn, M. (1909). Über einige bei Fischen beobachtete Geschwülste und Geschwülstartige Bildungen. *Ber. K. Bayerischen Biol. Versuchssta., München* **2**, 55–76.

Plehn, M. (1915). Fälle von multiplem Odontom bei der Bachforelle. *Z. Fisch. Hilfswiss.* **17**, 197–200.

Plehn, M. (1924). "Praktikum der Fischkrankheiten," pp. 301–479. Schweizerbartsche, Stuttgart.

Prince, E. E. (1892). Melanosarcoma in a haddock. *Report of the Fishery Board of Scotland* **10**, 320.

Prince, E. E., and Steven, J. L. (1892). On two large tumours in a haddock and a cod. *Report of the Fishery Board of Scotland* **10**, 323–325.

Proewig, F. (1954). Die Beeinflussung des Wachstums bösartiger Tumoren von Zahnkarpfen. *Z. Krebsforsch.* **60**, 470–472.

Puente-Duany, N. (1930). Tumoración pariocular en un pescade de rió. *Bol. Liga Cancer* **5**, 240.

Raabe, H. (1939). Cas d'épithélioma des visceres chez le poisson *Mollienisia velifera* Reg. *Arch. Zool. Exp. Gen.* **81**, 1–8.

Radulescu, I. (1967). Tumori tegumentare la guvizii din Marea Neagra Tărmul Românesc. *Bull. Inst. Cerc. Pisc.* **26**, 36–40.

Radulescu, I., Vasiliu, D. G., Ilie, E., and Snieszko, S. F. (1968). Thyroid hyperplasia of the Eastern brook trout *Salvelinus fontinalis* in Romania. *Trans. Amer. Fish. Soc.* **97**, 486–488.

Rasquin, P., and Hafter, E. (1951). Response of a fish lymphosarcoma to mammalian ACTH. *Zoologica (New York)* **36**, 163–169.

Rasquin, P., and Rosenbloom, L. (1954). Endocrine imbalance and tissue hyperplasia in teleosts maintained in darkness. *Bull. Amer. Mus. Natur. Hist.* **104**, 359–426.

Rayer, P. (1843). Observations sur les maladies des poissons. Exposé succinct des principales observations faites jusqu'à ce jour sur les maladies et sur les anomalies des poissons. *Arch. Med. Comp.* **1**, 245–308.

Reed, H. D., and Gordon, M. (1931). The morphology of melanotic overgrowths in hybrids of Mexican killifishes. *Amer. J. Cancer* **15**, 1524–1546.

Reichenbach-Klinke, H. H. (1966). "Krankheiten und Schadigungen der Fische," pp. 250–251. Fischer, Stuttgart.

Reichenbach-Klinke, H. H., and Elkan, E. (1965). "The Principal Diseases of Lower Vertebrates," pp. 152–165. Academic Press, New York.

Robertson, O. H., and Chaney, A. L. (1953). Thyroid hyperplasia and tissue iodine content in spawning rainbow trout: A comparative study of Lake Michigan and California sea-run trout. *Physiol. Zool.* **26**, 328–340.

Rodricks, J. V., Henery-Logan, K. R., Campbell, A. D., Stoloff, L., and Verrett, M. J. (1968). Isolation of new toxin from cultures of aspergillus flavus. *Nature (London)* **217**, 668.

Roffo, A. H. (1924). Le sarcome des poissons. *Neoplasmes* **3**, 231–234.

Roffo, A. H. (1925). Sobre un tumor paradentario en la corvina. *Bol. Inst. Med. Exp. Estud. Trat. Cancer, B. Aires,* **2**, 28–42.

Roffo, A. H. (1926). Sarcomas fusocelulares de corvina. *Bol. Inst. Med. Exp. Estud. Trat. Cancer, Buenos Aires* **3**, 206–207.

Ronca, V. (1914). I. Tumori nei pesci. *Tumori* **4**, 61–71.

Rucker, R. R., Yasutake, W. T., and Wolf, H. (1961). Trout hepatoma—A preliminary report. *Progr. Fish Cult.* **23**, 3–7.

Russell, F. E., and Kotin, P. (1957). Squamous papilloma in the white croaker. *J. Nat. Cancer Inst.* **18**, 857–861.

Sagawa, E. (1925). Zur Kenntnis der Fischengeschwülste. *Gann* **19**, 14–15.

Sandeman, G. (1892a). On the multiple tumours in plaice and flounders. *11th Annual Report of the Fishery Board of Scotland* pp. 391–392.

Sandeman, G. (1892b). On a tumour from a tunny. *11th Annual Report of the Fishery Board of Scotland* pp. 392–394.

Sarkar, H. L., and Dutta-Chaudhuri, R. (1953). On the occurrence of an epidermal papilloma in Koi fish, *Anabas testudenius* (Bloch). *J. Indian Med. Ass.* **22**, 152–154.

Sarkar, H. L., and Dutta-Chaudhuri, R. (1958). On the occurrence of osteogenic fibroma on the pre-maxilla of an Indian catfish, *Wallogo attu* (Bloch and Schneider). *Gann* **49**, 65–68.

Sarkar, H. L., and Dutta-Chaudhuri, R. (1964). On the occurrence of adenoma in the gill apparatus of a trout, *Salmo fario. Trans. Amer. Microsc. Soc.* **83**, 93–96.

Sarkar, H. L., Kapoor, B. G., and Dutta-Chaudhuri, R. (1955). A study of leiomyoma, a mesenchymal tumour on the fins of an Indian catfish, *Mystus (Osteobagrus) seenghala* (Sykes). *Growth* **19**, 257–262.

Sathyanesan, A. G. (1962). On the basophilic tumor in the pituitary of the freshwater teleost *Mystus seenghala* (Sykes). *Sci. Cult.* **28**, 432–433.

Sathyanesan, A. G. (1963). On the functional thyroid tumour in the kidney of the freshwater teleost, *Barbus stigma,* in its natural habitat. *Sci. Cult.* **29**, 90–91.

Sathyanesan, A. G. (1966). The structure of the glomerular cystic tumor present in the tropical freshwater catfish, *Mystus vittatus* (Bloch). *Trans. Amer. Microsc. Soc.* **85**, 53–57.

Scarpelli, D. G. (1967). Ultrastructural and biochemical observations on trout hepatoma. In "Trout Hepatoma Research Conference Papers" (J. E. Halver and I. A. Mitchell, eds.). *Fish Wildl. Serv. (U.S.), Res. Rep.* **70**, 60–71.

Scarpelli, D. G., Greider, M. H., and Frajola, W. J. (1963). Observations on hepatic cell hyperplasia, adenoma, and hepatoma of rainbow trout (*Salmo gairdneri*). *Cancer Res.* **23**, 848–857.

Schamberg, J. F., and Lucké, B. (1922). Fibrosarcoma of the skin in a goldfish (*Carassius auratus*). *J. Cancer Res.* **7**, 151–161.

Schäperclaus, W. (1953). Die Blumenkohlkrankheit der Aale und anderer Fische der Ostsee. *Z. Fisch. Hilfswiss.* **2**, 105–124.

Schäperclaus, W. (1954). "Fischkrankheiten." Akademie Verlag, Berlin.

Schlumberger, H. G. (1949). Cutaneous leiomyoma of goldfish. I. Morphology and growth in tissue culture. *Amer. J. Pathol.* **25**, 287–299.

Schlumberger, H. G. (1950). Polycystic kidney (mesonephros) in the goldfish. *Arch. Pathol.* **50**, 400–410.

Schlumberger, H. G. (1951). Limbus tumors as a manifestation of von Reckling-Hausen's neurofibromatosis in goldfish. *Amer. J. Ophthalmol.* **34**, 415–422.

Schlumberger, H. G. (1952). Nerve sheath tumors in an isolated goldfish population. *Cancer Res.* **12**, 890–899.

Schlumberger, H.G. (1953). Comparative pathology of oral neoplasms. *Oral Surg., Oral Med. Oral Pathol.* **6**, 1078–1094.

Schlumberger, H. G. (1954). Spontaneous hyperplasia and neoplasia in the thyroid of animals. *In* "The Thyroid Gland." *Brookhaven Symp. Biol.* **7**, 169–191.

Schlumberger, H. G. (1955). Spontaneous goiter and cancer of the thyroid in animals. *Ohio J. Sci.* **55**, 23–43.

Schlumberger, H. G. (1957). Tumors characteristic for certain animal species. A review. *Cancer Res.* **17**, 823–832.

Schlumberger, H. G. (1958). Krankheiten der Fische, Amphibien und Reptilien. *In* "Pathologie der Laboratoriumstiere" (P. Cohrs, R. Jaffe and H. Meessen, eds.), pp. 714–761. Springer, Berlin.

Schlumberger, H. G., and Katz, M. (1956). Odontogenic tumors of salmon. *Cancer Res.* **16**, 369–370.

Schlumberger, H. G., and Lucké, B. (1948). Tumors of fishes, amphibians and reptiles. *Cancer Res.* **8**, 657–754.

Schmey, M. (1911). Über Neubildungen bei Fischen. *Frankfurt. Z. Pathol.* **6**, 230–253.

Schreibman, M. P. (1966). Hypophysial cyst in a teleost fish. *J. Exp. Zool.* **162**, 57–67.

Schreibman, M. P., and Charipper, H. A. (1962). The occurrence of pituitary cysts in a particular strain of platyfish (*Xiphophorus maculatus*). *Amer. Zool.* **2**, 556. (Abstr.)

Schreitmüller, W. (1924). Schilddrüsengeschwulst (*Struma maligna*) bei *Jordanella floridae* Goode et Bean. *Blättes Aquarien- Terrarienkunde* **35**, 83.

Schroeders, V. D. (1908). Tumors of fishes. Dissertation. St. Petersburg. (In Russ.) (Engl. Transl., Army Med. Library, Washington, D.C.)

Schubert, G. (1964). Elektronenmikroskopische Untersuchungen zur Pockenkrankheit des Karpfens. *Z. Naturforsch. B* **19**, 675–682.

Scolari, C. (1953). Contributo alla conoscenza degli adenocarcinomi epatici della trota iridea. *Atti Sco. Ital. Sci. Vet.* **7**, 599–605.

Scott, P. E. (1891). Notes on the occurrence of cancer in fish. *Trans. Proc. N.Z. Inst.* **24**, 201.

Semer, E. (1888). Über allgemeine Carcinose u. Sarkomatose und über multiple Fibrome u. Lipoma bei den Haustieren. *Deut. Z. Tiermed. Vergl. Pathol.* **14**, 245–247.

Simon, R. C., Dollar, A. M., and Smuckler, E. A. (1967). Descriptive classification on normal and altered histology of trout livers. *In* "Trout Hepatoma Research Conference Papers" (J. E. Halver and I. A. Mitchell, eds.). *Fish Wildl. Serv. (U.S.), Res. Rep.* **70**, 18–28.

Sims, R. (1967). Analysis of hepato-carcinogenic fish meal lipids. *In* "Trout Hepatoma Research Conference Papers" (J. E. Halver and I. A. Mitchell, eds.). *Fish Wildl. Serv. (U.S.), Res. Rep.* **70**, 171–181.

Sinnhuber, R. O. (1967). Aflatoxin in cotton seed meal and liver cancer in rainbow trout. *In* "Trout Hepatoma Research Conference Papers" (J. E. Halver and I. A. Mitchell, eds.). *Fish Wildl. Res. Rep.* **70**, 48–55.

Sinnhuber, R. O., Wales, J. H., Engebrecht, R. H., Amend, D. F., Kray, W. D., Ayres, J. L., and Ashton, W. E. (1965). Aflatoxins in cottonseed meal and hepatoma in rainbow trout. *Fed. Proc. Fed. Amer. Soc. Exp. Biol.* **24**, 627. (Abstr.)

Sinnhuber, R. O., Wales, J. H., and Lee, D. J. (1966). Cyclopropenoids, co-carcinogens for aflatoxin-induced hepatoma in trout. *Fed. Proc. Fed. Amer. Soc. Exp. Biol.* **25**, 555. (Abstr.)

Sinnhuber, R. O., Wales, J. H., Ayres, J. L., Engebrecht, R. H., and Amend, D. F. (1968a). Dietary factors and hepatoma in rainbow trout (*Salmo gairdneri*). I. Aflatoxins in vegetable protein feedstuffs. *J. Nat. Cancer Inst.* **41**, 711–718.

Sinnhuber, R. O., Lee, D. J., Wales, J. H., and Ayres, J. L. (1968b). Dietary factors and hepatoma in rainbow trout (*Salmo gairdneri*). II. Co-carcinogenesis by cyclopropenoid fatty acids and the effect of gossypol and altered lipids on aflatoxin-induced liver cancer. *J. Nat. Cancer Inst.* **41**, 1293–1301.

Smith, G. M. (1934). A cutaneous red pigmented tumor (erythrophoroma) with metastases in a flatfish (*Pseudopleuronectes americanus*). *Amer. J. Cancer* **21**, 596–599.

Smith, G. M. (1935). A hyperplastic epidermal disease in the Winter flounder infected with *Cryptocotyle lingua* (Creplin). *Amer. J. Cancer* **25**, 108–112.

Smith, G. M., and Coates, C. W. (1937). The histological structure of the normal and hyperplastic thyroid in *Rasbora lateristriata*. *Zoologica (New York)* **22**, 297–302.

Smith, G. M., Coates, C. W., and Strong, L. C. (1936). Neoplastic diseases in small tropical fishes. *Zoologica (New York)* **21**, 219–224.

Smith, H. M. (1909). Case of epidemic carcinoma of thyroid in fishes. *Wash. Med. Ann.* **8**, 313.

Snieszko, S. F. (1961). Hepatoma and visceral granuloma in trouts. *N.Y. Fish Game J.* **8**, 145–149.

Snieszko, S. F., and Miller, J. A. (1966). Selected hematological and biochemical tests performed with blood and serum of adult rainbow trout (*Salmo gairdneri*) with a high incidence of hepatoma. *Ann. N.Y. Acad. Sci.* **136**, 193–210.

Solomon, G., Jenson, R., and Tanner, H. (1965). Hepatic changes in rainbow trout (*Salmo gairdneri*) fed diets containing peanut, cottonseed and soybean meals. *Amer. J. Vet. Res.* **26**, 764–769.

Southwell, T. (1915). Notes from the Bengal Fisheries Laboratory, Indian Museum: No. 2. On some Indian parasites of fish with a note on the carcinoma in trout. *Rec. Indian Mus.*, **11**, 311–330.

Southwell, T., and Prashad, B. (1918). Notes from the Bengal Fisheries Laboratory, Indian Museum: No. 5. Parasites of Indian fishes with a note on the carcinoma in the climbing perch. *Rec. Indian Mus.* **15**, 341–355.

Stanton, M. F. (1965). Diethylnitrosamine-induced hepatic degeneration and neoplasia in the aquarium fish, *Brachydanio rerio*. *J. Nat. Cancer Inst.* **34**, 117–130.

Stanton, M. F. (1966). Hepatic neoplasms of aquarium fish exposed to *Cycas circinalis*. *Fed. Proc. Fed. Amer. Soc. Exp. Biol.* **25**, 661.

Starks, E. C. (1911). The osteological characters of the Scombroid fishes of the families *Gempylidae, Lepidopidae* and *Trichiuridae*. *Stanford Univ. Publ.* **5**, 17–26.

Steeves, H. R., III (1969). An epithelial papilloma of the brown bullhead, *Ictalurus nebulosus*. *In* "Neoplasms and Related Disorders of Invertebrate and Lower Vertebrate Animals" (C. J. Dawe and J. C. Harshbarger, eds.). *Nat. Cancer Inst. Monogr.* **31**, 215–218.

Stewart, H. L., and Snell, K. C. (1957). The histopathology of experimental tumours of the liver of the rat. *Acta Unio Int. Contra Cancrum* **13**, 770–803.

Stewart, M. J. (1931). Pre-cancerous lesions of the alimentary tract. *Lancet* **ii**, 565, 617, 669.

Stolk, A. (1953a). Tumours of fishes. I. An ovarian teratoma in the viviparous cyprinodont *Lebistes reticulatus* Peters. *Proc. Kon. Ned. Akad. Wetensch. Ser. C* **56**, 28–33.

Stolk, A. (1953b). Tumours of fishes. II. Chromophobe adenoma of the pituitary gland in the viviparous cyprinodont *Lebistes reticulatus* Peters. *Proc. Kon. Ned. Akad. Wetensch. Ser. C* **56**, 34–38.

Stolk, A. (1953c). Tumours of fishes. III. Carcinoma of the epidermis in the black variety of the viviparous cyprinodont *Xiphophorus hellerii* Heckel. *Proc. Kon. Ned. Akad. Wetensch. Ser. C* **56**, 143–148.

Stolk, A. (1953d). Tumours of fishes. IV. Carcinoma of the pharynx in the viviparous cyprinodont *Lebistes reticulatus* Peters. *Proc. Kon. Ned. Akad. Wetensch., Ser. C* **56**, 149–151.

Stolk, A. (1953e). Tumours of fishes. V. Melanoma of the skin in the cyprinid *Brachydanio rerio* (Hamilton-Buchanan). *Proc. Kon. Ned. Akad. Wetensch., Ser. C* **56**, 152–156.

Stolk, A. (1954). Tumours of fishes. VI. Mesenchymal tumour of the skin in the viviparous cyprinodont *Xiphophorus maculatus* Günther (red variety). *Proc. Kon. Ned. Akad. Wetensch., Ser. C* **57**, 652–658.

Stolk, A. (1955a). Tumours of fishes. VII. Congenital teratoma of the skin in the viviparous cyprinodont *Lebistes reticulatus* (Peters). *Proc. Kon. Ned. Akad. Wetensch., Ser. C* **58**, 190–194.

Stolk, A. (1955b). Hyperplasia and hyperplastic adenoma of the thyroid gland of the viviparous cyprinodont *Xiphophorus hellerii* Heckel and *Lebistes reticulatus* (Peters) after thiouracil treatment. *Proc. Kon. Ned. Akad. Wetensch., Ser. C* **58**, 313–327.

Stolk, A. (1956a). Changes in the pituitary gland of the cyprinid *Tanichthys alvonubes* Lin with a thyroidal tumour. *Proc. Kon. Ned. Akad. Wetensch., Ser. C* **59**, 38–49.

Stolk, A. (1956b). Tumours of fishes. VIII. Thyroidal tumour in the cyprinid *Tanichthys alvonubes* Lin. *Proc. Kon. Ned. Akad. Wetensch., Ser. C* **59**, 50–60.

Stolk, A. (1956c). Polycystic kidneys in the veiltail *Carassius auratus* var. Japonicus Bicaudatus, Zernecke. *Proc. Kon. Ned. Akad. Wetensch., Ser. C* **58**, 70–73.

Stolk, A. (1956d). Tumours of fishes. IXA and IXB. Epithelioma of the oral mucosa in the scylliid *Scylliorhinus catulus* (L.). *Proc. Kon. Ned. Akad. Wetensch., Ser. C* **59**, 196–210.

Stolk, A. (1956e). Tumours of fishes. X. Thyroidal tumour with infiltration of the gills in the cichlid *Cichlasoma biocellatum* (Regan). *Proc. Kon. Ned. Akad. Wetensch., Ser. C* **59**, 387–397.

Stolk, A. (1956f). Changes in the pituitary gland of the cichlid *Cichlasoma biocellatum* (Regan) with thyroidal tumour. *Proc. Kon. Ned. Akad. Wetensch., Ser. C* **59**, 494–505.

Stolk, A. (1956g). Polycystic kidneys in the characid *Moenkhausia pittieri*. *Proc. Kon. Ned. Akad. Wetensch., Ser. C* **59**, 506–519.

Stolk, A. (1956h). Tumours of fishes. XI. Carcinoma of the skin in the anabantid *Colis labiosa* (Day). *Proc. Kon. Ned. Akad. Wetensch., Ser. C* **59**, 624–633.

Stolk, A. (1957a). Tumours of fishes. XII. Carcinoma of the kidneys in the characid *Thayeria obliqua* Eigenmann. *Proc. Kon. Ned. Akad. Wetensch Ser. C* **60**, 31–40.

Stolk, A. (1957b). Tumours of fishes. XIII. Multiple fibromas of the skin in the malapterurid *Malapterurus electricus*. *Proc. Kon. Ned. Akad. Wetensch., Ser. C* **60**, 41–52.

Stolk, A. (1957c). Tumours of fishes. XIV. Fibroma of the heart in the viviparous cyprinodont *Lebistes reticulatus* (Peters). *Proc. Kon. Ned. Akad. Wetensch., Ser. C* **60**, 185–195.

Stolk, A. (1957d). Tumours of fishes. XV. Renal adenocarcinoma in the cyprinid *Barbus tetrazona* (Bleeker). *Proc. Kon. Ned. Akad. Wetensch., Ser. C* **60**, 196–211.

Stolk, A. (1957e). Multiple cysts in the central nervous system and optic nerves of the cichlid, *Cichlasoma facetum*. *Proc. Kon. Ned. Akad. Wetensch., Ser. C* **60**, 338–348.

Stolk, A. (1957f). Cerebral cysts, abnormal pituitary gland and changes in the thyroid gland in the viviparous cyprinodont, *Lebistes reticulatus* (Peters). *Proc. Kon. Ned. Akad. Wetensch., Ser. C* **60**, 349–363.

Stolk, A. (1957g). Tumours of fishes. XVI. Fibroma of the intestine in the viviparous cyprinodont *Lebistes reticulatus* (Peters). *Proc. Kon. Ned. Akad. Wetensch., Ser. C* **60**, 364–375.

Stolk, A. (1957h). Pharyngeal glands of the cichlid *Haplochromis multicolor* (Hilgendorf). *Proc. Kon. Ned. Akad. Wetensch., Ser. C* **60**, 567–577.

Stolk, A. (1957i). Tumours of fishes. XVII. Adenoma of the pharyngeal gland in the cichlid *Haplochromis multicolor* (Hilgendorf). *Proc. Kon. Ned. Akad. Wetensch., Ser. C* **60**, 640–649.

Stolk, A. (1957j). Tumours of fishes. XVIII. Adenoma of the swim bladder in the viviparous cyprinodont *Lebistes reticulatus* (Peters). *Proc. Kon. Ned. Akad. Wetensch., Ser. C* **60**, 650–657.

Stolk, A. (1957k). Tumours of fishes. XIX. Odontogenic tumour in the oviparous cyprinodont *Cyprinodon variegatus variegatus* Lacepede. *Proc. Kon. Ned. Akad. Wetensch., Ser. C* **60**, 658–665.

Stolk, A. (1958a). Tumours of fishes. XX. Myxoma of the skin in characid *Phenecogrammus interruptus* (Boulenger). *Proc. Kon. Ned. Akad. Wetensch., Ser. C* **61**, 101–106.

Stolk, A. (1958b). Tumours of fishes. XXI. Haemangioma of the operculum in the erythrinid *Chilodus punctatus* (Müller et Troschel). *Proc. Kon. Ned. Akad. Wetensch., Ser. C* **61**, 107–114.

Stolk, A. (1958c). Tumours of fishes. XXII. Epidermoid carcinoma of the upper lip in the characid *Ephippicharax orbicularis* (Valenciennes). *Proc. Kon. Ned. Akad. Wetensch., Ser. C* **61**, 201–206.

Stolk, A. (1958d). Tumours of fishes. XXIIIA and XXIIIB. Some cases of chromophobe adenoma in the viviparous cyprinodont *Mollienesia velifera* Regan. *Proc. Kon. Ned. Akad. Wetensch., Ser. C* **61**, 363–380.

Stolk, A. (1958e). Tumours of fishes. XXIV. Ocular melanoma in the characid *Anoptichthys jordani* Hubbes et Innes. *Proc. Kon. Ned. Akad. Wetensch., Ser. C* **61**, 382–394.

Stolk, A. (1958f). Tumours of fishes. XXV. Melanoma in the hybrid of the viviparous cyprinodont *Lebistes reticulatus* and *Mollienesia sphenops*. *Proc. Kon. Ned. Akad. Wetensch., Ser. C* **61**, 499–514.

Stolk, A. (1958g). Some species-specific tumours in fishes. *Experientia* **14**, 244.

Stolk, A. (1959a). Development of ovarial teratomas in viviparous toothcarps by pathological parthenogenesis. *Nature (London)* **183**, 763–764.

Stolk, A. (1959b). Tumours in fishes. XXVI. Erythrophoroma in the oviparous cyprinodont *Nothobranchius guentheri* (Pfeffer). *Proc. Kon. Ned. Akad. Wetensch., Ser. C* **62**, 59–67.

Stolk, A. (1959c). Tumours of fishes. XXVII. Guanophoroma in the characid *Cteno-*

brycon spilurus (Valenciennes). *Proc. Kon. Ned. Akad. Wetensch., Ser. C* **62**, 155–162.

Stolk, A. (1959d). Tumours of fishes. XXVIII. Xanthophoroma in the oviparous cyprinodont *Rivulus xanthonotus* Ahl. *Proc. Kon. Ned. Akad. Wetensch., Ser. C* **62**, 163–171.

Stolk, A. (1960a). Melanoma of the skin in the black angelfish *Pterophyllum scalare* Cuvier with some theoretical considerations concerning the melanoma in extremely pigmented fishes. I and II. *Proc. Kon. Ned. Akad. Wetensch., Ser. C* **63**, 87–118.

Stolk, A. (1960b). Tumours of fishes. XXXI. Epidermoid carcinoma in a strain of the cichlid *Etroplus maculatus* (Bloch). *Proc. Kon. Ned. Akad. Wetensch., Ser. C* **63**, 200–219.

Stolk, A. (1960c). Histochemical analysis of three dehydrogenase systems in the renal adenocarcinoma of the cyprinodont *Aplocheilus lineatus lineatus. Proc. Kon. Ned. Akad. Wetensch., Ser. C* **63**, 548–566.

Stolk, A. (1962). Tumours of fishes. XXXII. Adenoma of the pharyngeal glands in the mouthbreeding anabantid *Betta anabantoides* Bleeker. *Proc. Kon. Ned. Akad. Wetensch., Ser. C* **65**, 469–482.

Surbeck, G. (1917). Nouvelles observations, méthode de pêche et essais d'elevage. *Bull. Suisse Pêche Piscicult.* **10**, 149–155.

Takahashi, K. (1929). Studie über Fischtumoren. *Z. Krebsforsch.* **29**, 1–73. [All the tumors reported in the Japanese journals which follow are considered in detail in the above mentioned reference. *Gann* **19**, 5–8 (1925); *Trans. Soc. Pathol. Jap.* **14**, 274–276 (1924); *Trans. Soc. Pathol. Jap.* **15**, 294 (1925); *Trans. Soc. Pathol. Jap.* **16**, 212 (1926)].

Takahashi, K. (1934). Studies on tumours of fishes from Japanese waters. *Proc. 5th Pac. Sci. Congr., Victoria, Vancouver, B.C., 1933* **5**, 4151–4155.

Tavolga, W. N. (1951). Epidermal fin tumors of the gobiid fish, *Bathygobius soporator. Zoologica (New York)* **36**, 273–278.

Thomas, L. (1926). Epithelioma odontoblastique des maxillaries chez une morue. *Bull. Ass. Fr. Etude Cancer* **15**, 464–470.

Thomas, L. (1927a). Les sarcomes fibroblastiques chez la morue. *Bull. Ass. Fr. Etude Cancer* **16**, 78–89.

Thomas, L. (1927b). Sur un cas de ganglioneurome abdominal chez la morue. *Bull. Ass. Fr. Etude Cancer* **16**, 282–286.

Thomas, L. (1930). Contribution a l'étude des lésions precancéreuses chez les poissons. Les papillomes cutanés de la sole. *Bull. Ass. Fr. Etude Cancer* **19**, 91–97.

Thomas, L. (1931a). Les tumeurs des poissons (étude anatomique et pathogénique). *Bull. Ass. Fr. Etude Cancer* **20**, 703–760.

Thomas, L. (1931b). Adenome kystique de l'intestin moyen chez une truite pourpre. *Bull. Ass. Fr. Etude Cancer* **20**, 575–584.

Thomas, L. (1931c). Le tumeur thyroidienne des salmonides. Intérêt de ses donnees en pathologie générale. *Rev. Med. Fr. Colonies* **8**, 235–246.

Thomas, L. (1932a). Rhabdomyome chez un flet. *Bull. Ass. Fr. Etude Cancer* **21**, 225-233.

Thomas, L. (1932b). Deux cas de tumeurs osseuses chez des téléosteens. *Bull. Ass. Fr. Etude Cancer* **21**, 280–294.

Thomas, L. (1932c). Sur un case de stiboneuroépithélioblastome chez une daurade. *Bull. Ass. Fr. Etude Cancer* **21**, 385–396.

Thomas, L. (1932d). Chondromes symétriques chez un colin. *Bull. Ass. Fr. Etude Cancer* **21**, 537–546.

Thomas, L. (1932e). Papillome tégumentaire chez une truite. *Bull. Ass. Fr. Etude Cancer* **21**, 547–550.

Thomas, L. (1933a). Fibrome de l'intestin juxta-pyloric chez une morue. *Bull. Ass. Fr. Etude Cancer* **22**, 106–112.

Thomas, L. (1933b). Sur deux cas de tumeurs tégumentaires chez la rousette. *Bull. Ass. Fr. Etude Cancer* **22**, 306–315.

Thomas, L. (1933c). Sur un cas de leiomyome de l'estomac chez un hareng. *Bull. Ass. Fr. Etude Cancer* **22**, 361–376.

Thomas, L. (1933d). Sur un lipome abdominal chez un colin. *Bull. Ass. Fr. Etude Cancer* **22**, 419–435.

Thomas, L., and Oxner, M. (1930). Papillomes de la lèvre inférieure chez *Anguilla vulgaris. Bull. Ass. Fr. Etude Cancer* **19**, 708–714.

Thompson, D. W. (1947). "A Glossary of Greek fishes." Oxford Univ. Press, London.

van Duijn, C., Jr. (1967). "Diseases of Fish," 2nd Ed. Iliffe Books, London.

Vivien, J., and Ruhland-Gaiser, M. (1954). Étude préliminaire de goutres envalissants spontanés recontres chez un cyprinodonte, *Lebistes reticulatus, V. Ann. Endocrinol.* **15**, 585–594.

von Sallmann, L., Halver, J. E., Collins, E., and Grimes, P. (1966). Thioacetamide-induced cataract with invasive proliferation of the lens epithelium in rainbow trout. *Cancer Res.* **26**, 1819–1825.

Wadsworth, J. R. (1961). Neoplasia of captive zoo species. *Vet. Med.* **56**, 25–26.

Wago, H. (1922). A case of a fibroblastic myxoma in a goldfish. *Gann* **16**, 11–12.

Wahlgren, F. (1876). Beiträge zur Pathologie der wilden Tiere. *Z. Tiermed. Vergl. Pathol.* **2**, 232–235.

Wales, J. H. (1967). Degeneration and regeneration of liver parenchyma accompanying hepatomagenesis. *In* "Trout Hepatoma Research Conference Papers" (J. E. Halver and I. A. Mitchell, eds.). *Fish Wildl. Serv. (U.S.), Res. Rep.* **70**, 56–59.

Wales, J. H., and Sinnhuber, R. O. (1966). An early hepatoma epizootic in rainbow trout, *Salmo gairdneri. Calif. Fish Game* **52**, 85–91.

Walker, R. (1947). Lymphocystis disease and neoplasia in fish. *Anat. Rec.* **99**, 559–60.

Walker, R. (1958). Lymphocystic warts and skin tumors of walleyed pike. *Rensselaer Review of Graduate Studies* **14**, 1–5.

Wellings, S. R. (1969). Neoplasia and primitive vertebrate phylogeny: Echinoderms, prevertebrates and fishes—A review. *In* "Neoplasms and Related Disorders of Invertebrate and Lower Vertebrate Animals" (C. J. Dawe and J. C. Harshbarger, eds.). *Nat. Cancer Inst. Monogr.* **31**, 59–128.

Wellings, S. R., and Chuinard, R. G. (1964). Epidermal papillomas with virus-like particles in flathead sole, *Hippoglossoides elassodon. Science* **146**, 932–934.

Wellings, S. R., Bern, H. A., Nishioka, R. S., and Graham, J. W. (1963). Epidermal papillomas in the flathead sole. *Proc. Amer. Ass. Cancer Res.* **4**, 71. (Abstr.)

Wellings, S. R., Chuinard, R. G., Gourley, R. T., and Cooper, R. A. (1964). Epidermal, papillomas in the flathead sole, *Hippoglossoides elassodon,* with notes on the occurrence of similar neoplasms in other pleuronectids. *J. Nat. Cancer Inst.* **33**, 991–1004.

Wellings, S. R., Chuinard, R. G., and Bens, M. (1965). A comparative study of skin neoplasms in four species of pleuronectid fishes. *Ann. N.Y. Acad. Sci.* **126**, 479–501.

Wellings, S. R., Cooper, R. A., and Chuinard, R. G. (1966). Skin tumors of pleuronectid fishes in Puget Sound, Washington. *Bull. Wildl. Dis. Ass.* **2**, 68.

Wellings, S. R., Chuinard, R. G., and Cooper, R. A. (1967). Ultrastructural studies of normal skin and epidermal papillomas of the flathead sole, *Hippoglossoides elassodon. Z. Zellforsch. Mikrosk. Anat.* **78**, 370–387.

Wessing, A. (1959). Über einen bösartigen, virusbedingten Tumor bei tropischen Zierfischen. *Naturwissenschaften* **46**, 517–518.

Wessing, A., and Von Bargen, G. (1959). Untersuchungen über einen virusbedingten Tumor bei Fischen. *Arch. Ges. Virusforsch.* **9**, 521–536.

Williams, G. (1929). Tumorous growths in fish. *Proceedings and Transactions of the Liverpool Biological Society* **43**, 120–148.

Williams, G. (1931). On various fish tumours. *Proceedings and Transactions of the Liverpool Biological Society* **45**, 98–109.

Williamson, H. C. (1911). On diseases and abnormalities in fish of the cod (*Gadus*), flathead (*Pleuronectes*), salmon (*Salmo*), skate (*Raia*), etc. families. *Scientific Investigations of the Fishery Board of Scotland* **11**, 3–39.

Willis, R. A. (1962). "Pathology of the Tumours of Children." Butterworth, London.

Willis, R. A. (1967). "Pathology of Tumours," 4th Ed. Butterworth, London.

Winqvist, G., Ljungberg, O., and Hellstroem, B. (1968). Skin tumours of northern pike (*Esox lucius* L.) II. Viral particles in epidermal proliferations. *Bull. Off. Int. Epizoot.* **69**, 1023–1031.

Wogan, G. N. (1967). Isolation, identification and some biological effects of aflatoxins. *In* "Trout Hepatoma Research Conference Papers" (J. E. Halver and I. A. Mitchell, eds.). *Fish Wildl. Serv.* (*U.S.*), *Res. Rep.* **70**, 121–129.

Wolf, H., and Jackson, E. W. (1963). Hepatomas in rainbow trout: Descriptive and experimental epidermiology. *Science* **142**, 676–678.

Wolf, H., and Jackson, E. W. (1967). Hepatomas in Salmonids: The role of cottonseed products and species differences. *In* "Trout Hepatoma Research Conference Papers" (J. E. Halver and I. A. Mitchell, eds.). *Fish Wildl. Serv.* (*U.S.*), *Res. Rep.* **70**, 29–33.

Wolf, K. (1966). The fish viruses. *Advan. Virus Res.* **12**, 35–101.

Wolff, B. (1912). Über ein Blastom bei einem Aal (*Anguilla vulgaris*) nebst Bemerkungen zur vergleichenden Pathologie der Geschwülste. *Virchows Arch. Pathol. Anat. Physiol.* **210**, 365–385.

Wolke, R. E., and Wyard, D. S. (1969). Ocular lymphosarcoma of an Atlantic cod. *Bull. Wildl. Dis. Ass.*, **5**, 401–403.

Wood, E. M., and Larson, C. P. (1961). Hepatic carcinoma in rainbow trout. *Arch. Pathol.* **71**, 471–479.

Woodhead, A. D., and Ellett, S. (1967). A note on the development of thyroid tumours in the senile guppy, *Lebistes reticulatus* (Peters). *Exp. Gerontol.* **2**, 73–77.

Woodhead, G. S. (1884–1885). Caseous tumours found in the muscles of the hake. *3rd and 4th Reports of the Fishery Board of Scotland* pp. 76–78.

Worm, O. (1655). "Historia Rerum Rariorum." Lugduni Batavorum.

Yasutake, W. T., and Rucker, R. R. (1967). Nutritionally induced hepatomagenesis of rainbow trout. *In* "Trout Hepatoma Research Conference Papers" (J. E. Halver and I. A. Mitchell, eds.). *Fish Wildl. Serv. (U.S.), Res. Rep.* **70**, 39–47.

Young, G. A., and Olafson, P. (1944). *Neurilemmomas* in a family of brook trout. *Amer. J. Pathol.* **20**, 413–419.

Young, M. W. (1923). Muscle tumours in the European turbot. *J. Mar. Biol. Ass. U.K.* **13**, 910–913.

Young, P. H. (1964). Some effects of sewer effluents on marine life. *Calif. Fish Game* **50**, 33–41.

Paralytic Shellfish Poisoning: A Status Report[1]

Sammy M. Ray

MARINE LABORATORY,
TEXAS A&M UNIVERSITY,
GALVESTON, TEXAS

I. Introduction

Severe and often fatal human intoxications following the ingestion of bivalve molluscs occur sporadically in widely scattered areas throughout the world. This illness, generally referred to clinically as paralytic shellfish poisoning (PSP),[2] is most prevalent in temperate regions. Other

[1] This article is based on a paper presented at the Third International Congress of Food Science and Technology (SOS/70), August 9–14, 1970, Washington, D.C.

[2] The abbreviation PSP is used in this chapter to denote either paralytic shellfish poisoning or paralytic shellfish poison.

designations, such as mussel, clam, or gonyaulax poisoning, paresthetic shellfish poisoning, and mytilointoxication are used for the same clinical entity. Certain species of unicellular, phytoplanktonic organisms known as dinoflagellates, especially those belonging to the genus *Gonyaulax*, have been definitely established as a source of the toxin. Filter-feeding molluscs such as mussels, clams, oysters, scallops, and so on, accumulate the toxin without harm to themselves by ingesting toxic dinoflagellates. A number of reviews (McFarren *et al.*, 1960; Schantz, 1960; Halstead, 1965; Russell, 1965; Kao, 1966; Evans, 1969a; Quayle, 1969) of various aspects of PSP have appeared in recent years. Halstead (1965) provides an excellent and especially comprehensive review. Our report does not consider other types of shellfish poisoning: gastrointestinal or choleratic, erythematous or allergenic, venerupin, collistin, and minamata disease. General accounts of these forms of shellfish poisoning are presented by Halstead (1965). Consult Halstead (1967) for a brief account of and references dealing with minamata disease, which is caused by the ingestion of shellfish that have accumulated mercury. With the exception of minamata disease, the other types of shellfish poisoning do not cause paralysis or neurotoxic symptoms such as those that characterize PSP. This chapter is not intended to be an exhaustive review, but rather general background information for a brief survey of current information concerning known and suspected sources of PSP.

II. Symptoms and Treatment

The principal symptoms of PSP are summarized from Halstead (1965) and Quayle (1969). Symptoms usually develop within 30 minutes after the ingestion of toxic shellfish. Early effects such as a tingling or burning sensation of lips, gums, and tongue may occur within a few minutes, and paresthesia gradually progresses to neck, arms, and legs, causing a feeling of numbness. This is followed in severe cases by ataxia (inability to coordinate voluntary movements) and general motor incoordination. Victims often report a "feeling of lightness" as though they are floating in air. Other symptoms may include weakness, dizziness, drowsiness, headache, rapid pulse, slightly subnormal temperature, slight respiratory distress, and impairment of vision. Gastrointestinal symptoms, nausea, vomiting, diarrhea, and abdominal pain are less common and do not occur consistently. Mental processes do not appear to be affected, and most victims remain calm and conscious during the illness. Characteristically, in the later stages of the illness, muscular paralysis becomes progressively more severe. In fatal cases death results from respiratory paralysis between 3 and 12 hours after intoxication. Patients surviving the first 12 hours generally recover rapidly without permanent aftereffects.

Treatment of PSP is primarily symptomatic. No specific antidote is known for this poison. Digitalis and alcohol are not recommended. The stomach should be evacuated as soon as possible with an emetic, followed by a rapid-acting laxative. In cases of respiratory difficulty, artificial respiration should be applied promptly and continued as long as necessary. Treatment for primary shock may be required. Evans (1969a) has suggested that increased urine production hastens recovery.

III. Public Health and Economic Significance

Because of its relatively low incidence, PSP does not constitute a major public health concern. The sporadic and unpredictable nature of outbreaks, however, creates difficult and expensive problems for public health and fishery agencies charged with assuring the safety of vast quantities of shellfish consumed throughout the world. The economic losses that may result from temporary cessation of shellfish harvest during toxic periods and reduced consumption of shellfish as a result of apprehension regarding possible toxicity following outbreaks are difficult to estimate.

In several instances shellfish that have been consumed for many years from a particular area without evidence of toxicity have become toxic without any warning whatsoever. In other areas, however, certain species such as the butter clam (*Saxidomus giganteus*) may maintain a high level of toxicity throughout the year and from year to year (Chambers and Magnusson, 1950; Neal, 1967; Quayle, 1969; Schantz, 1969). In southeastern Alaska great quantities (conservatively estimated at approximately $2\frac{1}{2}$ million lb) of butter clams are not utilized because of persistent toxicity (Lehman, 1966), which cannot be economically reduced by cooking or processing.

According to Halstead (1965), more than 957 cases of PSP, which resulted in more than 222 deaths, have been reported to have occurred between 1793 and 1962 (a single case was reported from France in 1689). Three outbreaks that occurred prior to 1962 were not listed by Halstead. Six cases but no deaths occurred in Oslo, Norway (Anchersen, 1939; not seen by author, cited by Oftebro, 1965). In July 1948, 12 cases with one death occurred in Toyohashi City, Japan (Hashimoto *et al.*,

1950), following consumption of clams (*Venerupis semidecussata*). Several cases showing symptoms of PSP, with one death, followed the consumption of molluscs taken from a lagoon on the west coast of Portugal (dos Santos Pinto and de Sousa e Silva, 1956).

Several outbreaks in addition to those listed by Halstead (1965) have occurred within the past 10 years in such widespread areas as Japan, England, Canada, Chile, the United States, and Norway. Two outbreaks occurred in Japan. In May 1962, 20 persons became ill and 1 person died after eating shellfish (*Chlamys nipponensis*) from Ofunata Bay (Kawabata *et al.*, 1962). In the other Japanese incident, consumption of oysters from Miyazu Bay caused 42 cases of illness in February 1963 with no fatalities (T. Akiba, personal communication, Chugai Pharmaceutical, Tokyo, 1970). Canada has experienced three outbreaks in recent years. In British Columbia seven cases were reported in 1964 and five in 1965, resulting in one death in the latter incident (Quayle, 1969). In September 1969, 14 persons became ill and 4 of them died as a result of eating molluscs taken on the beaches of the St. Lawrence River Estuary in Quebec (J. C. Medcof, personal communication, St. Andrews, Canada, 1970). In 1964 two cases were reported in Oslo, Norway (Oftebro, 1965). In the summer of 1968, an epidemic involving more than 80 persons occurred in a 3- to 4-day period following the consumption of mussels taken on the northeast (Northumbrian) coast of England (Ingham *et al.*, 1968; McCollum *et al.*, 1968; Robinson, 1968). In the spring of 1970, an outbreak involving several individuals, two of whom died, was attributed to eating mussels grown by raft culture off the coast of Chile (J. V. Junemann, personal communication, Instituto de Formento Pesquero, Santiago, Chile).

There have been three confirmed incidences of PSP on the west coast of the United States in recent years. Fortunately, the outbreaks have been rather small and no fatalities have resulted. Four residents of Solano County, California, became ill on August 1, 1962 after consuming raw oysters purchased from a restaurant on the coast about 50 mi north of San Francisco (Link, 1962). The oysters were harvested from a commercial oyster bed in Drakes Bay, Marin County, California. Two separate outbreaks occurred in California in 1969 (Anonymous, 1969a,b,c). Three individuals in Redway became ill on September 21 following the consumption of stewed mussels collected in Shelter Cove, Humboldt County. The second 1969 episode, September 27, involved 12 persons from the Livermore Valley who ate stewed mussels harvested from Mendocino Bay, Mendocino County. In 1969 the toxin levels along the northern coast of California were so high that the annual mussel quarantine period—May 1 to October 21—was extended to December 31.

The National Communicable Disease Center (Anonymous 1969d) cited an incident of shellfish poisoning of unknown etiology involving three individuals who became mildly ill after consuming raw oysters in a restaurant in Englewood, Colorado, on October 7, 1969. The oysters were harvested from the Gulf of Mexico, probably from Plaquemine Parish, Louisiana. After this outbreak Dr. John C. Breckinridge (unpublished report dated December 4, 1969, to the State of Colorado Department of Health) suggested that *Gymnodinium breve* was the cause of the poisonings since the oysters came from the Gulf of Mexico. *Gymnodinium breve* toxin was not detected in a very small sample of meats from the same shipment, but not the same sack, of the incriminated oysters (Nevis E. Cook, personal communication, Food and Drug Administration, New Orleans). Moreover, no other illnesses were reported among individuals who had consumed oysters from the same shipment. We seriously doubt that *G. breve* was the source of poisoning in this incident since the salinity is generally too low in the New Orleans area for the development of blooms of this organism.

The majority of the victims of PSP, especially in North America, are tourists and picknickers harvesting shellfish for personal consumption on outings to beaches and estuaries (Medcof *et al.*, 1947, 1966; McFarren *et al.*, 1960). Visitors and new residents to an endemic area are often either unaware of the fact that normally edible shellfish may be toxic in certain areas at certain times of the year, or they tend to disregard the posted warning against poisonous shellfish (Medcof, 1960; Medcof *et al.*, 1966). Generally, residents of an endemic area are aware of such danger. Commercially harvested shellfish have seldom been involved in PSP outbreaks because of the stringent monitoring and quarantine measures carried out by fisheries and public health agencies when dealing with shellfish from endemic or suspected areas of endemicity. In the 1968 outbreak in England, most of the victims had purchased cooked mussels (*Mytilus edulis*) from a local seafood shop (McCollum *et al.*, 1968). In view of the high level of toxicity shown by the incriminated molluscs, the practice of discarding liquor from cooked mussels is credited with reducing the severity of this epidemic.

IV. Geographical and Seasonal Distribution

PSP is definitely a problem of the temperate regions of the world (Fig. 1). Halstead (1965) records only two outbreaks (Vera Cruz, Mexico, in 1797 and Manus Island, New Guinea, in 1962) as occurring in subtropical and tropical regions (between lat. 30° N and lat. 30° S).

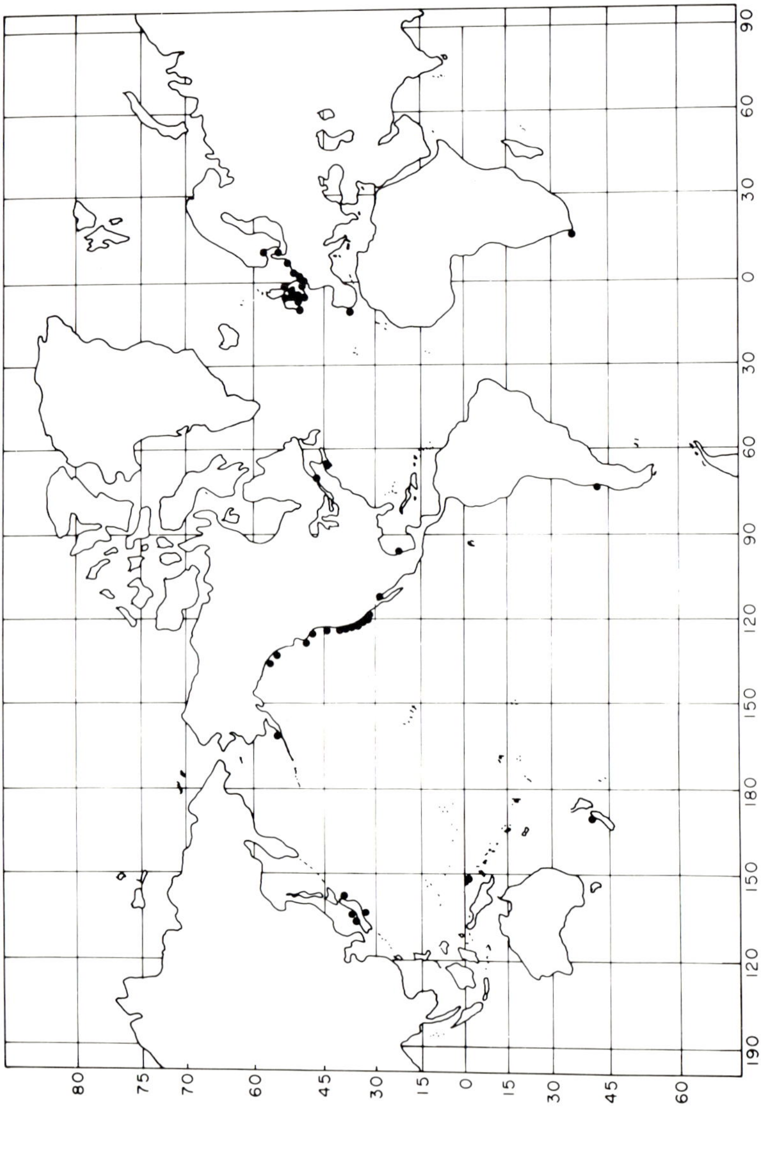

Fig. 1. Map showing world distribution of reported outbreaks of PSP (adapted from Halstead, 1965).

Since the Vera Cruz outbreak was attributed to the eating of fish, its classification as PSP is open to serious question, to say the least. Perhaps the poisonings resulted from ciguatera. The only other case of PSP listed by Halstead (1965) in which fish were incriminated occurred in Table Bay, South Africa, in 1837. Grindley and Sapeika (1969) suggest that this epidemic may have been gastroenteritis resulting from the eating of decaying fish rather than PSP. Prior to the 1927 outbreak in the vicinity of San Francisco, California, most cases were reported from northern Europe. Subsequently, most incidents have occurred in North America. Quayle (1966) is of the opinion that PSP is on the increase in British Columbia.

In North America the Pacific coastline between central California and the Aleutian Islands has suffered from this plague at various times. A small outbreak occurred in the Gulf of California in 1937 (Halstead, 1965). On the Atlantic coast occurrence of PSP has been limited to the St. Lawrence River Estuary and the Bay of Fundy in Canada. Halstead (1965) lists two outbreaks (1943 and 1954) of PSP as occurring in Maine (Bay of Fundy area). He cites McFarren *et al.* (1957) as the descriptive source of these poisonings. A search of the papers by McFarren *et al.* (1957, 1960) failed to reveal references to a 1954 outbreak in Maine. The 1943 incident of PSP, involving 26 cases in Maine, reported by the U.S. Fish and Wildlife Service (unpublished report of a conference on mussel poisoning, August 6, 1946), appears to be unfounded according to Goggins (1958). The illness occurred among workers in a mussel cannery, but there was no evidence that they had eaten any mussels. Although the toxicity in mussels (*M. edulis*) exceeded quarantine levels at some stations in Maine (Bay of Fundy area) in 1958, 1959, and 1961, Goggins (1961) states that thus far no confirmed cases of PSP have been reported in that state.

A number of European countries have had PSP outbreaks, including England, Wales, France, Scotland, Germany, Norway, Ireland, Belgium, Denmark, and Portugal. On the continent of Africa, only South Africa (principally the west coast) has experienced outbreaks. The coastal areas of Japan appear to be the only areas in the Orient from which PSP has been reported. In addition to the previously noted occurrence in Manus Island, New Guinea, and South Africa, New Zealand is the only other locality in the Southern Hemisphere from which PSP has been recorded in the literature available to us. Although occasional investigators have mentioned the occurrence of PSP in Australia without citing a particular outbreak, there appear to be no confirmed published reports from that country (Cleland and Southcott, 1965; Halstead, 1965; R.

Endean, personal communication, University of Queensland, 1970). Perhaps these authors were referring to the 1951 outbreak in New Zealand, which was cited by Halstead (1965).

There appear to be no recorded reports of the occurrence of PSP in South America. The apparent absence of PSP from South America is somewhat surprising since the water temperatures, especially along the west coast of Chile and Peru, appear to be suitable (sufficiently low) to support growth of toxic dinoflagellates such as *Gonyaulax catenella.* Very recently, however, we received a verbal report (J. V. Junemann, personal communication, Instituto de Formento Pesquero, Santiago, Chile) of the outbreak of PSP previously mentioned. The toxic molluscs (mussels) were grown in rafts maintained along the Chilean coast (lat. 41°–42° S).

A few cases of mild human illness have been associated with consumption of oysters and clams taken during red tide outbreaks caused by *G. breve* on the west coast of Florida (Eldred *et al.*, 1964; McFarren *et al.*, 1965). The symptoms observed were similar to the early symptoms of PSP, but according to McFarren *et al.* (1965) the toxin was more similar to ciguatera, which is found in certain fishes in tropical areas, than to PSP. The Florida shellfish toxin differs from PSP in that it is insoluble in water but is readily soluble in organic solvents such as ethyl ether, acetone, and chloroform.

PSP is most prevalent during the warm months—May through October inclusive (Meyer *et al.*, 1928; Sommer and Meyer, 1937; Medcof *et al.*, 1947; Prakash and Medcof, 1962). Quayle (1969) noted that PSP may develop along the British Columbia coast any time from April to November inclusive. Except for butter clams, which are capable of storing poison in the siphon throughout the year, the molluscs of British Columbia contain virtually no toxin during the winter.

Sribhibhadh (1963) studied the seasonal development and geographical distribution of toxicity in the California mussel (*Mytilus californianus*) and Pacific oyster (*Crassostrea gigas*) in the Strait of Juan de Fuca, Washington, from April 1961 to October 1962. Both species showed a similar pattern of toxicity with maximum levels occurring in midsummer. Moreover, toxicity appeared initially in shellfish at the most seaward station and then spread progressively to the more inland waters. This pattern of delay in seasonal onset, as well as decreasing intensity of toxicity in a progressive manner from the most seaward stations to more inland areas, has been noted by several observers (Sommer and Meyer, 1937; Medcof *et al.*, 1947; McFarren *et al.*, 1960; Prakash, 1963; Bourne, 1965).

The more recent cases in Japan have occurred in May, July, and February (Hashimoto *et al.*, 1950; Kawabata *et al.*, 1962; T. Akiba, personal communication, Chugai Pharmaceutical, Tokyo, 1970), and those in South Africa during April, May, and December (Grindley and Sapeika, 1969).

V. Transvectors

The consumption of bivalve molluscs, especially mussels and clams, is the most common cause of recorded incidents of PSP (Halstead, 1965). Of these two groups of bivalves, by far the greatest number of human poisonings have been traced to various species of mussels; hence the common usage of "mussel poisoning" in referring to such intoxications, especially among Europeans. The most frequent transvectors are the blue or bay mussel (*M. edulis*) and the California or sea mussel (*M. californianus*). Although both species occur on the west coast of the United States, it is of interest to note that in California only *M. californianus* is known to cause PSP (Sommer and Meyer, 1937). This condition is related to the distribution of toxic dinoflagellates. *Gonyaulax catenella* is more prevalent along open coasts and straits than in protected bays and estuaries. *Mytilus californianus* inhabits open, unprotected coastlines of California, whereas *M. edulis* is found in more protected areas such as bays. Nonetheless, *M. edulis* has been frequently involved in PSP outbreaks in other areas of the world. In North America open coasts and straits have a greater tendency to harbor toxic molluscs than more inland areas.

A number of other molluscan species, oysters, scallops, predatory and filter-feeding gastropods and some nonmolluscan invertebrates, filter-feeding crustaceans (barnacles and sand crabs), and a starfish are known to accumulate PSP (Sommer and Meyer, 1937; Goggins, 1961; Halstead, 1965; Quayle, 1969). Goggins (1961) reported the occurrence of PSP in a crab (*Cancer borealis*) in Maine. Because of their great filter-feeding capacity, bivalve molluscs are unquestionably the most serious cause of poisoning. Nonetheless, the potential danger of consuming any organisms that accumulate PSP should not be disregarded.

Predatory gastropods deserve some mention in this respect since they may accumulate PSP by feeding on toxic bivalves (Goggins, 1961; Medcof *et al.*, 1966; Ingham *et al.*, 1968; Quayle, 1969). The rough whelk (*Buccinum undatum*) from the north shore of the St. Lawrence

Estuary has been tentatively confirmed as causing 12 mild cases of PSP in 1938 or 1939 (Medcof *et al.*, 1966).

Rates of accumulation and loss of toxin by molluscs, as well as its anatomical distribution, vary from species to species (Sommer *et al.*, 1937; Sommer and Meyer, 1937; Medcof *et al.*, 1947; Quayle, 1969). Nontoxic organisms have been known to become toxic within a day or two under both natural and experimental conditions (Meyer *et al.*, 1928; Prakash, 1963). Generally, the digestive glands ("hepatopancreas," "liver," or "dark gland") accumulate the greatest concentration of the poison, and it appears to be eliminated without appreciable accumulation in other organs. In some species, however, organs such as gills and siphons become the principal storage sites of PSP following initial accumulation in the digestive glands (Medcof *et al.*, 1947; Quayle, 1969). Such a condition is most marked in the butter clam (*S. giganteus*). In this species most of the toxin becomes localized primarily in the siphon, as much as one-half to three-fourths of it occurring in this organ, which constitutes about 20% of the total meat weight.

The muscular tissues (white meat) of molluscs (mantle muscle, adductor muscles, foot, and body—exclusive of digestive glands) tend to store relatively small amounts of poison (Medcof *et al.*, 1947; Bourne, 1965; Quayle, 1969). This is a fortunate circumstance and it can be and is used to reduce the dangers of ingesting toxic levels of PSP. Scallops may become highly toxic for long periods (Medcof *et al.*, 1947; Bourne, 1965), but since only the adductor muscle is marketed, human intoxication is unlikely unless the entire animal is eaten.

Fortunately, except for butter clams and scallops which may remain toxic throughout the year, most molluscs, including both siphonated (clams) and nonsiphonated (mussels and oysters) species, lose the poison rather rapidly. Thus the poisonous condition is transitory in most cases (Medcof *et al.*, 1947; Schantz and Magnusson, 1964; Halstead, 1965; Quayle, 1969), lasting from a few days to a few weeks (2 months). Quayle (1969) studied the rate of toxin loss in eight species of bivalves; most species including both siphonated and nonsiphonated lost most of the toxin in a few weeks, whereas approximately 2 years were required for butter clams. The nonsiphonated forms, bay or black mussels (*M. edulis*) and the Pacific oyster (*C. gigas*), lost the toxin very rapidly. Oysters and cockles (*Clinocardium nuttallii*) accumulated far less toxin than the other species examined. In the Strait of Juan de Fuca, California mussels (*M. californianus*) became toxic earlier and accumulated higher levels of poison than Pacific oysters; both species accumulated and lost toxin at rapid rates (Sribhibhadh, 1963). In studies conducted near

Ketchikan, Alaska, Neal (1967) compared the levels of PSP in four species of bivalve molluscs. Mussels (*M. edulis*) accumulated and released toxin rapidly, whereas littleneck clams (*Protothaca staminea*) and Pacific oysters accumulated only small amounts of poison. Butter clams, however, accumulated toxin rapidly but released it very slowly; thus they were toxic throughout the year. Since old clams were more toxic than young ones, this species apparently accumulates toxin from year to year.

Although oysters are consumed in large quantities throughout the world, this relatively low capacity for storing PSP probably accounts for the low frequency with which they have been involved in causing PSP. In this connection it is of interest to note that oysters apparently have not been involved in lethal cases of PSP. A possible, but highly questionable, lethality attributed to the eating of oysters is listed by Halstead (1965) as having occurred in Austria in 1896.

Brief mention should be made of xanthid crabs which contain a toxin that is similar, if not identical, to PSP or saxitoxin (Konosu *et al.*, 1968; Noguchi *et al.*, 1969). Lethal human intoxications of a paralytic type attributed to consumption of xanthid crabs have been reported from the Ryukyu and Amami Islands (Hashimoto *et al.*, 1967, 1969; Inoue *et al.*, 1968). The poison, which has been isolated from at least three xanthid crabs that inhabit coral reefs, is located primarily in the exoskeleton and muscles of the appendages. The source of the toxin is unknown. There was no evidence of algal blooms or red tides in the areas from which the toxic crabs were obtained. Presently, marine algae on coral reefs are being screened for the toxin since the crabs seem to be herbivorous rather than carnivorous (Y. Hashimoto, personal communication, University of Tokyo, 1970). Consideration of algae as a possible source of the crab toxin was stimulated by the recent demonstration by Jackim and Gentile (1968) that toxic fractions isolated from a freshwater blue-green alga (*Aphanizomenon flos-aquae*) appear to be similar, if not identical, to saxitoxin.

VI. Prevention and Control

The surveillance of edible molluscs for toxicity during potential danger periods constitutes the most effective means of preventing PSP. The mouse bioassay, first developed by Sommer and Meyer (1937) and later modified by Medcof *et al.* (1947), is the standard method for monitoring the safety of shellfish. Details of the procedure for quantitating PSP by the mouse bioassay are available from a number of sources (Medcof *et al.*, 1947; McFarren, 1959; McFarren *et al.*, 1960; Halstead, 1965; Anonymous, 1970). A mouse unit is defined as the amount of poison injected intraperitoneally that will kill a 20-gm mouse in 15 minutes with typical symptoms of paralysis and respiratory failure. Concentrations of less than 200 mouse units/100 gm of shellfish cannot be accurately measured by this method. A chemical method for quantitating PSP, based on the Jaffe test, has been developed by McFarren *et al.* (1958), and a serological test has been developed by Johnson and Mulberry (1966). Pringle (1966) concluded that the mouse bioassay is still the most suitable method developed thus far to quantitate PSP.

With purification of clam and mussel toxins (Mold *et al.*, 1957; Schantz *et al.*, 1957), Schantz *et al.* (1958) recommended the use of purified clam toxin to standardize the mouse bioassay. The purified clam toxin is known as saxitoxin[3] since it is extracted from siphons of butter clams (*S. giganteus*). Thus the amount of toxin may be reported by weight (micrograms) rather than in mouse units. According to McFarren *et al.* (1960), the average conversion factor (CF) obtained by several laboratories gave an average value of 0.191 μg of poison per mouse unit. Using this average CF value, the previously accepted tolerance level of 400 mouse units/100 gm of shellfish was converted to 80 μg/100 gm (Jensen, 1959). Despite the recommendation that toxicity be reported by weight, most workers continue to report in mouse units.

The public health and fisheries agencies of the United States and Canada have cooperated extensively in developing a certification program to insure the safety of interstate shipments of fresh or canned shellfish. In the United States and Canada, growing areas are quarantined when the toxicity is known to reach 400 mouse units (80 μg)/100 gm of shellfish or more (McFarren *et al.*, 1960; Quayle, 1969). According to McFarren *et al.* (1960), the U.S. Food and Drug Administration does not permit the marketing of fresh, frozen, or canned clams when the average toxicity exceeds 400 mouse units/100 gm, and no individual package may exceed 2000 mouse units; minced or chopped clams must have an average toxicity of less than 2000 mouse units/100 gm, and individual packages may not exceed 2000 mouse units. While adherence

[3] The Army Chemical Corps has made a limited supply of saxitoxin available to the U.S. Public Health Service for use in assay standardization and research (Schantz *et al.*, 1958; McFarren *et al.*, 1960). Requests for PSP standard solution (100 μg/ml) should be submitted to Division of Criteria and Standards, Bureau of Water Hygiene, ECA, 12720 Twinbrook Parkway, Rockville, Maryland.

to the above standards may cause appreciable economic losses to the shellfish industry, their strict enforcement by United States and Canadian authorities may be credited with the notable lack of human intoxications traceable to commercially processed shellfish.

Aside from strict quarantine of commercial harvest and interstate shipment of poisonous shellfish, a number of other precautionary measures are employed to control PSP. Signs are posted in shellfish growing areas and on beaches to warn the general public of the potential dangers in consuming toxic shellfish. The news media, newspapers, television, and radio, are used extensively to warn picknickers and tourists as well as local residents of the hazards of PSP during the danger season. Such use of the news media to issue prompt warnings of PSP outbreaks is credited by McCollum *et al.* (1968) with preventing an even greater epidemic than was actually experienced in England in 1968.

The eating of whole, uncooked shellfish from endemic areas may be extremely dangerous. Cooking does not completely destroy PSP since it is rather heat stable. Nevertheless, cooking in any form reduces the toxicity by more than 70% of the concentration found in raw shellfish (Medcof *et al.*, 1947). Because of its water solubility, much of the poison is concentrated in the nectars or liquors produced by cooking. All such fluids should be discarded. Despite the high level of toxicity among mussels in the 1968 outbreak in England, no deaths resulted from more than 80 intoxications. The common practice of discarding the liquor from cooked mussels is credited by McCollum *et al.* (1968) with reducing the severity of the epidemic. Moreover, the discarding of certain portions of the shellfish, such as siphons (butter clams), digestive glands, and gills, prior to cooking further reduces the hazards of intoxication.

Commercial canning of shellfish is more effective than ordinary cooking in reducing toxicity. Medcof *et al.* (1947) showed that precooking fairly toxic clams (*Mya arenaria*) with steam for 10 minutes reduces the poison content by about 90%. Considerable effort has been made to develop processes to render the highly toxic butter clams in southeastern Alaska safe for human consumption. Dassow (1966) reports that trimming the siphons from shucked meats and steaming the meats for 10 minutes, followed by retorting at 250°F for 75 minutes, reduces the poison content of butter clams by as much as 93% without affecting the quality of the product. The Alaskan shellfish industry, however, has not used the process since it is considered unprofitable. The apparent ease with which PSP can be extracted from molluscan tissues prompted consideration by the U.S. Bureau of Commercial Fisheries (Anonymous, 1966) of pretreating butter clams in a mild acid solution to reduce toxicity. No reduction in PSP was noted in butter clams (live and chopped meats) held in acid solutions of pH 5.0–6.0 for periods up to 17 hours.

The monitoring of vast areas of shellfish growing waters in British Columbia and southeastern Alaska presents an expensive and formidable task (Quayle, 1969). As pointed out by Schantz (1969) and others (see Felsing, 1966), one of the most important problems facing the shellfish industry is the need for an economical commercial process that can reliably reduce the toxicity of butter clams from Alaska and British Columbia to safe levels. Numerous efforts to develop commercially feasible means of detoxifying raw butter clams, including transplanting live animals to nonendemic waters and storage in air, on ice, and in a frozen state, as well as irradiation, have been unsuccessful (McFarren *et al.*, 1960).

Since outbreaks of PSP are directly related to the occurrence of toxic dinoflagellates (Sommer *et al.*, 1937; Needler, 1949; Prakash, 1963; Wood, 1968), the systematic search for dinoflagellate blooms as indicated by discolored water (red tides or red water) and plankton sampling for toxic dinoflagellates may be used to determine where and when poisonous shellfish are likely to occur. Clark (1968) has suggested that biological events such as the presence of sick and dying sea birds and sand eels, and luminescence at night, which preceded the 1968 English outbreak, might serve as useful warnings of impending PSP.

VII. Source of PSP

The mystery of the cause of PSP was finally solved by the brilliant research of Sommer and his colleagues (Sommer *et al.*, 1937), while investigating various aspects of a series of outbreaks that began on the west coast of the United States in 1927. These workers proved that the dinoflagellate *G. catenella* was the primary source of the toxin in this region. Since that time additional species belonging to the genus *Gonyaulax* and other genera as well either have been shown to be the source or have been implicated as such in various areas of the world (Table I). Some of the poison-bearing dinoflagellates are shown in Fig. 2. *Gonyaulax catenella,* a chain-forming species, and *G. tamarensis,* a nonchain-forming species, are the most commonly known causes of PSP and probably represent the most poisonous of the dinoflagellates.

Gonyaulax catenella is probably the primary cause of PSP along the

TABLE I
KNOWN AND SUSPECTED SOURCES OF PSP

Source	Region	Reference
Gonyaulax catenella	Pacific coast, North America	Sommer *et al.* (1937); Sparks and Sribhibhadh (1961); Neal (1967); Hsu (1967)
Gonyaulax tamarensis	North Atlantic coast, North America	Needler (1949); Prakash (1963); Medcof *et al.* (1966)
	Oslo, Norway	Oftebro (1965)
	Northeast coast, England	Wood (1968); Robinson (1968)
	West coast, Portugal	de Sousa e Silva (1963)
Gonyaulax acatenella	Pacific coast, British Columbia	Prakash and Taylor (1966)
Gonyaulax polyedra	West coast, Southern California	Schradie and Bliss (1962)
Pyrodinium phoneus[a]	Belgium	Koch (1939); Woloszynska and Conrad (1939)
Prorocentrum micans	West coast, Portugal	dos Santos Pinto and de Sousa e Silva (1956)
Glenodinium foliaceum	West coast, Portugal	de Sousa e Silva (1963)
Exuviaella baltica	West coast, Portugal	de Sousa e Silva (1963)
Exuviaella mariae-lebouriae[b]	Lake Hamana, Japan	Nakazima (1965a,b,c, 1968)
Gymnodinium breve[c]	West coast, Florida	Eldred *et al.* (1964); McFarren *et al.* (1965); Ray and Aldrich (1965, 1967); Morton and Burklew (1969); Cummins *et al.* (1968); Cummins and Stevens (1970)

[a] *Pyrodinium phoneus* is probably synonymous with *G. tamarensis* (T. Braarud, personal communication, Institutt for Marin Biologi, Oslo, 1970).

[b] Suspected cause of venerupin shellfish poisoning in Japan, previously reported as a *Prorocentrum* sp. by Nakazima (1965a,b,c).

[c] Shellfish poisoning caused by this organism differs from the typical PSP.

Pacific coast between central California and the Aleutian Islands. Although this dinoflagellate is most likely the source in Alaskan waters, there is still some question in this regard because of the extremely low *G. catenella* densities encountered thus far (Schantz and Magnusson, 1964; Neal, 1967; Sparks, 1966). Nevertheless, the fact that the chemical

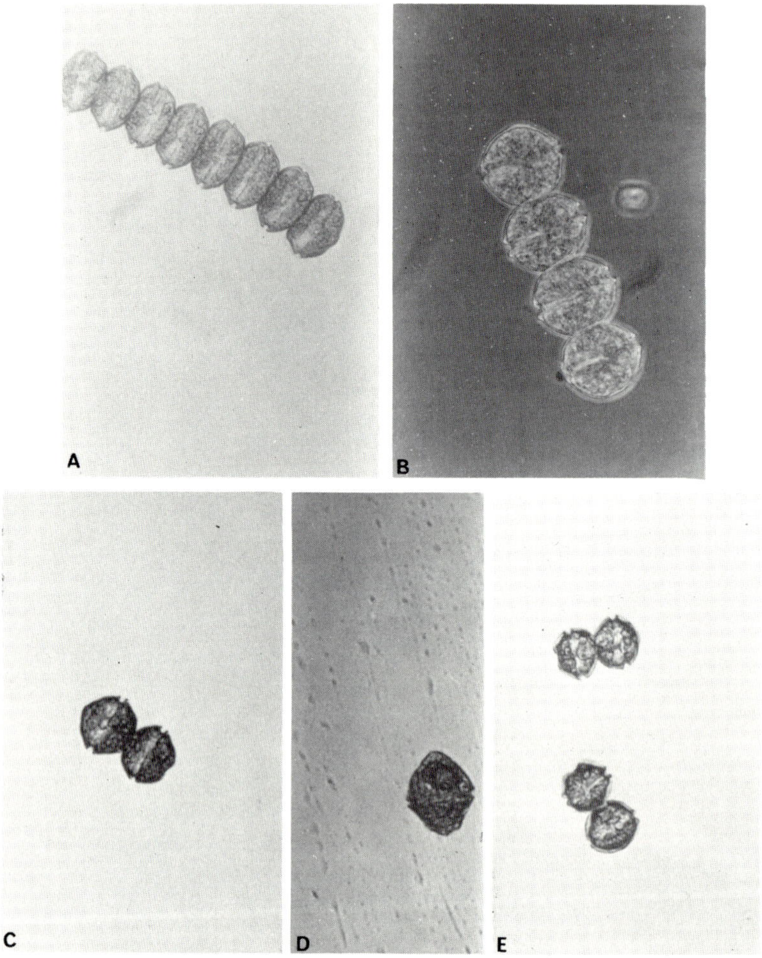

Fig. 2. Phase-contrast photomicrographs of various species of *Gonyaulax* implicated as toxin producers. (A) *Gonyaulax monilata.* (B) *Gonyaulax acatenella.* (C) *Gonyaulax catenella.* (D) *Gonyaulax polyedra.* (E) *Gonyaulax tamarensis.* Magnifications approximately 400×, except (B), which is approximately 750×. All specimens are from cultures grown in artificial seawater media.

and physical properties (Schantz *et al.*, 1966; Schantz, 1969) of purified clam toxin are identical to those of *G. catenella* poison strongly implicates this organism as the primary source in Alaska. Oddly enough, Schantz and Magnusson (1964) found that mussels (*M. edulis*) showed very low levels of toxicity even when taken from the general vicinity of areas containing highly toxic butter clams. Moreover, a lack of toxicity in extracts of total net phytoplankton from endemic areas suggests the absence of significant concentrations of any other toxic species in the phytoplankton. The explanation of the Alaskan situation, according to Schantz (1969), is probably related to the rapid manner in which mussels eliminate poison in contrast to its extended persistence in butter clams, especially in the siphon.

Neal (1967) reported that uptake of toxin by mussels (*M. edulis*) held in trays near Ketchikan was closely correlated with the presence of *G. catenella* at two stations, and with that of an unidentified species of *Gonyaulax* at the other three stations. The uptake of toxin by butter clams, however, did not always coincide with the periods of uptake by the other species (littleneck clams, Pacific oysters, and bay mussels). Neal suggested that butter clams may obtain toxin from bottom sediments, organic debris, or encysted *G. catenella* cells rather than active *G. catenella* cells.

A chain-forming species of *Gonyaulax,* probably *G. catenella,* has been associated with shellfish toxicity in several areas of the state of Washington (Sparks and Sribhibhadh, 1961; Hsu, 1967). Hsu (1967) considered that the organisms from Washington, although closely related to *G. catenella* as described by Whedon and Kofoid, showed certain morphological characteristics that indicated it to be an undescribed species. He assigned the name *Gonyaulax washingtonensis* to these dinoflagellates. After further study, B. C. Hsu and A. K. Sparks (Sparks, personal communication, Bureau of Commercial Fisheries, Galveston, 1970) considered it a variety of *G. catenella* and are preparing to describe it as *G. catenella* var. *washingtonensis.*

Recently, *G. catenella* was shown by Grindley and Sapeika (1969) to be the source of PSP on the west coast of South Africa.

In 1965 a bloom of *Gonyaulax acatenella,* a species previously considered nontoxic, was demonstrated to be the cause of an outbreak of PSP in the Strait of Georgia, British Columbia, by Prakash and Taylor (1966). These investigators mentioned that *G. acatenella* and *G. catenella* possibly are conspecific, that is, *G. acatenella* may be a morphological variation of *G. catenella.* In any case, Quayle (1969) has pointed out that this observation represents the first specific source to be documented for PSP in British Columbia despite its long history with this problem. Quayle also noted that *G. catenella* had not been recorded from British Columbia.

Gonyaulax tamarensis, as shown by Needler (1949) and confirmed by Prakash (1963), is the cause of PSP in the Bay of Fundy and most likely is the source in the St. Lawrence River Estuary (Prakash, 1963; Medcof *et al.*, 1966). The evidence that this species caused the 1968 outbreak in England is most substantial (Wood, 1968; Robinson, 1968). *Gonyaulax tamarensis* and associated toxic shellfish occurred again in 1969 on the northeast coast of England, but at a lower level than in 1968 (P. C. Wood, personal communication, Burnham-on-Crouch, 1970).

During both 1968 and 1969, toxic shellfish and concentrations of *G. tamarensis* were observed over an extensive length of the coastline and extending several miles from shore. In this respect this most recent occurrence in the western North Sea differs from most of the early European outbreaks, which generally have been reported from more-or-less stagnant, brackish water areas such as estuaries, harbors, and canals (Sommer and Meyer, 1937; Gemmill and Manderson, 1960; Halstead, 1965). There has been speculation by some investigators that the source of PSP in brackish areas is different from that in open areas.

In Belgium, *Pyrodinium phoneus,* described as a new species by Woloszynska and Conrad (1939), is considered the source of PSP (Koch, 1939; Woloszynska and Conrad, 1939). Since *P. phoneus* was associated with PSP attributed to eating mussels from a brackish water canal in the 1938 outbreak, some workers believed this species to be the probable cause of PSP in other brackish water areas of northern Europe. Some question, however, regarding the validity of considering *P. phoneus* a separate species from *G. tamarensis* has been raised by Trygve Braarud (personal communication, Institutt for Marin Biologi, Oslo, 1970), who "considers it most probable that *Pyrodinium phoneus* is identical with the Oslofjord *G. tamarensis* as well as the Bay of Fundy *G. tamarensis*."

Although not definitely established, *G. tamarensis* by virtue of its occurrence is probably the cause of PSP in Norway (Oftebro, 1965); and it is perhaps one of several sources in a small lagoon (Óbidos) on the west coast of Portugal (de Sousa e Silva, 1963).

Results of comparative studies dealing with toxin production by the Canadian (Bay of Fundy) and the English (Tamar River Estuary, near Plymouth, England) forms of *G. tamarensis* in cultures (Prakash, 1963) give cause to question that these two forms are identical. Prakash found that extracts of unialgal cultures of the English form were nontoxic, whereas those of the Canadian form were highly toxic. Nevertheless, Prakash indicated that there was insufficient morphological evidence to warrant separation of these two forms at present. He suggested that the English and Canadian forms represent different strains of the same species.

In view of strong evidence that *G. tamarensis* was the cause of the

1968 outbreaks of PSP on the northeastern English coast, there can be little doubt that toxic forms of this species occur in England. Moreover, Schantz (personal communication, Dept. of the Army, Frederick, Md., 1970) found that toxin extracted from mussels collected during the 1968 outbreak in England behaved chemically and physically in the same manner as poison extracted from scallops taken from the Bay of Fundy. Perhaps the results observed by Prakash are attributable to vagaries of the cultures. Variations in toxin production have been noted in both unialgal and axenic cultures of *G. catenella* by Burke *et al.* (1960).

Preliminary attempts have been made by Prakash (1963, 1966) to compare the relative toxin production per cell of the three North American sources of PSP. He suggests that *G. tamarensis* is more toxic than *G. catenella* and *G. acatenella*. No comparison was made between the two last-mentioned species in these reports. However, Quayle (1969) comments on the relative toxicity of these three species of dinoflagellates: "From cell extract studies, Sommer *et al.* (1937) and Prakash (MS, 1967) concluded that *G. tamarensis* is more toxic than *G. catenella*, which in turn is more toxic than *G. acatenella*." Although *G. tamarensis* and *G. catenella* toxins are similar in biological action, according to Schantz (1969), there are indications that there may be some differences in their chemical and physical properties.

Blooms or red tides of *Gonyaulax polyedra*, another nonchain-forming species, often occur in the warmer waters along the Pacific coast south of Point Conception, California (Schradie and Bliss, 1962), and in other areas of the world. Although no cases of PSP have been attributed to this organism, mass mortalities of fish and invertebrates have occurred during some blooms but such is not always the case. It is generally believed that such mortalities are related to oxygen deficiencies resulting from decomposition of large quantities of organic matter and not attributable to toxins produced by this organism. Schradie and Bliss (1962) extracted a toxic substance from the cells of *G. polyedra* grown in axenic culture, however. The pharmacological and chemical nature of this toxin appears to be similar to purified shellfish (clam) poison and *G. catenella* toxin. These investigators implied that *G. polyedra* might be the cause of PSP in outbreaks that have occurred in the warmer waters south of Point Conception. The observations by Schradie and Bliss suggest that this organism is a potential source of PSP; consumption of shellfish taken during blooms of this organism may be hazardous.

Several species of dinoflagellates belonging to genera other than *Gonyaulax* have been associated with PSP in Óbidos Lagoon on the west coast of Portugal (dos Santos Pinto and de Sousa e Silva, 1956; de Sousa e Silva, 1963). In 1955 high densities of *Prorocentrum micans* coincided with the occurrence of highly toxic cockles (*Cardium edule*) and several illnesses and one death were attributed to eating cockles (dos Santos Pinto and de Sousa e Silva, 1956). Interestingly enough, mussels (*M. edulis*) in the same area were much less toxic than cockles and they apparently did not cause poisonings.

de Sousa e Silva (1963), in a later study in the same area, showed that shellfish toxicity was associated with high densities of three dinoflagellates: *Exuviaella baltica, G. tamarensis,* and *Glenodinium foliaceum.* Although four species of dinoflagellates are suspected as sources in Portugal, *G. tamarensis* is the only proven producer of PSP among them.

Two other toxic dinoflagellates have been strongly incriminated as causes of shellfish poisonings that differ from typical PSP. These organisms are worthy of mention since they produce toxins that are obviously different from PSP.

A serious form of nonparalytic shellfish poisioning, thus far limited to Kanagawa and Schizuoka Prefectures in Japan, is known as venerupin poisoning. According to Halstead (1965), the first recorded outbreak occurred in 1887 and there were 81 cases of intoxication with 54 deaths. No other outbreaks were reported until 1941. Between 1941 and 1950 there were several incidents involving more than 500 individuals, of whom about one-third succumbed. All poisonings were traced to the consumption of oysters (*C. gigas*) and Japanese littleneck clams (*Tapes semidecussata*). The latter mollusc is a member of the family Veneridae, hence the name venerupin poison.

Nakazima (1965a,b,c) provided convincing evidence that a dinoflagellate, originally reported as a *Prorocentrum* sp. but later identified (Nakazima, 1968) as *Exuviaella mariae-lebouriae,* was the source of venerupin poison. When administered to mice, cells of *E. mariae-lebouriae,* extracts of such cells, and extracts of the digestive glands of shellfish that had fed on cultured cells of this species induced the same type of pathological damage noted in human poisonings.

Along the west coast of Florida, a few cases of mild human illness have been associated with consumption of oysters and clams taken during red tide outbreaks caused by the naked dinoflagellate *G. breve* (Eldred *et al.*, 1964; McFarren *et al.*, 1965). According to McFarren *et al.*, the Florida shellfish poisonings had the initial symptoms of PSP, however, the toxin produced is similar to ciguatoxin found in certain fishes in tropical areas. This organism has been definitely established as the source of the Florida shellfish toxin (Ray and Aldrich, 1965, 1967; Morton and Burklew, 1969; Cummins *et al.*, 1968; Cummins and Stevens, 1970).

VIII. Nature of PSP

PSP, a nonprotein substance of low molecular weight, is one of the most potent human poisons known. The purified clam (saxitoxin) and mussel poisons (95–100% pure) have a toxicity of 5500 $\pm$ 500 mouse units per milligram of dry solids (Mold *et al.*, 1957; Schantz, 1969). According to Schantz (1969), based on data provided by Bond and Medcof (1958), oral ingestion of 2000–3000 mouse units (0.2–0.3 mg) may be lethal to man. In terms of purified toxin, 100 μg by oral ingestion is considered a lethal dose to humans (Schantz, 1966).

The toxin is a metabolic product of dinoflagellates and appears to be bound in molluscan tissues without undergoing change (Schantz *et al.*, 1966). Dupuy (1968) suggested that the substance produced by *Gonyaulax* spp. and accumulated in shellfish is not actually a toxin but a larger molecule (precursor) which, when hydrolyzed by acid, is activated to become a toxin.

Poisons extracted from mussels (*M. californianus*), clams (*S. giganteus*), and axenic cultures of *G. catenella* have been purified (Mold *et al.*, 1957; Schantz *et al.*, 1957, 1966; Schantz, 1967). Studies conducted by Burke *et al.* (1960) indicated that mussel poison and *G. catenella* toxin from axenic cultures have similar chemical and physical properties. Moreover, mice showed the same symptoms when injected intraperitoneally with these two poisons. Schantz *et al.* (1966) and Schantz (1969) confirmed the identical nature of mussel, clam (saxitoxin), and *G. catenella* poisons by comparative study of the chemical, physical, and toxicity characteristics of purified material from these three sources. Since the *G. catenella* toxin was extracted from bacteria-free cultures, there can be no doubt that this organism is the direct source of mussel poison as originally proclaimed by Sommer *et al.* (1937).

The biochemical and physical properties of these poisons have been extensively studied by Schantz and co-workers (Schantz, 1960, 1967). The general properties of PSP are summarized by Schantz (1960): "The poisons are basic nitrogenous substances soluble in water and lower alcohols and insoluble in all lipid solvents. They are stable in acid solutions, but labile in alkaline solutions. The molecular formula is

$C_{10}H_{17}N_7O_4 \cdot 2HCl$ (molecular weight 372). The molecule is readily reduced with hydrogen to form a nontoxic dihydro derivative. Various oxidizing and hydrolytic agents yield guanidopropionic acid, guanidine, urea, ammonia, and carbon dioxide."

Kao (1966) considers that the molecular formula of saxitoxin may be $C_{10}H_{15}N_7O_4$ instead of $C_{10}H_{17}N_7O_4$ as generally believed. Rapoport *et al.* (1964, not seen by author, cited by Schantz, 1966; and Evans, 1969a), have suggested a structural formula for this poison (see Schantz, 1966; and Evans, 1969a, for proposed structure of saxitoxin). Evans (1969a) states that the empirical formula ($C_{10}H_{17}N_7O_4$) is incompatible with the structural formula proposed by Rapoport *et al.* Additional structures for clam toxin as proposed by Bannard (1962) are presented by Baslow (1969).

The availability of saxitoxin (purified clam poison) has prompted numerous studies of the toxicological and pharmacological properties of this poison (Murtha, 1960; Kao, 1966, 1967; Evans, 1967, 1969a,b; Bull and Pringle, 1968). Kao (1966) presents an excellent review on this subject. Likewise, Baslow (1969) reviews this topic in his book on marine pharmacology. Saxitoxin and tetrodotoxin (puffer poison) have provided an extremely valuable tool in the study of neuromuscular physiology (Kao, 1966; Evans, 1969a). Although of different biological origin, both saxitoxin and tetrodotoxin have a direct paralyzing action on striated (skeletal) muscle and nerve fibers, reducing membrane permeability to sodium ions (or ions that may substitute for sodium) by blockage of sodium channels (Kao, 1966; Evans, 1969a).

IX. Discussion

Extensive blooms of dinoflagellates, commonly referred to as red tides or red water since the water may develop a brownish to reddish discoloration because of great densities of organisms, occur from time to time in various areas of the world, especially in estuarine and marine waters. The literature concerning this phenomenon is too extensive to be covered in this chapter. For a general reference the reader is referred to Brongersma-Sanders (1948). Blooms of dinoflagellates are often accompanied by spectacular displays of luminescence or phosphorescence at night; this feature is reported by Quayle (1969) to have been used by the Indians along the Pacific coast of North America as a warning of shellfish toxicity.

Ecological factors responsible for such blooms are poorly understood. A number of factors such as upwelling, tides and currents, salinity and freshwater influx, amount of sunshine and light penetration, wind intensity and direction, water temperature and turbulence (degree of calmness), introduction of nutrients and growth factors (including pollutants) from land drainage, abundance of dinoflagellate predators (ciliates) and competitors (diatoms), and so on, have been considered by various observers. The role and interaction of the various factors are not sufficiently understood, however, to permit prediction of dinoflagellate blooms with any degree of accuracy.

Blooms are caused by numerous dinoflagellate species; mortalities of aquatic organisms occur in some incidents, but not always. Such mortalities may result either from indirect effects such as oxygen deficiency and attendant deleterious substances resulting from decomposing masses of dinoflagellates, or from toxins produced by the blooming organisms. In the latter case several species, *Gymnodinium breve* (Gunter *et al.*, 1948; Ray and Wilson, 1957; Ray and Aldrich, 1967; Sievers, 1969), *Gymnodinium veneficum* (Abbott and Ballantine, 1957), and *Gonyaulax monilata* (Connell and Cross, 1950; Gates and Wilson, 1960; Aldrich *et al.*, 1967; Ray and Aldrich, 1967; Sievers, 1969), have been shown to produce substances that are toxic to fish and some invertebrates. Another species, *Gonyaulax grindleyi*, appears to have caused mortality of numerous invertebrates, including molluscs, with little evidence of fish mortality along the west coast of South Africa (Grindley and Nel, 1968; Grindley and Sapeika, 1969). Since there was no evidence of mass decay of plankton, one may suspect that *Gonyaulax grindleyi* produces a toxin. The toxins produced by the above organisms appear to have different specificities. Both *Gymnodinium breve* and *Gymnodinium veneficum* are toxic to fish and mice; and generally these species show little or no toxicity to invertebrates. *Gonyaulax monilata* is toxic to fish and a number of invertebrates including molluscs, but shows little evidence of toxicity to mice and chicks. In this respect *Gonyaulax grindleyi* appears to be similar to *Gonyaulax monilata* except for the apparent lack of toxicity of the former organism to fish. Extracts of *Gonyaulax grindleyi* proved nontoxic to mice (Grindley and Nel, 1968; Grindley and Sapeika, 1969). As a general rule, the mortality of aquatic organisms has been notably absent during blooms of dinoflagellates associated with PSP outbreaks. The 1968 outbreak along the northeast English coast, however, was a notable exception in that extensive mortality of sand eels (*Ammodytes* sp.), birds (especially shags, *Phalacrocorax aristotelis,* which had fed on the eels), some bivalves (primarily noncommercial species), and other animals that feed upon mussels occurred shortly before and during the outbreak (Adams *et al.*, 1968; Clark, 1968; Coulson *et al.*, 1969; Ingham *et al.*, 1968). Most of the bivalves harvested for human consumption such as mussels (*Mytilus*), scallops (*Pecten*), and queens (*Chamys*) accumulated large quantities of toxin without apparent harmful effects as reported by Adams *et al.* (1968) and Clark (1968). These investigators noted that other molluscs such as cockles (*Cardium*), clams (*Venus, Tellina, Macoma*), and starfish (*Asterias*) suffered considerable mortality in some areas. The restriction of fish mortality to sand eels suggests that ingestion of a toxin through the food chain rather than an indirect effect such as oxygen deficiency was the cause of death among the eels. Assuming that the noncommercial bivalves were not killed by some indirect cause, it appears that some molluscs are more sensitive to *Gonyaulax tamarensis* toxin than others.

There remain numerous problems related to the causative organisms of PSP and the ecological conditions responsible for the development of massive populations of these organisms. The solution of some problems requires integrated field and laboratory investigations concerning taxonomic status and distribution of various species, physical and nutritional requirements, toxin-producing capability and specificity of such toxins, physical and chemical nature of the toxins, and toxicological and pharmacological characteristics, as well as ecological and physiological relationships between causative and transvector organisms. Most of the studies mentioned above require development of pure cultures of known and suspected causative organisms. The various studies may be patterned after those conducted thus far with *G. catenella*, beginning with the pioneering work of Sommer and his co-workers. With the proper identification and isolation of known causative organisms, knowledge of their nutritional and physical requirements, as well as the ecological interaction of such factors, may be used in developing means for predicting the timing and location of the occurrence of toxic shellfish. Moreover, information regarding the toxicological, pharmacological, and chemical nature of various toxins may lead to the development of a satisfactory antidote for human poisonings.

Acknowledgments

The preparation of this report was supported in part by research grant No. FD-00151 from the Food and Drug Administration, U.S. Public Health Service and National Science Foundation Sea Grant Program, Institutional Award GH-59 made to Texas A&M University.

References

Abbott, B. C., and Ballantine, D. (1957). The toxin from *Gymnodinium veneficum* Ballantine. *J. Mar. Biol. Ass. U.K.* **36**, 169–189.

Adams, J. A., Seaton, D. D., Buchanan, J. B., and Longbottom, M. R. (1968). Biological observations associated with the toxic phytoplankton bloom off the east coast. *Nature (London)* **220**, 24–25.

Aldrich, D. V., Ray, S. M., and Wilson, W. B. (1967). *Gonyaulax monilata:* population growth and development of toxicity in cultures. *J. Protozool.* **14**, 636–639.

Anchersen, P. (1939). Blaskjellforgiftning, *Nord. Med.* **3**, 2538–2540.

Anonymous (1966). Acid pre-treatment to remove paralytic shellfish poison from butter clams, *Saxidomus giganteus. U.S. Fish Wildl. Serv., Tech. Rep.* **72**, 4 pp. (Processed report.)

Anonymous (1969a). Shellfish poisoning alert. California Morbidity, 2 pp. State Dep. Pub. Health, Bur. Communicable Dis. Contr., Sacramento, California.

Anonymous (1969b). Did mussel poisoning do-in Molly Malone? *Calif. Health* **27**, 11.

Anonymous (1969c). Paralytic shellfish poisoning. Communicable Diseases, pp. 27 and 46. State Dep. Pub. Health, Sacramento, California.

Anonymous (1969d). Annual Summary of Foodborne Outbreaks. Nat. Communicable Dis. Center, Atlanta, Georgia.

Anonymous (1970). Bioassay for shellfish toxins. *In* "Recommended Procedures for the Examination of Sea Water and Shellfish," 4th Ed., pp. 57–66. Amer. Pub. Health Ass., New York.

Bannard, R. A. B. (1962). Clam poison. VI. Summary of investigations related to structural analysis of clam poison 1954–60 (U). *Def. Res. Bd. Can. Def. Res. Chem. Lab., Rep.* **368**, 39.

Baslow, M. H. (1969). "Marine Pharmacology." Williams & Wilkins, Baltimore, Maryland.

Bond, R. M., and Medcof, J. C. (1958). Epidemic shellfish poisoning in New Brunswick, 1957. *Can. Med. Ass. J.* **79**, 19–24.

Bourne, N. (1965). Paralytic shellfish poison in sea scallops (*Placopecten magellanicus* Gmelin). *J. Fish. Res. Bd. Can.* **22**, 1137–1149.

Brongersma-Sanders, M. (1948). The importance of upwelling water to vertebrate paleontology and oil geology. *Verh. Kon. Ned. Akad. Wetensch., Sect. 2* **45**, 1–112.

Bull, R. J., and Pringle, B. H. (1968). Saxitoxin as an example of biologically active marine substances. *In* "Drugs from the Sea," Trans. of the Drugs from the Sea Symp., Univ. of Rhode Island, 1967 (H. D. Freudenthal, ed.), pp. 73–86. Mar. Technol. Soc., Washington, D.C.

Burke, J. M., Marchisotto, J., McLaughlin, J. J. A., and Provasoli, L. (1960). Analysis of the toxin produced by *Gonyaulax catenella* in axenic culture. *Ann. N.Y. Acad. Sci.* **90**, 837–842.

Chambers, J. S., and Magnusson, H. W. (1950). Seasonal variations in toxicity of butter clams from selected Alaska beaches. *U.S. Fish Wildl. Serv.,* **53**, 1–9. *Spec. Sci. Rep., Fish.*

Clark, R. B. (1968). Biological causes and effects of paralytic shellfish poisoning. *Lancet* **ii**, 770–772.

Cleland, J. B., and Southcott, R. V. (1965). Injuries to man from marine invertebrates in the Australian region. *National Health and Medical Research Council, Special Report Series* **12**, 282 pp.

Connell, C. H., and Cross, J. B. (1950). Mass mortality of fish associated with the protozoan *Gonyaulax* in the Gulf of Mexico. *Science* **112**, 359–363.

Coulson, J. C., Potts, G. R., Deans, I. R., and Fraser, S. M. (1968). Mortality of shags and other sea birds caused by paralytic shellfish poison. *Nature (London)* **220**, 23–24.

Cummins, J. M., and Stevens, A. A. (1970). Investigations on *Gymnodinium breve* toxins in shellfish. *U.S. Public Health Service, Environmental Health Service, Gulf Coast Water Hygiene Laboratory, Dauphin Island, Alabama* 76 pp.

Cummins, J. M., Stevens, A. A., Huntley, B. E., Hill, W. F., Jr., and Higgins, J. E. (1968). Some properties of *Gymnodinium breve* toxin(s) determined bioanalytically in mice. *In* "Drugs from the Sea," Trans. of the Drugs from the Sea Symp., Univ. of Rhode Island, 1967 (H. D. Freudenthal, ed.), pp. 213–228. Mar. Technol. Soc., Washington, D.C.

Dassow, J. A. (1966). Processing detoxification. *In* "Proceedings, Joint Sanitation Seminar on North Pacific Clams," Juneau, Alaska, 1965 (W. A. Felsing, Jr., ed.), p. 12. Alaska Dep. Health and Welfare, U.S. Pub. Health Serv., Washington, D.C.

de Sousa e Silva, E. (1963). Les "red waters" a la Lagune D'Óbidos. Ses causes probables et ses rapports avec la toxicité des bivalves. *Proc. 4th Int. Seaweed Symp. Biarritz, 1961* pp. 265–275.

dos Santos Pinto, J., and de Sousa e Silva, E. (1956). The toxicity of *Cardium edule* L. and its possible relation to the dinoflagellate *Prorocentrum micans* Ehr. *Notas e Estudos Instituto Biologia Maritima* **12**, 20 pp.

Dupuy, J. L. (1968). Isolation, culture and ecology of a source of paralytic shellfish toxin in Sequim Bay, Washington. Ph.D. Thesis, Univ. of Washington, Seattle, Washington.

Eldred, B., Steidinger, K., and Williams, J. (1964). Preliminary studies of the relation of *Gymnodinium breve* counts to shellfish toxicity. *In* "A Collection of Data in Reference to Red Tide Outbreaks During 1963," pp. 23–52. Mar. Lab., Fla. Bd. of Conserv., St. Petersburg, Florida.

Evans, M. H. (1967). Block of sensory nerve conduction in the cat by mussel poison and tetrodotoxin. *In* "Animal Toxins" (F. E. Russell and P. R. Saunders, eds.), pp. 97–108. Macmillan (Pergamon), New York.

Evans, M. H. (1969a). Mechanism of saxitoxin and tetrodotoxin poisoning. *Brit. Med. Bull.* **25**, 263–267.

Evans, M. H. (1969b). Spinal reflexes in cat after feeding intravenous saxitoxin and tetrodotoxin. *Toxicon* **7**, 131–138.

Felsing, W. A., Jr., ed. (1966). "Proceedings, Joint Sanitation Seminar on North Pacific Clams," Juneau, 1965. Alaska Dep. Health and Welfare, U.S. Pub. Health Serv., Washington, D.C.

Gates, J. A., and Wilson, W. B. (1960). The toxicity of *Gonyaulax monilata* Howell to *Mugil cephalus*. *Limnol. Oceanogr.* **5**, 171–174.

Gemmill, J. S., and Manderson, W. B. (1960). Neurotoxic mussel poisoning. *Lancet* **ii**, 307–309.

Goggins, P. L. (1958). Paralytic shellfish survey, Maine—1958. *In* "Proceedings, 1958 Shellfish Sanitation Workshop" (E. T. Jensen, ed.), Appendix G, pp. 59–63. U.S. Pub. Health Serv., Washington, D.C.

Goggins, P. L. (1961). Paralytic shellfish poison. *In* "Proceedings, 1961 Shellfish Sanitation Workshop" (E. T. Jensen, ed.), Appendix W, pp. 252–265. U.S. Pub. Health Serv., Washington, D.C.

Grindley, J. R., and Nel, E. (1968) Mussel poisoning and shellfish mortality on the west coast of South Africa. *S. Afr. J. Sci.* **64**, 420–422.

Grindley, J. R., and Sapeika, N. (1969). The cause of mussel poisoning in South Africa. *S. Afr. Med. J.* **43**, 275–279.

Gunter, G., Williams, R. H., Davis, C. C., and Smith, F. G. W. (1948). Catastrophic mass mortality of marine animals and coincident phytoplankton bloom on the west coast of Florida, November 1946 to August 1947. *Ecol. Monogr.* **18**, 309–324.

Halstead, B. W. (1965). "Poisonous and Venomous Marine Animals of the World; Invertebrates," Vol. 1, 994 pp. U.S. Govt. Printing Office, Washington, D.C.

Halstead, B. W. (1967). "Poisonous and Venomous Marine Animals of the World; Vertebrates," Vol. 2, 1070 pp. U.S. Govt. Printing Office, Washington, D.C.

Hashimoto, Y., Kanna, K., and Shiokawa, A. (1950). On shell-fish poisons. II. Paralytic poison (preliminary report). *Nippon Suisan Gakkaishi* **15**, 771–776.

Hashimoto, Y., Konosu, S., Yasumoto, T., Inoue, A., and Noguchi, T. (1967). Occurrence of toxic crabs in Ryukyu and Amami Islands. *Toxicon* **5**, 85–90.

Hashimoto, Y., Konosu, S., Inoue, A., Saisho, T., and Miyake, S. (1969). Screening of toxic crabs in the Ryukyu and Amami Islands. *Nippon Suisan Gakkaishi* **35**, 83–87.

Hsu, B. C. C. (1967). Study of paralytic shellfish toxicity causative organisms in the State of Washington, 129 pp. M.S. Thesis, Univ. of Washington, Seattle, Washington.

Ingham, H. R., Mason, J., and Wood, P. C. (1968). Distribution of toxin in molluscan shellfish following the occurrence of mussel toxicity in north-east England. *Nature (London)* **220**, 25–27.

Inoue, A., Noguchi, T., Konosu, S., and Hashimoto, Y. (1968). A new toxic crab, *Atergatis floridus*. *Toxicon* **6**, 119–123.

Jackim, E., and Gentile, J. (1968). Toxins of a blue-green alga: similarity to saxitoxin. *Science* **162**, 915–916.

Jensen, E. T., ed. (1959). "Proceedings of the Shellfish Sanitation Workshop," 72 pp. U.S. Pub. Health Serv.; Washington, D.C.

Johnson, H. J., and Mulberry, G. (1966). Paralytic shellfish poison: serological assay by passive haemagglutination and bentonite flocculations. *Nature (London)* **211**, 747–748.

Kao, C. Y. (1966). Tetrodotoxin, saxitoxin and their significance in the study of excitation phenomena. *Pharmacol. Rev.* **18**, 997–1049.

Kao, C. Y. (1967). Comparison of the biological actions of tetrodotoxin and saxitoxin. *In* "Animal Toxins" (F. E. Russell and P. R. Saunders, eds.), pp. 109–114. Macmillan (Pergamon), New York.

Kawabata, T., Yoshida, T., and Kubota, Y. (1962). Paralytic shellfish poison. I. A note on the shellfish poisoning occurred in Ofunato City, Iwate Prefecture in May, 1961. *Nippon Suisan Gakkaishi* **28**, 344–351.

Koch, H. J. (1939). La cause des Empoisonnements Paralytiques Provoqués par les Moules. *Ass. Franc. Avan. Sci., 63rd Sess., Seances Sect., Liége.*

Konosu, S., Inoue, A., Noguchi, T., and Hashimoto, Y. (1968). Comparison of crab toxin with saxitoxin and tetrodotoxin. *Toxicon* **6**, 113–117.

Lehman, C. (1966). Clam resources of Alaska. *In* "Proceedings, Joint Sanitation

Seminar on North Pacific Clams," Juneau, 1965 (W. A. Felsing, Jr., ed.), p. 34. Alaska Dep. Health and Welfare, U.S. Pub. Health Serv., Washington, D.C.

Link, V. B. (1962). Epidemiological report: paralytic shellfish poisoning from oysters—California. *Morbidity and Mortality Weekly Report* **11**, 256. Nat. Communicable Dis. Center, Atlanta, Georgia.

McCollum, J. P. K., Pearson, R. C. M., Ingham, H. R., Wood, P. C., and Dewar, H. A. (1968). An epidemic of mussel poisoning in northeast England. *Lancet* **ii**, 767–770.

McFarren, E. F. (1959). Report on collaborative studies of the bioassay for paralytic shellfish poison. *J. Ass. Offic. Agr. Chem.* **42**, 263–271.

McFarren, E. F., Schafer, M. L., Campbell, J. E., Lewis, K. H., Jensen, E. T., and Schantz, E. J. (1957). Public health significance of paralytic shellfish poison: a review of literature and unpublished research. *Proc. Nat. Shellfish. Ass.* **47**, 114–141.

McFarren, E. F., Schantz, E. J., Campbell, J. E., and Lewis, K. H. (1958). Chemical determination of paralytic shellfish poison in clams. *J. Ass. Offic. Agr. Chem.* **41**, 168–177.

McFarren, E. F., Schafer, M. L., Campbell, J. E., Lewis, K. H., Jensen, E. T., and Schantz, E. J. (1960). Public health significance of paralytic shellfish poison. *Advan. Food Res.* **10**, 135–179.

McFarren, E. F., Tanabe, H., Silva, F. J., Wilson, W. B., Campbell, J. E., and Lewis, K. H. (1965). The occurrence of a ciguatera-like poison in oysters, clams and *Gymnodinium breve* cultures. *Toxicon* **3**, 111–123.

Medcof, J. C. (1960). Shellfish poisoning—another North American ghost. *Can. Med. Ass. J.* **82**, 87–90.

Medcof, J. C., Leim, A. H., Needler, A. B., and Needler, A. W. H. (1947). Paralytic shellfish poisoning on the Canadian Atlantic Coast. *Bull., Fish. Res. Bd. Can.* **75**, 32 pp.

Medcof, J. C., Morin, N., Nadeau, A., and Lachance, A. (1966). Survey of incidence and risks of paralytic shellfish poisoning in the Province of Quebec. *Fish. Res. Bd. Can., Misc. Rep. Ser.* (*Biol.*) **886**.

Meyer, K. F., Sommer, H., and Schoenholz, P. (1928). Mussel poisoning. *J. Prev. Med.* **2**, 365–394.

Mold, J. D., Bowden, J. P., Stanger, D. W., Maurer, J. E., Lynch, J. M., Wyler, R., Schantz, E. J., and Riegel, B. (1957). Paralytic shellfish poison. VII. Evidence of the purity of the poison isolated from toxic clams and mussels. *J. Amer. Chem. Soc.* **79**, 5235.

Morton, R. A., and Burklew, M. A. (1969). Florida shellfish toxicity following blooms of the dinoflagellate *Gymnodinium breve. Florida Department of Natural Resources, Technical Series* **60**, 26 pp.

Murtha, E. F. (1960). Pharmacological study of poisons from shellfish and puffer fish. *Ann. N.Y. Acad. Sci.* **90**, 615–950.

Nakazima, M. (1965a). Studies on the source of shellfish poison in Lake Hamana. I. Relation of the abundance of a species of dinoflagellata, *Prorocentrum* sp. to shellfish toxicity. *Nippon Suisan Gakkaishi* **31**, 198–203.

Nakazima, M. (1965b). Studies on the source of shellfish poison in Lake Hamana. II. Shellfish toxicity during the "Red-Tide." *Nippon Suisan Gakkaishi* **31**, 204–207.

Nakazima, M. (1965c). Studies on the source of shellfish poison in Lake Hamana.

III. Poisonous effects of shellfishes feeding in *Prorocentrum* sp. *Nippon Suisan Gakkaishi* **31**, 281–285.

Nakazima, M. (1968). Studies on the source of shellfish poison in Lake Hamana. IV. Identification and collection of the noxious dinoflagellates. *Nippon Suisan Gakkaishi* **34**, 130–132.

Neal, R. A. (1967). Fluctuations in the levels of paralytic shellfish toxin in four species of Lamellibranch molluscs near Ketchikan, Alaska, 1963–1965. 149 pp. Ph.D. Thesis, Univ. of Washington, Seattle, Washington.

Needler, A. B. (1949). Paralytic shellfish poisoning and *Goniaulax tamarensis*. *J. Fish. Res. Bd. Can.* **7**, 490–504.

Noguchi, T., Konosu, S., and Hashimoto, Y. (1969). Identity of the crab toxin with saxitoxin. *Toxicon* **7**, 325–326.

Oftebro, T. (1965). Occurrence of paralytic shellfish poison in mussels (*Mytilus edulis* L.) from Norwegian waters, 1964. *Nord. Veterinaermed.* **17**, 467–477.

Prakash, A. (1963). Source of paralytic shellfish toxin in the Bay of Fundy. *J. Fish. Res. Bd. Can.* **20**, 983–996.

Prakash, A. (1966). Physiological ecology of the causative organism including mechanisms of toxin accumulation in shellfish. *In* "Proceedings, Joint Sanitation Seminar on North Pacific Clams," Juneau, 1965 (W. A. Felsing, Jr., ed.), p. 34. Alaska Dep. Health and Welfare, U.S. Pub. Health Serv., Washington, D.C.

Prakash, A., and Medcof, J. C. (1962). Hydrographic and meteorologic factors affecting shellfish toxicity at Head Harbour, New Brunswick. *J. Fish. Res. Bd. Can.* **19**, 101–112.

Prakash, A., and Taylor, F. J. R. (1966). A "red water" bloom of *Gonyaulax acatenella* in the Strait of Georgia and its relation to paralytic shellfish poisoning. *J. Fish. Res. Bd. Can.* **23**, 1265–1270.

Pringle, B. H. (1966). Analytical procedures for paralytic shellfish poison. *In* "Proceedings, Joint Sanitation Seminar on North Pacific Clams," Juneau, 1965 (W. A. Felsing, Jr., ed.), pp. 16–17. Alaska Dep. Health and Welfare, U.S. Pub. Health Serv., Washington, D.C.

Quayle, D. B. (1966). Seasonal and geographic distribution of toxin in Alaska and British Columbia clams. *In* "Proceedings, Joint Sanitation Seminar on North Pacific Clams," Juneau, 1965 (W. A. Felsing, Jr., ed.), pp. 7–8. Alaska Dep. Health and Welfare, U.S. Pub. Health Serv., Washington, D.C.

Quayle, D. B. (1969). Paralytic shellfish poisoning in British Columbia. *Bull., Fish. Res. Bd. Can.* **168**, 68 pp.

Rapoport, H., Brown, M. S., Oesterlin, R., and Schuett, W. (1964). Papers of the 147th National Meeting of the American Chemical Society, Philadelphia, Pennsylvania, April (Abstr.)

Ray, S. M., and Aldrich, D. V. (1965). *Gymnodinium breve:* induction of shellfish poisoning in chicks. *Science* **148**, 1748–1749.

Ray, S. M., and Aldrich, D. V. (1967). Ecological interactions of toxic dinoflagellates and molluscs in the Gulf of Mexico. *In* "Animal Toxins" (F. E. Russell and P. R. Saunders, eds.), pp. 75–83. Macmillan (Pergamon), New York.

Ray, S. M., and Wilson, W. B. (1957). Effects of unialgal and bacteria-free cultures of *Gymnodinium brevis* on fish. *U.S. Fish Wildl. Serv., Fish. Bull. 123* **57**, 469–496.

Robinson, G. A. (1968). Distribution of *Gonyaulax tamarensis* Lebour in the western North Sea in April, May and June 1968. *Nature (London)* **220**, 22–23.

Russell, F. E. (1965). Marine toxins and venomous and poisonous marine animals. *Advan. Mar. Biol.* 3, 255–384.

Schantz, E. J. (1960). Biochemical studies on paralytic shellfish poisons. *Ann. N.Y. Acad. Sci.* **90**, 843–855.

Schantz, E. J. (1966). Chemical studies on shellfish poisons. *In* "Proceedings, Joint Sanitation Seminar on North Pacific Clams," Juneau, 1965 (W. A. Felsing, Jr., ed.), pp. 18–21. Alaska Dep. Health and Welfare, U.S. Pub. Health Serv., Washington, D.C.

Schantz, E. J. (1967). Biochemical studies on purified *Gonyaulax catenella* poison. *In* "Animal Toxins" (F. E. Russell and P. R. Saunders, eds.), pp. 91–95. Macmillan (Pergamon), New York.

Schantz, E. J. (1969). Studies on shellfish poisons. *Agr. Food Chem.* **17**, 413–416.

Schantz, E. J., and Magnusson, H. W. (1964). Observations on the origin of the paralytic poison in Alaska butter clams. *J. Protozool.* **11**, 239–242.

Schantz, E. J., Mold, J. D., Stanger, D. W., Shavel, J., Riel, F. J., Bowden, J. P., Lynch, J. M., Wyler, R., Riegel, B., and Sommer, H. (1957). Paralytic shellfish poison. VI. A procedure for the isolation and purification of the poison from toxic clam and mussel tissues. *J. Amer. Chem. Soc.* **79**, 5230.

Schantz, E. F., McFarren, E. F., Schafer, M. L., and Lewis, K. H. (1958). Purified shellfish poison for bioassay standardization. *J. Ass. Offic. Agr. Chem.* **41**, 160–168.

Schantz, E. J., Lynch, J. M., Vayvada, G., Matsumoto, K., and Rapoport, H. (1966). The purification and characterization of the poison produced by *Gonyaulax catenella* in axenic culture. *Biochemistry* **5**, 1191–1195.

Schradie, J., and Bliss, C. A. (1962). The cultivation and toxicity of *Gonyaulax polyedra*. *Lloydia* **25**, 214–221.

Sievers, A. M. (1969). Comparative toxicity of *Gonyaulax monilata* and *Gymnodinium breve* to annelids, crustaceans, molluscs and a fish. *J. Protozool.* **16**, 401–404.

Sommer, H., and Meyer, K. F. (1937). Paralytic shell-fish poisoning. *Arch. Pathol.* **24**, 560–598.

Sommer, H., Whedon, W. F., Kofoid, C. A., and Stohler, R. (1937). Relation of paralytic shell-fish poison to certain plankton organisms of the genus *Gonyaulax*. *Arch. Pathol.* **24**, 537–559.

Sparks, A. K. (1966). Physiological ecology of the causative organisms including mechanisms of toxin accumulation in shellfish. *In* "Proceedings, Joint Sanitation Seminar on North Pacific Clams," Juneau, 1965 (W. A. Felsing, Jr., ed.), pp. 10–11. Alaska Dep. Health and Welfare, U.S. Pub. Health Serv., Washington, D.C.

Sparks, A. K., and Sribhibhadh, A. (1961). Status of paralytic shellfish toxicity studies in Washington. *In* "Proceedings of the Shellfish Sanitation Workshop," (E. T. Jensen, ed.), pp. 266–269. U.S. Pub. Health Serv., Washington, D.C.

Sribhibhadh, A. (1963). Seasonal variations of paralytic shellfish toxicity in the California mussel, *Mytilus californianus* Conrad, and the Pacific oyster, *Crassostrea gigas* (Thunberg), along the Strait of Juan de Fuca and in Willapa Bay. 157 pp. Ph.D. Thesis, Univ. of Washington, Seattle, Washington.

Woloszynska, J., and Conrad, W. (1939). *Pyrodinium phoneus* n. sp., agent de la Toxicité des Moules du Canal Maritime de Bruges à Zeebrugge. *Bull. Mus. Hist. Natur. Belg.* **15**, 1–5.

Wood, P. C. (1968). Dinoflagellate crop in the North Sea. *Nature* (*London*) **220**, 21–27.

Small, Free-Living Amebas: Cultivation, Quantitation, Identification, Classification, Pathogenesis, and Resistance

Shih L. Chang[1]

ENVIRONMENTAL CONTROL ADMINISTRATION,
PUBLIC HEALTH SERVICE,
U.S. DEPARTMENT OF HEALTH, EDUCATION, AND WELFARE,
CINCINNATI, OHIO

[1] Present address: Environmental Protection Agency, Division of Water Hygiene, 5555 Ridge Avenue, Cincinnati, Ohio.

I. Introduction

Small, free-living amebas attracted little attention in the period between the establishment of families under the order Amoebida (Wenyon, 1926) and the systematic treatment on a phylogenic basis by Singh (1952). It is worth noting that Singh's important taxonomic work exerted very little influence on authors describing this group of amebas in textbooks and reference books on protozoa in general and Sarcodina in particular prior to 1968.

Some excitement resulted when free-living amebas, loosely named *Acanthamoeba,* were found to contaminate tissue cultures (Jahnes *et al.,* 1957; Chi *et al.,* 1959), and a similar isolate was found to produce meningoencephalitis in mice and monkeys (Culbertson *et al.,* 1959). Clinical interests were aroused by the isolation of *Hartmannella* spp., including *Acanthamoeba,* in tissue cultures used in the survey of children's throats for viruses (Wang and Feldman, 1961, 1967). Some "virus" isolates of throat origin were later identified as amebas of the *Acanthamoeba* genus (Armstrong and Pereira, 1967; Chang *et al.,* 1966; Little and Chang, 1968).

Public health significance was established when three cases of primary meningoencephalitis were reported from Orlando, Florida (Butt, 1966), with one more case added later (Butt *et al.,* 1968). The significance attained worldwide recognition when 6 similar cases were reported from South Australia (Fowler and Carter, 1965; Carter, 1968) and 17 cases from Czechoslovakia (Červa and Novăk, 1968; Červa *et al.,* 1969).

The series of episodes reached a climax in 1968–1969 with the occurrence of three cases of amebic meningoencephalitis in the Richmond, Virginia area (Callicott *et al.,* 1968; Duma *et al.,* 1969), and a disclosure of nine more cases in the same area between 1951 and 1966 in a retrospective study of hospital records (Nelson, personal communication, 1969). Four additional cases were added to the list after further study of case records (Duma, Virginia Medical College, Richmond, personal communication). Very recently, a fatal case of primary amebic meningoencephalitis was reported (McCroan *et al.,* 1970) to have occurred in a 7-year-old boy in Atlanta, Georgia. The case had a history of swimming in both a municipal pool and a lake prior to the onset of the disease, and amebas were found in the brain abscess at autopsy.

Symmers (1969) briefly reviewed the occurrence of amebic meningoencephalitis and reported three probable cases in Britain. Two cases were disclosed in a retrospective study of hospital records and pathological specimens, one in an Essex boy in 1909 and the other in a Belfast girl in 1937. He mentioned a third case (report in Times, 13 August 1969) in one of two brothers who developed meningitis and recovered on amphotericin B, but *Naegleria gruberi* was isolated from the cerebrospinal fluid of one of them. Appley *et al.* (1970) further reported three cases, two of which were the brothers mentioned in Symmer's report and the third one, a boy who lived three doors away from the two brothers. The younger brother died after 15 days of illness, and *Naegleria* ameba was isolated from his cerebrospinal fluid and a very small ameba from brain substance obtained at autopsy. The elder brother was hospitalized two days after his brother. *Naegleria* amebas were isolated from his C.S.F. on the eighth day of illness but he recovered after amphotericin B therapy. The third case was hospitalized six days after the first case and recovered on amphotericin B treatment without evidence of amebic infection. Warhurst *et al.* (1970) reported on the *Naegleria* sp. isolated from the C.S.F. of the first case, but indicated that the very small ameba isolated from the brain material could be a contaminant.

Several points of interest in these episodes deserve mention. First, all cases gave a history of swimming in small, warm lakes (Orlando and Richmond), a polluted warm estuary (South Australia), or an indoor swimming pool (Czechoslovakia). A case of *Acanthamoeba* meningoencephalitis was reported (Padras and Andujar, 1966) to have developed in a hospital patient who suffered liver damage after a tooth extraction. This infection was likely a complication when resistance was greatly reduced.

Second, *Acanthamoeba* was believed to be the causative agent in those episodes reported in and before the early part of 1968; this belief was apparently influenced by the pathological findings obtained in laboratory animals inoculated with *Acanthamoeba* or *Hartmannella* amebas

(Culbertson *et al.*, 1958, 1959; Culbertson, 1961). In all the cases reported in and after the latter part of 1968, *Naegleria gruberi* was shown to be the etiological agent. It is generally believed that all the swimming-associated cases of amebic meningoencephalitis so far reported were caused by this ameba.

Third, the swimming-associated cases of meningoencephalitis were all fatal. The incubation period was not well defined in most cases, but was 7 days in the two Richmond, Virginia cases (Callicott *et al.*, 1968; Duma *et al.*, 1969). The clinical course was amazingly consistent in that 4–5 days elapsed between onset of symptoms and death. Antibiotics were ineffective in altering the course of the disease (Butt *et al.*, 1968; Carter, 1968; Callicott *et al.*, 1968; Cĕrva *et al.*, 1969), as were antiamebic chemotherapeutic drugs (Carter, 1968; Duma *et al.*, 1969).

Fourth, most investigators revealed diving activities in the history of the swimming-associated cases of meningoencephalitis and were led to the belief that introduction of *N. gruberi*–laden water into the upper nasal cavity and subsequent cranial invasion via nasal mucosa and cribriform plate constituted the likely route of infection. In fact, Carter (1968) observed inflammation and ulceration of the nasal olfactory mucosa and the presence of amebas in nasal discharge, and Callicott and his associates (1968) reported that the nasal olfactory mucosa was focally hemorrhagic and infiltrated with lymphocytes and plasma cells. Penetration into nasal olfactory mucosa by amebas was also observed in mice after nasal instillation of the latter (Culbertson *et al.*, 1959, 1966).

Many factors remain to be ascertained in understanding the "cluster" occurrence of cases of this disease in four geographic areas. In numerous examinations of surface waters and sewage effluents, small, free-living amebas were found to be the largest single group of nonpigmented microfauna and, of this group two species, namely, *Acanthamoeba rhysodes* and *N. gruberi,* were the most frequently encountered (S. L. Chang, unpublished observations). Of particular interest was the recovery of these two amebas in two outdoor swimming pools in the Cincinnati area in August 1969 (also S. L. Chang, unpublished observations). The density of *A. rhysodes* ranged from 2 to 30/gal of water and that of *N. gruberi* from 1 to 10/gal; their densities in surface waters in the same area were at least 20 times as high.

What factors existing in the four areas were responsible for the occurrence of clusters of cases? Do there exist pathogenic and nonpathogenic strains of *N. gruberi?* Could cases of meningoencephalitis have occurred among a much larger number of asymptomatic cases of nasopharyngeal infection, somewhat analogous to that of poliovirus? What ecological factors existed in the lakes in Orlando and Richmond and in the South Australian estuary were responsible for the disease? Why should an indoor swimming pool be involved in the occurrence of the disease unless the pool was improperly operated and free-living amebas were growing on the pool wall? Is there a critical *N. gruberi* density in water above which the chances of precipitating a nasal infection become great? Can other free-living amebas, especially those in the Schizopyrenidae family, also become pathogenic to man?

To carry out studies that can answer these and related questions, methods are required for isolating, enumerating, cultivating, and identifying free-living amebas recovered from various waters and in a nasopharyngeal survey. A practical classification is required for identification to avoid the use of different names for the same ameba. Different strains of *N. gruberi* and other species of amebas so isolated, if necessary, should be studied for their pathogenicity in both cell cultures and laboratory animals.

This chapter describes the methods that have been developed in our laboratory for such studies and presents the data obtained with these methods. In addition, it describes studies made on cultural characteristics, cytopathogenicity in cell cultures, pathogenesis in laboratory animals, and resistance to antibiotics and chemical agents of different strains and species of small, free-living amebas to see if any of these characteristics can be used to supplement the limited morphological and cytological criteria of ameba identification and classification. Based on the findings of these studies, the classification proposed by Singh (1952) has been modified and the modified classification is presented.

II. Materials and Methods

A. *Free-Living Amebas*

Four wild and four pathogenic strains of *N. gruberi*, two strains of *A. rhysodes*, and one strain each of *Schizopyrenus erythaenusa*, *Hartmannella gelbae*, *H. agricola*, and *Singhella* (*Hartmannella*) *leptocnemus* were employed in this study. In addition, six strains of a small schizopyrenid, tentatively identified as *Schizopyrenus russelli* (SR_1, SR_2, SR_3, SR_4, SR_5, and SR_6), were received from Dr. R. J. Duma of the Virginia Medical College in April 1970 and were included in the study.

Naegleria gruberi strain NG_2 was isolated from water from a Mississippi well in 1962 and had been maintained on buffered sucrose tryptose (BST) agar in association with *Aerobacter aerogenes* ever since. Its flagellate-transforming capacity had, however, been retained in the original state by refrigeration of well-developed cultures and making transfers at 3- to 4-month intervals. Strains NG_4, NG_6, and NG_7 were isolated from outdoor swimming pools in Greater Cincinnati in August 1969.

Three pathogenic strains of *Naegleria gruberi* (HB_1, HB_2, and HB_3) were obtained through the courtesy of Dr. C. G. Culbertson of the Lilly Research Laboratories. Strains HB_1 and HB_2 were isolated from patients in Orlando (Butt, 1966; Butt *et al.*, 1968), and had been carried in MK cell cultures for 2½ and 1½ years, respectively, before they were received in December 1969. Strain HB_3 was isolated from a patient in Czechoslovakia (Červa *et al.*, 1969) and had been grown in MK cell cultures for less than 1 year at the Lilly Research Laboratories.

The fourth pathogenic strain (NG_8) was obtained through the courtesy of Dr. R. J. Duma; it was isolated from a patient in July 1969 (Duma *et al.*, 1969). The bacterium associate in the culture on inorganic agar was identified as *Bordetella bronchoseptica* by Mr. B. Kenner of the Cincinnati Water Research Laboratory. When this strain was introduced into MK cell cultures in December 1969, it grew poorly because of the lack of cytopathic effect (CPE) to lyse MK cells for food and lack of encystment to tide over the long waiting period prior to autolytic degeneration. By adding a few drops per tube of a filtrate from a culture of strain HB_1 at the time of transfer, better growth of the amebas was obtained after each transfer. After the fourth transfer rich cultures were maintained with morphology and CPE indistinguishable from those of the HB strains.

One strain of *A. rhysodes*, AR_1, was isolated in 1959 by Dr. S. S. Wang of the Syracuse University Medical Center (Wang and Feldman, 1961) and sent to us for identification. It has been maintained in a calf serum–casein fluid medium (Chang *et al.*, 1960) ever since. The other strain AR_2, was received in 1967 from Dr. R. S. Chang, then of the Harvard School of Public Health, and was also carried in the same fluid medium. This strain was first described as a "lipovirus–ameba cell" complex (Chang *et al.*, 1966; Liu and Rodina, 1966) but later was referred to as a strain of *Acanthamoeba* (Little and Chang, 1968). Cultural, cytological, and fluorescent antibody (FA)–staining studies made in our laboratory identified it as a strain of *A. rhysodes*.

The strain of *S. erythaenusa* was isolated from a river water sample collected in Pennsylvania in the summer of 1969. The species was established from the schizopyrenid type of mitosis (see Section III,C), and the reddish pigment developed in cultures on BST agar grown with a number of gram-negative bacillary species of bacteria, not just with non-nutrient agar with *A. aerogenes* as reported by Singh (1952).

The strain of *H. glebae* has been described elsewhere (Chang, 1960). The strain of *H. agricola* was isolated in March 1969 from a river water sample collected in Pennsylvania. The strain of *S. leptocnemus* was isolated in February 1969 from scum scraped off the surface of a water tank supplying a small California town. The criteria for establishment of both species of amebas are given in Section III,C.

Six plate cultures of amebas were received from Dr. R. J. Duma in April 1970. They were isolated in March 1970 from Lake Chester where two cases of meningoencephalitis occurred in July 1969. Five of the isolates were apparently strains of a single species of ameba characterized by very small size (trophozoites 8–12 μ and cysts 7–10 μ), limax formation, high motility, no flagellate transformation, nucleolus origin of polar bodies, and lack of interzonal bodies in mitosis. Hence they were identified as *S. russelli* (see Section III,C). The strains were designated SR_P, SR_2, SR_3, SR_4, SR_6, and SR_7 (P for pier and numerals for the distances from the pier where the samples were taken). The plate culture from which strain SR_2 was isolated contained another ameba which was identified as *A. rhysodes*. Only the SR strains were included in the study.

Stock cultures of all species of amebas used in the study were maintained on BST agar with one bacterium associate or another, and cultures showing mass encystment were refrigerated to preserve the original characteristics of the amebas.

Cultivation of the three HB strains of *N. gruberi* in MK cell cultures has continued since their arrival in December 1969. The fourth pathogenic strain of *N. gruberi* (NG_8) and the six strains of *S. russelli* have been carried in MK cell cultures since March 1970. The four wild strains of *N. gruberi* (NG_2, NG_4, NG_6, and NG_7) have been maintained in MK cell cultures since April 1970.

B. Bacterium Associates

A strain each of a *Pseudomonas* sp., *Zooglea ramigera* (both of sewage effluent origin), *Escherichia coli, Alcaligenes faecalis* (Chang, 1960), *Sarcina lutea* (Chang, 1958a), and *B. bronchoseptica* (original bacterium associate of *N. gruberi* strain NG_8) were used at one time or another as associates in plate cultures of amebas. They were also employed in determining ameba concentrations by the plaque-count method.

C. Cell Cultures

MK cell cultures were prepared with both African green and rhesus monkey kidney cells in roller and Leighton tubes. The procedure for preparing tube cultures has been described elsewhere (Chang *et al.*, 1958). HeLa cells were obtained through the courtesy of Dr. R. Sullivan, Milk Sanitation Research Section, Food and Drug Administration, Public Health Service, and cultures were also prepared in both roller and Leighton tubes using medium L-25 with 10% fetal calf serum in the growth medium and 2% in the maintenance medium. Penicillin, streptomycin, and tetracycline were used in all cell culture media at concentrations of 50 μg each per milliliter.

D. BST Agar

The preparation of BST agar has been previously described (Chang, 1958a). In essence, it is a phosphate-buffered agar containing 1% sucrose and 0.2% tryptose (pH 7.4–7.5). Higher concentrations of tryptose are tolerated by *A. rhysodes* but are growth inhibiting to all other small, free-living amebas. To minimize the drying effect on prolonged incubation, plates were poured with 25 ml of the agar per dish.

A serum–fresh yeast extract–antibiotic BST (SYEABST) agar was used to obtain bacteria-free amebas for seeding cell cultures and for preparing axenic cultures in fluid media. The medium was prepared in the following manner.

Equal volumes of fresh calf serum, heated calf serum (80° C for 1 hour to coagulate proteins), and fresh yeast extract (obtainable commercially as a 25% frozen solution) are mixed with enough penicillin, streptomycin, and tetracycline to give final concentrations of 500 μg each per ml. When plates are poured with 2.5 ml of the mixture and 25 ml of melted BST agar per petri dish, the final concentrations of the antibiotics become 45 μg each per milliliter.

A serum–casein fluid (SCF) medium, which was prepared for axenic cultivation of free-living nematodes (Chang *et al.*, 1960) and contained 1 part of heated calf serum (75° C for $\frac{1}{2}$ hour) and 9 parts of phosphate-buffered 0.2% casein solution, was modified by replacing the serum with the serum–yeast extract mixture described above. This modification, abbreviated SYECF, was dispensed in 8-ml amounts in 25-cm^2 culture T flasks.

E. Procedures

The various procedures used in isolation, cultivation, enumeration, identification, determining CPE, FA staining, growth rate determination, and ascertaining resistance to antiamebic agents are described in the following discussion.

F. Isolation, Cultivation, and Enumeration

Small, free-living amebas grow well on BST agar in association with many gram-negative species of bacillary bacteria (Chang, 1960). Samples of small sizes—1 or 2 liters—were concentrated by the membrane filter technique (Chang and Kabler, 1956); the filtration rate could be greatly increased by replacing the HA-type membrane with one of 5-μ-pore size. The fiberglass prefilter was found equally satisfactory for concentrating small amebas. Large samples, as in the case of swimming pool water, were concentrated with a 5-μ membrane or fiberglass prefilter 90–142 mm in diameter. Samples of highly turbid water were prestrained through a 25-μ metal strainer to remove large particulate matter and organisms.

After the filtration process was completed, each membrane was removed from the holder and placed on the wall of a sterile beaker of suitable size; the membrane was flushed repeatedly with sterile dilution water with the aid of a capillary pipet; 5, 10, and 25 ml of water were used for washing membranes 47-, 90-, and 142-mm in diameter, respectively. When ameba concentrations were low, the washings were centrifuged at 1000 rpm for 15 minutes and the sediments were suspended in suitable amounts of water. A direct microscopic examination of 1 drop or more of each final concentrate was made as a preliminary survey of both density and types of amebas.

For accurate determination of ameba density and for isolation of individual species, a plaque count method has been developed. It is based on the fact that when a mixed suspension containing a high concentration of bacteria and a small number of amebas is smeared uniformly on a BST agar plate the amebas develop into a colony by multiplying and feeding on the bacteria. When the bacteria supply is so consumed by the amebas as to leave an area cleared (not completely) of bacterial cells, a plaque is formed. The clearness of the plaque, the incubation time required for the formation of plaques, and the outline and shape of plaques depend on the species of bacteria and the growth and motility characteristics of individual amebas. Using a single species of bacteria, the plaque characteristics can be used as preliminary criteria for differentiating different genera or even species. For instance, the appearance of a reddish pigment in a plaque indicates the ameba to be S. *erythaenusa.*

To prepare for plaque count, an ameba concentration is diluted with a thick suspension of bacteria to give a final ameba density of 10 to 30 per drop from a calibrated capillary pipet; 1, 2, 3, and 4 drops of the mixture are pipetted separately onto four poured BST agar plates. Drops of the same bacterial suspension but without the amebas are pipetted in a reversed order so that each plate receives a total of 5 drops. The inocula are evenly smeared over the entire surface of the plates with sterile glass rods shaped as golf clubs. After about 1 hour's standing to allow absorption of excessive fluid, the plates are inverted and incubated at 25° or 35° C. Examination of plates for the appearance of plaques is made daily, and enumeration of plaques is made with a Quebec counter.

Similar to virus plaques, ameba plaques do not all appear at once; but by marking the plaques as they are counted, errors introduced by coalescence can be avoided (Berg *et al.*, 1963). The density of each ameba identifiable by plaque appearance in the original sample is obtained by multiplying the average number of specific plaques per drop by the number of drops per milliliter and dividing the product by the concentration factor (number of liters per milliliter of concentrate).

To isolate individual amebas in pure cultures, plaques were examined directly under a microscope (100 to 125×) for morphological characteristics of the amebas, and those showing a different morphology were picked separately with sterile glass rods from the center of each plaque. Each inoculum was placed in the center of a BST agar plate presmeared with a selected bacterium associate. Subsequent transfers made with growth materials removed from the periphery of plates thus prepared yielded pure cultures of a single species of ameba and a single species of bacterium (Chang, 1958a).

G. Preparation of Cell Cultures of Amebas

Bacteria-free inocula were prepared by placing in the center of a SYEABST agar plate a small amount of growth material from a known plate culture of amebas. As the trophozoites moved away from the area of inoculation, the antibiotic-inhibited bacteria were left behind. While there was usually limited growth of the amebas on this enriched agar, enough organisms were generally found in the periphery. About $\frac{1}{2}$ ml of the maintenance medium was pipetted from a tube culture of MK cells and placed on the agar plate held at a 45° angle. With due precaution to avoid the center area, the amebic growth was washed off the agar surface below the center by repeated, gentle flushing, with the aid of a capillary pipet. The washing was then returned to the cell culture tube and incubated at 35° C for growth of the amebas.

H. Determination of the Nature of the CPE of Amebas

Most free-living amebas exhibit a CPE in HeLa cell cultures, and it is related to contact of the cells with trophozoites. HeLa cell cultures are not suitable for studying the CPE of these amebas. MK cells, however, are resistant to this effect, and their cultural life is unaffected by the presence of these amebas, except that cells that have phagocytized large numbers of amebic cysts may undergo autodegeneration a little earlier than those free of a heavy cyst burden (Chang, 1960).

As discussed later, this is not true of the pathogenic strains of *N. gruberi*, which exhibit marked a cytolytic effect on MK cells. In such cases it is essential to determine the origin and nature of the CPE. This was done by seeding MK cell cultures with varying numbers of amebas and parallel cultures with varying amounts of a filtrate (obtained with a Swinnex syringe) of the same culture from which the amebas were harvested. Unseeded MK cell cultures were used as controls. Both test and control cultures were examined daily for CPE.

The stability of the CPE agent to heat and on storage at room and refrigeration temperature, and in a frozen state, was ascertained by subjecting the culture material to the respective conditions and testing its CPE at various times during each treatment. Chemical identification of the agent was hampered by the rapid loss of the CPE when the culture material was subject to any separation process to isolate the agent.

I. Determination of Growth Rates of Amebas

Determination of the growth rate of each species of ameba in plate cultures on BST agar was made easier by using the plaque-count technique rather than the method used previously (Chang, 1958a). The procedure is as follows.

Eight plaque count plates are prepared with each species of ameba and a *Pseudomonas* sp., which makes the enumeration of amebas a little easier than with *B. bronchoseptica,* with each plate having not more than 20 amebas. The plates are examined under a microscope, and one ameba is selected in each plate for its suitable location and identified with a china pencil mark on the bottom of the dish. Four plates are incubated at 25° C and the other four at 35° C. Both incubators are saturated with moisture to avoid a drying effect. Enumeration of amebas is made twice a day for 2 days and daily thereafter for 2 days or more, depending on the rate of growth of the amebas.

The counts obtained from each of the four plates are averaged and the mean count is plotted against the respective time on semilog graph paper. The linear section of each growth curve is used to compute the growth rate constant k and the generation time g by equations described elsewhere (Chang and Negherbon, 1947). The standard deviations of the mean counts are computed by the conventional equation:

$$\text{D.S.} = \sqrt{\frac{E(\bar{x} - x)^2}{N}},$$

where $\bar{x}$ is the mean count, x is individual count, and N is the number of plates counted.

The growth rates of amebas in MK cell cultures were determined by seeding Leighton tube (without a thin slide) cultures in triplicate per strain with known numbers of amebas per inoculum. After 2 hour's standing to allow the amebas to settle and attach to the cell sheet on the rectangular area, the tubes were examined under a microscope to determine the number of organisms per rectangular area. During the period of incubation at 35° C, tubes that were seeded with the pathogenic strains of *N. gruberi* were enumerated daily for 5–6 days; tubes of all other strains were enumerated every other day for 2–3 weeks. The values of k and g and their standard deviations were computed in the same manner as those obtained for plate cultures.

J. Cytological Examination

In cytological examination of the pathogenic strains of *N. gruberi,* the thin slides in the Leighton tube cultures were removed at the peak of growth. Smears of all the other strains of amebas were prepared with growth material from BST agar plate cultures at their peak growth. Fresh preparations were examined immediately under a phase-contrast microscope, and dried smears were fixed in Schaudinn fluid, put through ethanol in decreasing concentration, and stained with either iron alum–hematoxylin or Feulgen stain (Gurr, 1962). All stained smears were examined under oil immersion for nuclear changes in mitosis.

K. *Flagellate Transformation*

Since flagellate transformation capacity of *N. gruberi* is at a peak in the cystic stage after a period of refrigeration (Chang, 1958b), all tests for this activity were made by suspending in water cysts of a strain of ameba that had been stored in a refrigerator for at least several days. Observations were made daily for flagellate transformation activity over a period of 2 weeks.

L. *FA Staining*

The FA-staining procedure was described in detail by Liu and Rodina (1966) in a study of the "lipovirus–ameba cell" complex which was later identified as a strain of *A. rhysodes,* as explained in a later report by Little and Chang (1968). In brief, it consists of obtaining hyperimmune antiserum in rabbits, separating globulin fractions by ammonium sulfate precipitation, and conjugating the globulin with fluorescein isocyanate.

To prepare amebas for FA staining, the thin slides in seeded Leighton tube cell cultures were removed at scheduled times during incubation. The slides were dried in a warm-air chamber and fixed in acetone. To the fixed slides was added the fluorescein-labeled antibody and, after a 30-minute staining at room temperature and a 10-minute rinsing with phosphate-buffered saline, the slides were mounted under cover slips with glycerin buffered at pH 7.0. They were then ready for examination under a fluorescent microscope.

M. *Resistance of Amebas to Antibiotics and Antiamebic Agents*

All tests were conducted on amebas grown in MK cell cultures. Antibiotics or antiamebic agents were added separately to cell culture tubes in a series of scheduled dilutions. After the ineffective agents were excluded, parallel tests were made with the promising ones at minimum effective concentrations. Cell culture tubes without antibiotics or antiamebic agents were used as controls.

In one set of tests antibiotics or antiamebic agents were added separately to the maintenance fluid before the tubes were seeded with amebas. In another set each antibiotic or antiamebic agent was added to the culture at the peak of amebic growth. Daily examinations of both test and control tubes were made to ascertain the effect of the agents on amebas as well as on MK cells. Cultures in the first set showing absence of antiamebic effects were subcultured twice in cell cultures prepared with the same antibiotic-incorporated maintenance medium to determine if protracted exposure to these agents would produce a CPE.

N. Determination of Pathogenicity

Only preliminary tests have been carried out so far with the wild strain of *N. gruberi* (NG_2). Mice were tied onto a board with faces up and received through their nostrils 4 drops per animal of an amebic suspension containing about 1000 organisms per drop. After 15–30 minutes the mice were released and observed for development of cerebral symptoms for 2 weeks. Healthy mice were sacrificed and autopsied for possible mild, localized infection.

Dr. C. G. Culbertson of the Lilly Research Laboratories is currently conducting an experimental study of the pathogenicity of NG_8 and wild strains of *N. gruberi* and other species of amebas including those sent to us recently by Dr. Duma.

III. Experimental Data

A. Cultivation

1. Isolation

With the membrane-filter method and the plaque-count technique described in the preceding section, field examinations were conducted on three outdoor swimming pools in the Cincinnati area, two rivers, and one resort lake in northern Kentucky during the summer of 1969. In examining swimming pool water, as much as 50 gal were processed at a time. The results obtained in these examinations are presented in Table I.

Table I shows that *A. rhysodes* is the most common and most predominant small ameba encountered in examination of outdoor swimming

TABLE I
SMALL FREE-LIVING AMEBAS RECOVERED IN EXAMINATION OF SWIMMING POOLS AND NATURAL SURFACE WATERS

Source of sample collected	Species of amebas identified	Concentration of amebas per gallon determined
Swimming pool no. 1	*Acanthamoeba rhysodes*	15 ± 5
	Naegleria gruberi	3 ± 2
Swimming pool no. 2	*Acanthamoeba rhysodes*	18 ± 6
	Naegleria gruberi	2 ± 1
	Hartmannella agricola	1 ± 1
Swimming pool no. 3	*Acanthamoeba rhysodes*	10 ± 4
	Naegleria gruberi	1 ± 1
Missouri River near Kansas City, Mo.	*Acanthamoeba rhysodes*	500 ± 78
	Naegleria gruberi	55 ± 10
	Hartmannella glebae	10 ± 4
	Schizopyrenus erythaenusa	5 ± 2
Ohio River near Cincinnati, Ohio	*Acanthamoeba rhysodes*	200 ± 55
	Naegleria gruberi	44 ± 10
	Singhella leptocnemus	8 ± 3
Lake Falmouth, Kentucky	*Acanthamoeba rhysodes*	650 ± 120
	Naegleria gruberi	63 ± 15
	Schizopyrenus russelli	45 ± 12
	Hartmannella agricola	35 ± 10

pools and surface waters. Next on the list is *N. gruberi,* whose concentration is only a fraction of that of *A. rhysodes.* The other species occur irregularly and in smaller numbers. Examination of a small sample of soil removed from the ground near one of the sampled swimming pools revealed *A. rhysodes, N. gruberi, Hartmannella* spp., and *Schizopyrenus* spp. in concentrations much higher than those found in the pool water. These findings indicate that the ground surrounding outdoor swimming pools is likely to be a source of the amebas found in the pool water.

2. CULTIVATION IN BACTERIAL ASSOCIATION

Most, if not all, small, free-living amebas grow well on BST agar in association with many species of gram-negative bacillary bacteria and with the micrococcus *S. lutea* (Chang, 1958a, 1960). For development of the plaque-count method to quantitate amebas in water or other fluids, the cultural features of amebas grown with several bacterium associates have been studied for their possible use in plaque

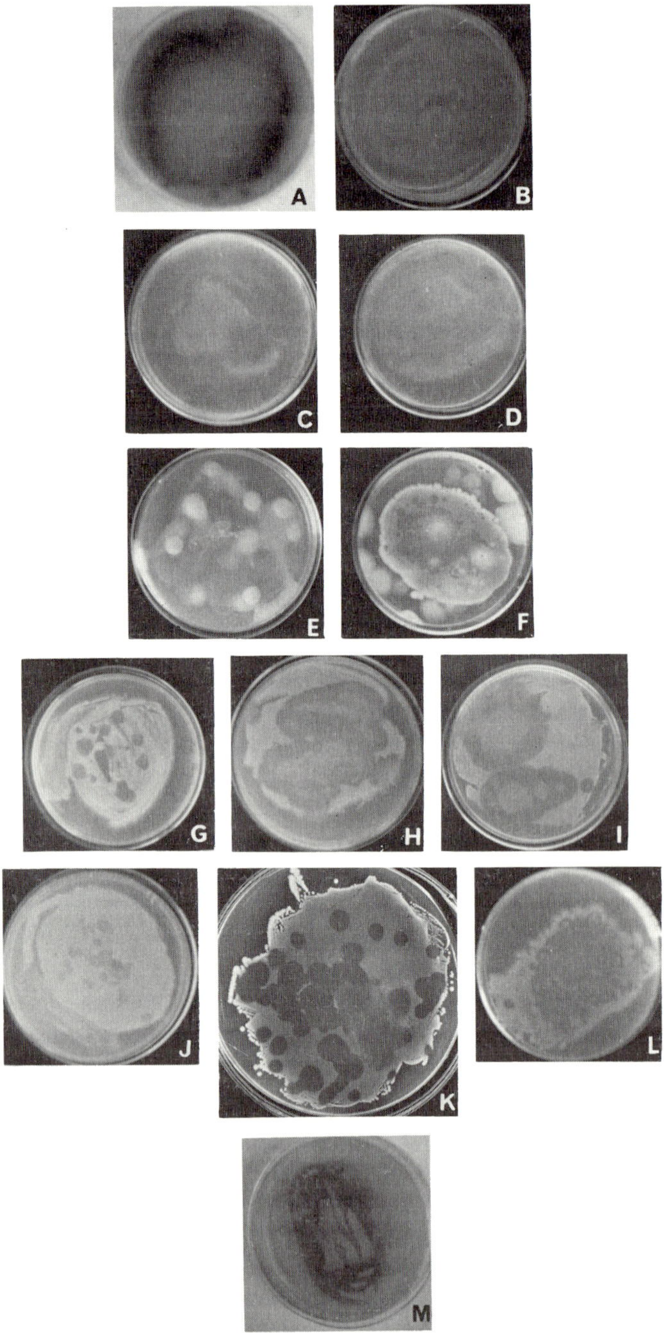

counting. The findings of this study are illustrated by the photographs of representative cultures shown in Fig. 1.

Several interesting points related to Fig. 1 deserve mention. First, the *Pseudomonas* sp. supported good growths of both wild and pathogenic strains of *N. gruberi* (Fig. 1A and H), and of *S. leptocenmus* (Fig. 1D) and *S. erythaenusa* (Fig. 1M). The growth of strain NG_7 was so rich in 4 days of cultivation that the packed cysts produced a dark hue (Fig. 1A), which was absent in moderate growth in association with *Z. ramigera* (Fig. 1B). Second, *B. bronchoseptica* supported equally good, if not better, growths of *N. gruberi* NG_8 (Fig. 1I) and HB_3 (Fig. 1J), *H. agricola* (Fig. 1G), and *H. glebae* (Fig. 1K). Third, the toxic effect of the yellow pigment of *S. lutea* was demonstrated by the relatively poor growth of *N. gruberi* NG_7 (Fig. 1C) and the formation of small plaques without coalescence by HB_3 (Fig. 1L).

The fourth point of interest is the formation of plaques by the slow-

---

Fig. 1. Appearance of cultures of different species of amebas on BST agar plates in association with different species of bacteria at 25° C. (A) *Naegleria gruberi* NG_7 with a *Pseudomonas* sp. Dark color in periphery not attributable to pigment but to densely packed cysts; 4 days old. (B) *Naegleria gruberi* NG_7 with *Z. ramigera.* Thin layer of bacterial growth supported moderate amebic growth; no dark color; 4 days old. (C) *Naegleria gruberi* NG_7 with *S. lutea.* Amebic growth similar to that in (B) not attributable to poor bacterial growth but to weak toxic effect of yellow pigment in early association; 11 days old. (D) *Shinghella leptocnemus* with a *Pseudomonas* sp. Faint plaques noticeable in bacterial growth attributable to slow growth of amebas; 9 days old. (E) *Naegleria gruberi* NG_7 with *A. aerogenes.* Rich mucoid bacterial growth supporting a rich amebic growth for several days; 4 days old. (F) *Hartmannella agricola* with *S. lutea.* Slow growth and motility of amebas resulting formation of plaques coalesced in center area and scattered in periphery; many years of association eliminated toxic effect of pigment; 9 days old. (G) *Hartmannella agricola* with *B. bronchoseptica.* Appearance similar to that in (F); presence of small number of medium-sized plaques without coalescence because of poor inoculum; 18 days old. (H) *Naegleria gruberi* NG_8 with *Pseudomonas* sp. Note the coalescence of several large plaques with leftover of bacterial growth in center; 18 days old. (I) *Naegleria gruberi* NG_8 with *B. bronchoseptica.* Appearance similar to that in (H) but plaques have clearer outline; note also leftover bacterial growth in plaque center; 18 days old. (J) *Naegleria gruberi* HB_1 with *B. bronchoseptica.* Note small plaques after 9 days of incubation; leftover bacterial growth giving plaques ring appearance. (K) *Hartmannella glebae* with *B. bronchoseptica.* Note the well-outlined, clear plaques resulting from slow but rich amebic growth; 12 days old. (L) *Naegleria gruberi* HB_3 with *S. lutea.* Numerous small plaques formed together as a result of slow growth of a good inoculum; very small-sized plaques attributable to weak toxic effect of bacterial pigment; 18 days old. (M) *Schizopyrenus erythaenusa* with a *Pseudomonas* sp. Note reddish pigment; clear patches result from uneven smearing of inoculum; 11 days old.

growing amebas in association with either *B. bronchoseptica* or *Pseudomonas;* but the plaques formed with the former (Fig. 1G, I, J, and K) were clearer and sharper than those formed with the latter (Fig. 1D and H). Clear and sharp plaques were also formed with *S. lutea* by amebas that had had long associations with it and had developed a tolerance to the toxic effect of the pigment (Fig. 1F).

The fifth interesting point is the production of a reddish pigment by *S. erythaenusa* with the *Pseudomonas* (Fig. 1M). Singh (1952) reported the phenomenon with this ameba grown on non-nutrient agar supplied with *A. aerogenes.* Our observations indicated that the reddish pigment can be produced on BST agar in association with *Salmonella* and *Shigella* spp., *E. coli,* and *A. aerogenes* as well as *Pseudomonas.* Preliminary tests made with this pigment revealed that it is insoluble in water but quite soluble in ethanol, chloroform, ethyl ether, and acetone and exhibits an antibiotic effect on gram cocci and bacilli.

The six strains of *S. russelli* received in early April 1970 were found to grow into rich cultures on BST agar in association with the species of bacteria employed in this study. Their growth with *S. lutea* also showed a weak toxic effect of the yellow pigment.

Some essential growth characteristics associated with these plate cultures should be considered. The growth of the amebas in association with *A. aerogenes* in the mucoid growth of the bacteria was rich, but mass encystment was delayed and trophozoites were found in fair numbers over 2 weeks when cultures were kept at room temperature. The fast-growing amebas (*S. russelli, S. erythaenusa,* and wild strains of *N. gruberi*) did not undergo massive encystation until 5–6 days had elapsed. The slow-growing hartmannellids required 2–3 weeks for the appearance of mass encystment, while the very slow-growing pathogenic strains of *N. gruberi* grew very poorly in the mucoid material and formed few cysts.

In association with the *Pseudomonas* sp., *B. bronchoseptica,* or *Z. ramigera,* the fast-growing schizopyrenids and the wild strains of *N. gruberi* covered the entire smeared agar surface with trophozoites in 2 days of incubation (Figs. 2B and 3A) and with a sheet of cysts in 4 days (Figs. 2A and 3B). The slow-growing hartmannellids grew in isolated patches resulting in the formation of plaques, and the plaques were covered with rich growth, cysts in the center and trophozoites in the periphery. A similar but slower growth pattern was observed with all pathogenic strains of *N. gruberi.* In plaques formed by these strains, the cysts were scattered in the midst of trophozoites which were never packed together (Figs. 4A and 5A and B).

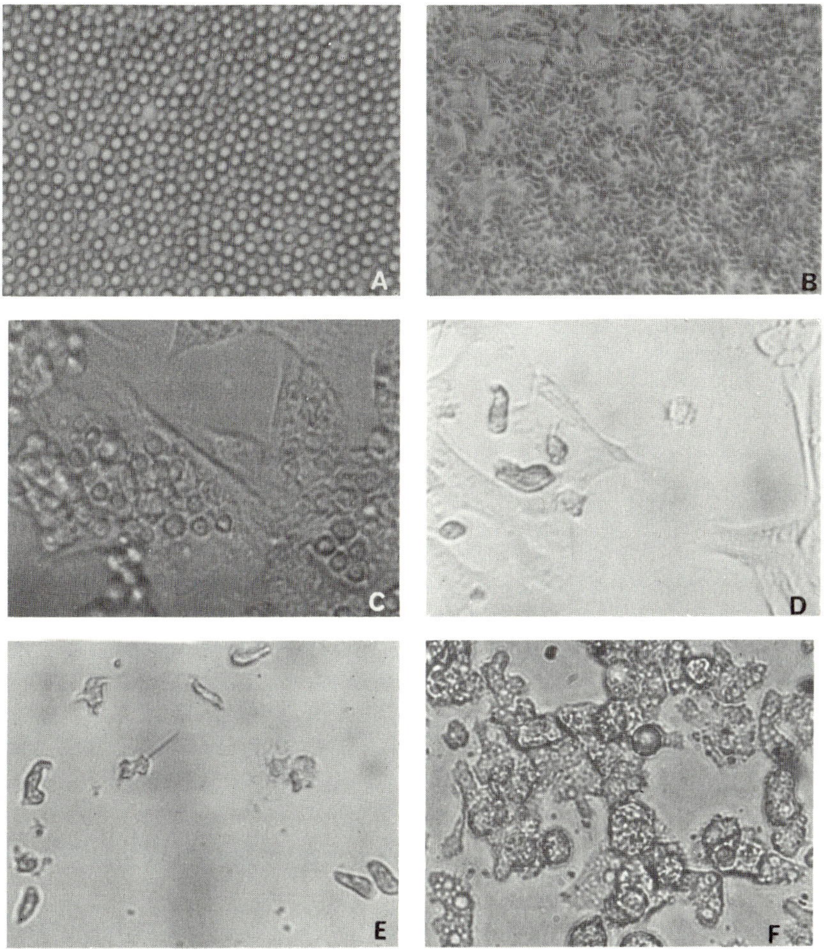

Fig. 2. Photomicrographs of *N. gruberi* NG_7 and *A. rhysodes.* (A) Photomicrographs of a plate culture of NG_7 grown with a *Pseudomonas* sp. on BST agar; 4 days old. Note the packed cysts. 174×. (B) Photomicrograph of the same culture shown in (A) taken at peak growth; 2 days old. Note the packed trophozoites. 87×. (C) Photomicrograph of NG_7 in MK cell culture; 6 days old. Note the large number of cysts phagocytized by MK cells with many ingested cysts digested. 218×. (D) Photomicrograph of the same culture shown in (C) taken 4 days later with appearance of trophozoites. Note the trophozoites gliding on top of the MK cells without CPE. 218×. (E) Photomicrograph of the same culture shown in (C) taken 10 days later. Note the difference in appearance between these trophozoites and those of HB strains and strain NG_8. (F) Photomicrograph of *A. rhysodes* AR_2 in MK cell cultures at peak of growth; 16 days old. Note the "vacuolated" appearance of the cytoplasm and the polygonlike shape of the trophozoites, which are strikingly different from the appearance of *N. gruberi* trophozoites. 218×.

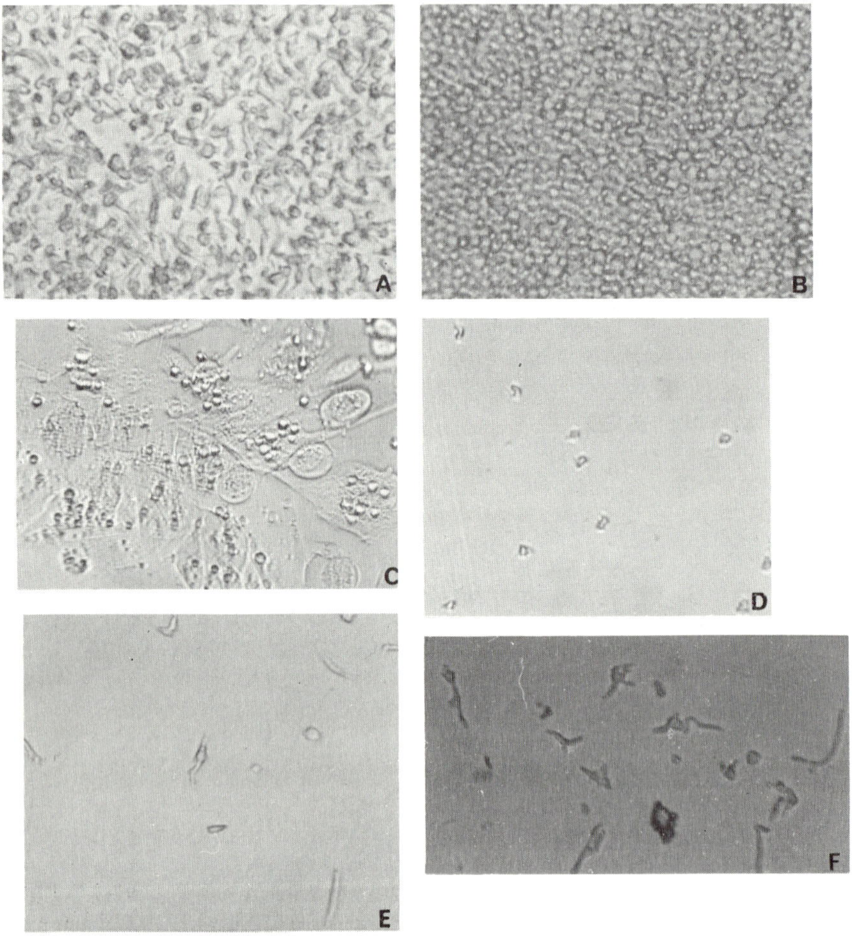

Fig. 3. Photomicrographs of *S. russelli* strain P. (A) Photomicrograph of a plate culture grown with *B. bronchoseptica;* 2 days old. Note the "slug"-shaped trophozoites. 200×. (B) Photomicrograph of the same plate culture shown in (A) taken 2 days later. Note the packed small cysts. 200×. (C) Photomicrograph of a MK cell culture 24 hours after seeding with material from the first MK cell culture established for this strain. Note that most of the cysts were phagocytized by MK cells. 200×. (D) Photomicrograph of the same culture shown in (C) taken 10 days later. Note the small trophozoites. 200×. (E) Photomicrograph of strain P after three transfers in MK cell cultures; 12 days old. Note the slight increase in size and "slug"-shaped appearance of trophozoites. 200×. (F) Photomicrograph of strain P after the fifth transfer in MK cell cultures. Note the further increase in size of the trophozoites and the appearance quite similar to the pathogenic strains of *N. gruberi.* 200×.

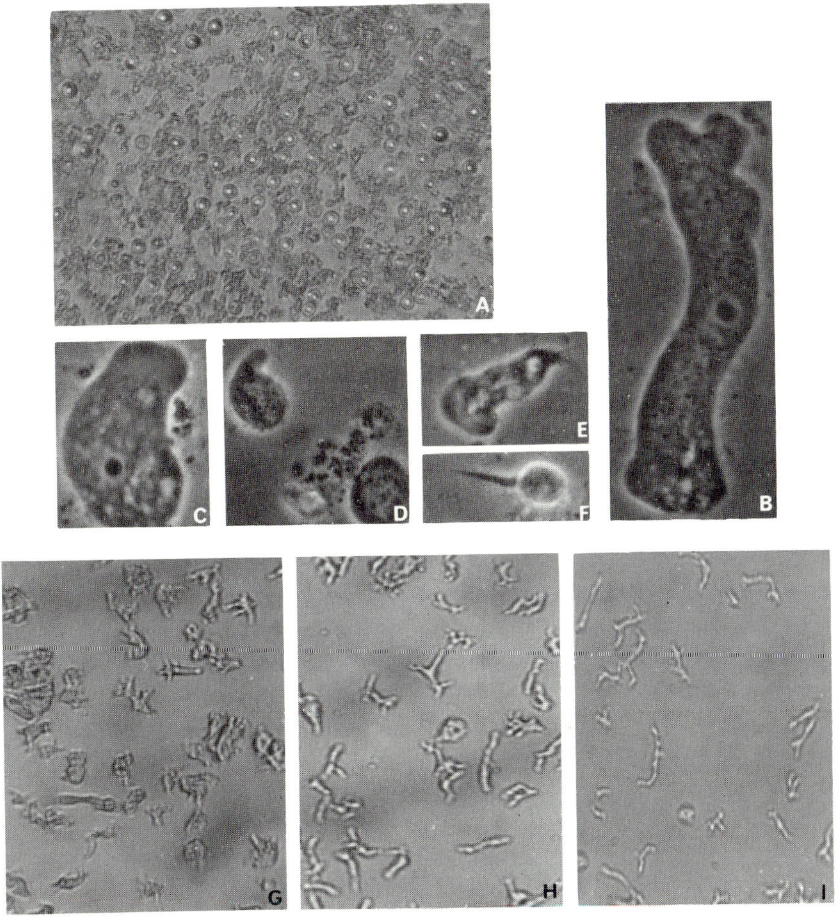

Fig. 4. Photomicrographs of HB strains of *N. gruberi.* (A) Photomicrograph of a plate culture of strain HB in association with *B. bronchoseptica* incubated at 25° C; 18 days old. Note the scattered cysts among the trophozoites. 140×. (B, C, and D) Phase-contrast photomicrographs of trophozoites of strain HB_1 removed from MK cell culture at the peak of cytolysis. Note the tremendous difference in size between the trophozoites in (B) and those in (D) and also between nucleoli. 875×. (E and F) Phase-contrast micrographs of flagellate forms of HB_3 in a water suspension prepared with material from a plate culture containing cysts. (E) Beginning of flagellate transformation. (F) Fully transformed flagellate. 700×. (G) Photomicrograph of trophozoites of strain HB_3 in MK cell culture at peak of cytolysis; 4 days old. Note the granular appearance of organisms as a result of large amounts of cell debris ingested. 175×. (H) Photomicrograph of trophozoites of strain HB_2 in MK cell culture after peak growth with cell debris disappearing; 6 days old. 175×. (I) Photomicrograph of trophozoites of strain HB_1 in MK cell culture with cell debris mostly consumed; 7 days old. 175×.

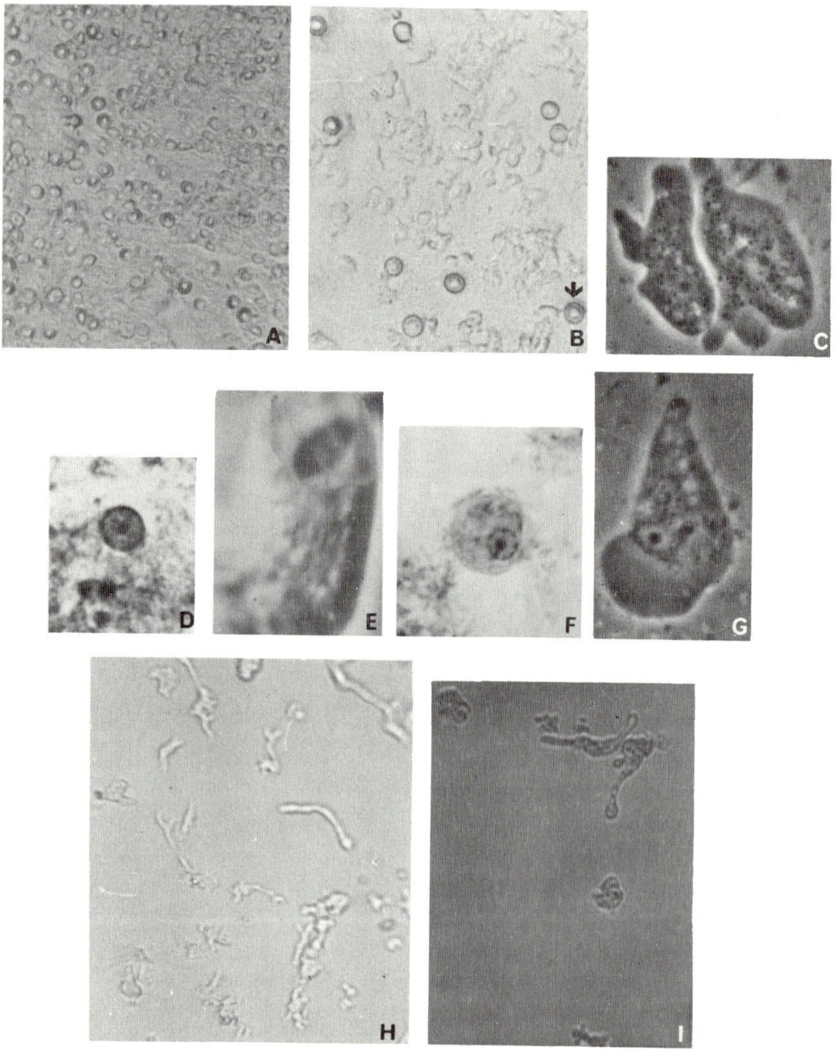

Fig. 5. Photomicrographs of *N. gruberi* strain NG_s (pathogenic). (A) Photomicrograph of a plate culture grown with *B. bronchoseptica;* 16 days old. Encystment somewhat richer than that of HB strains. 154×. (B) Photomicrograph of the same plate culture shown in (A) but under higher magnification. Arrow points to a double-walled cyst. 385×. (C) Phase-contrast photomicrograph of two trophozoites removed from MK cell culture after the strain had developed a CPE. Note the large amounts of cell debris ingested. 770×. (D) Photomicrograph of a hematoxylin-stained cyst. Note the prominent nucleolus and chromatin material under the nuclear membrane. 960×. (E) Photomicrograph of a hematoxylin-stained trophozoite during mitosis. Note the interzonal bodies at the equator. 1920×. (F) Photomicrograph of a hematoxylin-stained trophozoite in resting stage. Note the chromatin material under the nuclear membrane and threadlike structures radiating from nucleolus. 770×. (G) Phase-contrast photomicrograph of a trophozoite about to undergo flagellate transformation. Note the small cytoplasmic protrusion at the

3. Axenic Cultivation without Tissue Cells

Attempts were made to grow bacteria-free amebas obtained in SYEABST agar axenically in both SCF and SYECF media. The pathogenic strains of *N. gruberi* survived three transfers at weekly intervals, while the wild strains survived only two transfers. The slightly longer survival of the pathogenic strains apparently was attributable to cell debris carried by the inocula into the fluid media, which apparently supported a very limited amount of growth in the first transfer. Results obtained with the schizopyrenids and hartmannellids (excluding *A. rhysodes* which grew into rich cultures in both fluid media) were essentially the same as those obtained with the wild strains of *N. gruberi*. These failures were attributed to lack of enough settled food particles to feed the amebas, since the coagulated serum proteins remained mostly in a suspended state.

When the amebas on SYEABST agar were transferred to the same agar but with the antibiotics omitted, moderate growths of the HB and NG_8 strains ensued; less growth was observed with all the other strains and species, including *A. rhysodes*. This was attributed to the fact that lack of encystment of the former facilitated a longer growing period, while the latter underwent encystation in a relatively dry environment. The difficulty encountered in maintaining axenic cultures on this enriched BST agar was traced to a lack of enough organisms per inoculum during the transfer from plates where growths never consisted of more than scattered organisms separated by wide spaces.

4. Growth in MK Cell Cultures

a. HB Strains in MK Cell Cultures and the CPE. HB strains were, as stated early, carried in MK cell cultures without interruption. These strains exhibited marked CPE on MK cells, and the degree of CPE depended on the size of inoculum and, to a less extent, the age of culture. Since the differences in CPE did not follow a definite pattern, it appears that these differences were not attributable to strain differences in cytopathogenicity but rather to differences in cultural conditions at the time when transfers were made.

Generally, when 4–5 drops of culture fluid were drawn at or shortly after the peak of amebic growth and seeded into a tube of cell culture, about 20% of the cell sheet showed signs of early degeneration in 24 hours with very little increase in the number of amebas. After another 24 hours disintegration of small numbers of cells was observed; amebas

---

pointed end. 960×. (H) Photomicrograph of trophozoites in MK cell culture with an appearance not unlike that of HB strains. 154×. (I) Photomicrograph of trophozoites in MK cell culture taken toward end of culture life. Note the large-sized trophozoites. 154×.

gathered in areas of cell disintegration showed signs of active growth, since the density was considerably higher than that in general. By the fourth day most of the cells had been replaced by trophozoites highly granular in appearance because of the large amounts of cell debris ingested (Fig. 4B and G). By the fifth to sixth days, most trophozoites showed clear cytoplasm as a result of the digestion of ingested cell debris and exhaustion of this food supply (Fig. 4H). In another day or two, a decrease in number and size of trophozoites occurred, resulting from starvation (Fig. 4I). Unless transfers were made within 48 hours, such cultures generally died out.

To determine the nature and origin of the CPE agent, washed trophozoites and filtrate were prepared from a batch of cell cultures at the peak growth of each strain by the procedure described in Section II. Cell cultures were seeded, in duplicate, with known numbers of trophozoites; parallel cultures were prepared with known amounts of the filtrate. Unseeded cultures were used as controls. The test and control cultures were examined daily for 1 week for CPE. The results obtained in these experiments are presented in Table II.

Table II demonstrates that the CPE agent is bound to the filtrate and requires a minimum concentration of 3% (1 drop/ml) to exert a noticeable CPE in MK cells. Additional experiments made with filtrates obtained from HB cultures at different times of incubation yielded results indicating that the amount of CPE agent correlated directly with the growth activity of the amebas; very little CPE agent was found in 24-hour cultures, and less was found in those when the trophozoites were dying of "old age."

The growth pattern of the washed trophozoites indicated that the latter are able to liberate very small amounts of the CPE agent in these cell cultures, and when enough of them are gathered in one area, enough of the agent may be liberated to cause a focal cell degeneration, which can serve as a starting point of amebic growth. If too few trophozoites are introduced into a cell culture in the absence of extraamebic CPE agent, the ameba may even fail to establish itself in the new environment.

Preliminary experiments made on filtrates obtained from cultures of the HB strains at their peak growth indicated the following features: (1) The CPE agent is unstable on storage at room temperature; most of its CPE is destroyed in 4–5 days. (2) It is rapidly inactivated at temperatures between 50° and 60° C. (3) It is inactivated in less than 24 hours at room temperature and pH 4.5 or 9.5. (4) It withstands freezing and thawing three times if the temperature remains below 10° C.

TABLE II

Cytopathic Effects of Trophozoites of HB Strains of *N. gruberi* and of Their MK Cell Culture Filtrates

Inoculum	Number of trophozoites or drops of filtrate per inoculum	CPE in MK cell cultures of stated strains		
		HB_1	HB_2	HB_3
Trophozoites	100	No CPE in 1 week; tubes negative after 2 weeks; no growth in subcultures	No CPE in 6 days; 1 tube negative; 1 barely positive after 2 weeks	No CPE in 6 days; fair to good growth in both tubes after 2 weeks
	1000	No CPE in 4 days; growth fair after 9 days; patches of degenerating cells	No CPE in 4 days; growth fair after 6 days; patches of degenerating cells	No CPE in 4 days; fair to good growth after 8 days; many patches of degenerating cells
	5000	No CPE in 2 days; growth good after 8 days; patches of degenerating cells	No CPE in 2 days; growth good after 1 week; patches of degenerating cells	No CPE in 2 days; good growth after 6 days; many patches of degenerating cells
Filtrate	2	Few rounded and fewer granular cells after 24 hours; slightly larger number of changed cells after 48 hours; no further changes		
	5	20–25% of cells rounded and granular after 24 hours; 30–35% of cells after 48 hours; few cells disintegrated after 72 hours; no further changes		
	10	Over 75% of cells rounded and granular after 24 hours; over 30% of cells disintegrated after 48 hours; over 50% of cells disintegrated after 72 hours; 10–15% of cells remained after 210 hours		

(5) It slowly loses its CPE on storage at 3°–5° C, and only about one-half of its activity is retained after 2 weeks. (6) The CPE is preserved for at least 2 months storage in a frozen state at —70° C. Its chemical nature was not studied on account of its unstability in any separation process used for its isolation. It is speculated that the agent is of an enzyme nature capable of causing a cytolytic effect.

b. NG_8 and Nonpathogenic Amebas. By using bacteria-free amebas obtained from SYEABST agar plates to seed MK cell cultures, establishment of amebic growths in these cultures was successful in one or more trials. Difficulty was encountered with the NG_8 strain as a result of its failure to form cysts or exert a CPE in cell cultures. Most of the trophozoites died during the long waiting period prior to autolytic cell degeneration. By the time cell degeneration started to take place, there were so few live trophozoites that poor growth ensued.

By adding 4–5 drops of a filtrate obtained from an active culture of strain HB_1 to the inoculum per tube of cell culture, it was possible to produce good cultures in 6–8 days through the CPE effect of the filtrate. After several consecutive transfers with decreasing amount of the filtrate until the latter was completely withdrawn from the inoculum, the NG_8 developed its own CPE and behaved in cell cultures in a manner indistinguishable from that of the HB strains. During the active growing period, the trophozoites ingested large amounts of cell debris (Fig. 5G) and assumed the elongated forms (Fig. 5H and I) typical of HB strains. Occasionally, a trophozoite undergoing flagellate transformation (Fig 1I), or a flagellate (which cannot be photomicrographed without immobilization), was seen in an examination of early cultures. This phenomenon was not seen in later cultures of this strain or in any cell cultures of HB strains.

The growth characteristics of the wild strains of *N. gruberi* and other species of amebas (including *A. rhysodes*) employed in the study were essentially the same as those reported earlier for *N. gruberi* NG_1 and *H. agricola* (Chang, 1960). Briefly, no CPE was observed; most of the cysts introduced were phagocytized by MK cells within 24 hours, and trophozoites formed cysts, which in turn became phagocytized (Figs. 2C and 3C). Cells having a heavy cyst burden began to degenerate at much earlier times than normal, and the cysts that survived the intracellular stay excysted. The metacystic amebas fed on cell debris and increased in number. These new trophozoites glided around on the cell sheet (Fig. 2D) or open areas (Figs. 3D and E) in search of food. When there was lack of cell debris, some formed cysts, which again became phagocytized. This process repeated itself until most of the cells were gone, generally lasting a period of $2\frac{1}{2}$–3 weeks. During the course "pockets" of trophozoites were found in areas where cells had disintegrated (Figs. 2E and 3F). Interestingly, trophozoites of a wild strain of *N. gruberi* (Fig. 2E) appeared quite different from, while those of *S. russelli* (Fig. 3F) resembled, those of the pathogenic strain of *N. gruberi* and the HB strains.

The two strains of *A. rhysodes* (AR_1 and AR_2), being able to grow in SCF and SYECF media as well as in the maintenance medium without additional food, attained good growths in the MK cell cultures when the cells were in a healthy state. The formation of cysts and phagocytosis of the cysts prevented the amebas from developing rich cultures until the latter period of incubation when most calls were gone and had been replaced by amebas. The "mosaic" appearance of their trophozoites and their irregularly outlined cysts made it relatively simple to identify them (Fig. 2F).

Of particular significance was the failure to induce the wild strains of *N. gruberi* and other species of amebas to exhibit CPE by the same procedure applied to strain NG_8. In every case there was a significant increase in the growth of amebas in cell cultures; but as soon as the HB culture filtrate was withdrawn, the growths of these amebas returned to the original state.

These observations strongly indicate that the CPE on MK cells is inherent or can be induced only in pathogenic strains that have potentiality for such activity. This point is stressed later in this chapter.

5. Growth Rates

From the study of growth characteristics of these amebas both on BST agar plates in bacterial association and in MK cell cultures, it is quite clear that, with the exception of the pathogenic strains of *N. gruberi,* schizopyrenids grow considerably faster on bacteria food than do hartmannellids. There is also indication that the former grow faster in MK cell cultures than the latter, although both groups lack CPE. The very slow-growing pathogenic strains of *N. gruberi* in bacterial association have their growth rates reversed in MK cell cultures owing to their CPE and their ability to adapt better to feeding on cell debris than on bacteria.

To determine how much the growth rates of these amebas differ from one another under these two cultural conditions, the growth of each ameba in plate culture in association with *B. bronchoseptica* at 25°

and 35° C and in MK cell cultures at 37° C were studied by the procedure described in Section II. The mean of each quadruple plate count obtained for one strain or species at each temperature was plotted against the respective incubation time in hours on semilog graph paper. The linear section of each growth curve was used to compute the growth rate constant k (per hour), from which the generation time g (in hours) was derived by the equations described in an early report on the growth of hemoflagellates (Chang and Negherbon, 1947). When more than one strain was used, and when the values of k and g were not significantly different, the mean was computed from them to represent the growth rate of a species. The standard deviations of these values were calculated with the conventional equation given in books on statistics. The results thus obtained are tabulated in Table III.

The same quantitative treatment was applied to data obtained with the MK cell cultures at 35° C. Results of this treatment are also presented in Table III.

Of particular interest is the fact that the schizopyrenids, excluding pathogenic strains of *N. gruberi*, grew about twice as fast as the hartmannellids at both 25° and 35° C. In bacterial association in plate cultures, the pathogenic strains of *N. gruberi* grow five times slower than the wild strains. The growth rate of the pathogenic strains of *N. gruberi* in MK cell cultures, however, was three times as fast as the wild strains. The two species of *Schizopyrenus* and the wild strains of *N. gruberi* grew almost twice as fast as the two species of *Hartmannella* and *S. leptocnemus*. The two strains of *A. rhysodes* grew even faster than the schizopyrenids as a result of their ability to grow in the absence of cell degeneration.

While it is intended in this chapter to treat small, free-living amebas (excluding *N. gruberi* because of its distinct pathogenic and nonpathogenic strains) at the species level, we wish to stress the existence of strains that show qualitative resemblance to one another but quantitative differences in physiological and serological characteristics. Differences between pathogenic and wild strains have already been demonstrated in *N. gruberi*.

In a recent study made to identify the "lipovirus–ameba cell" complex as a strain of *A. rhysodes* (AR_2 in this discussion), a comparison was carried out between this strain and another strain of *A. rhysodes* (AR_1 in this discussion) in growth pattern and in FA-staining properties (S. L. Chang and Liu, unpublished observations). Although the growth pattern was ascertained then in the SYECF medium while that in this study was made on BST agar in bacterial association, the relative growth

TABLE III
GROWTH RATES OF SMALL, FREE-LIVING AMEBAS ON BST AGAR PLATES WITH *B. bronchoseptica* AND IN MK CELL CULTURES

Family, genus, and species of ameba	Growth rate constants[a]			
	Value of k at 25° C (per hour)	Value of k at 35° C (per hour)	Value of g at 25° C (hours)	Value of g at 35° C (hours)
In plate cultures:				
Schizopyrenidae				
Schizopyrenus russelli (six strains)	0.079 ± 0.013	0.140 ± 0.021	3.8 ± 0.6	2.1 ± 0.3
Schizopyrenus erythaenusa	0.071 ± 0.009	0.131 ± 0.018	4.2 ± 0.5	2.3 ± 0.3
Naegleria gruberi (wild strains)	0.068 ± 0.011	0.122 ± 0.016	4.4 ± 0.7	2.5 ± 0.3
Naegleria gruberi (HB and NG_8 strains)	0.015 ± 0.002	0.027 ± 0.005	19.0 ± 2.5	11.1 ± 1.8
Hartmannellidae				
Hartmannella glebae	0.022 ± 0 004	0.040 ± 0.008	13.7 ± 2.5	7.5 ± 1.5
Hartmannella agricola	0.020 ± 0 004	0.038 ± 0.007	15.0 ± 3.0	7.9 ± 1.5
Acanthamoeba rhysodes (two strains)	0.026 ± 0 007	0.045 ± 0.011	11.5 ± 3.1	6.7 ± 1.6
Singhella leptocnemus	0.031 ± 0.005	0.047 ± 0.012	9.7 ± 1.6	7.2 ± 1.8
In MK cell cultures:				
Schizopyrenidae				
Schizopyrenus russelli (six strains)	—	0.031 ± 0.005	—	9.7 ± 1.6
Schizopyrenus erythaenusa	—	0.026 ± 0.004	—	11.5 ± 1.8
Naegleria gruberi (wild strains)	—	0.029 ± 0.004	—	10.3 ± 1.4
Naegleria gruberi (HB and NG_8 strains)	—	0.083 ± 0.012[b]	—	3.6 ± 0.5[b]
Hartmannellidae				
Hartmannella glebae	—	0.017 ± 0.002	—	17.7 ± 2.1
Hartmannella agricola	—	0.019 ± 0.003	—	15.8 ± 2.6
Singhella leptocnemus	—	0.016 ± 0.002	—	18.8 ± 2.5
Acanthamoeba rhysodes (two strains)	—	0.041 ± 0.009	—	7.3 ± 1.6

[a] Computed from amebic density during the log growth phase.
[b] Computed from amebic density ascertained after MK cells were affected by a CPE.

rates should be comparable. To show how much difference existed between these two strains in growth rates, the growth curves obtained in the earlier study are shown in Fig. 6.

From these growth curves the values of k (per hour) and g (in hours) at 25° and 35° C for AR_1 and AR_2 were computed to be 0.024

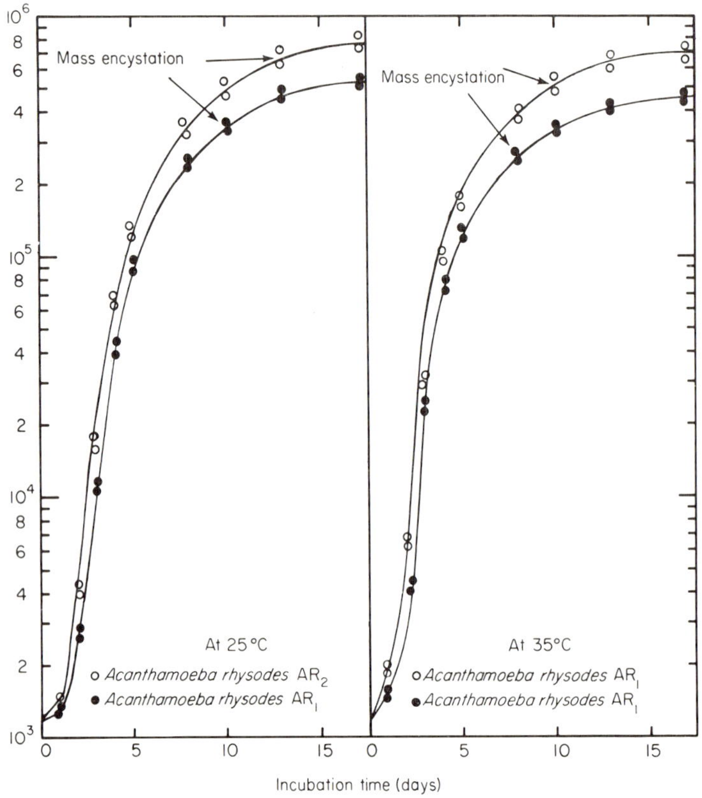

Fig. 6. Comparison of growth rate of *A. rhysodes* strains AR_1 and AR_2 in SYCEF medium at 25° and 35° C.

and 12.5 hours and 0.028 and 10.7 hours, respectively, at 25° C, and 0.042 and 7.1 hours and 0.048 and 6.3 hours, respectively, at 35° C. The AR_2 strain grows about 13% faster than strains AR_1. As is seen later, there is also a difference in degree of intensity in FA staining between these two strains. Interestingly, these values are very close to those obtained for the same two strains in this study.

B. Quantitation of Amebas by the Plaque Count Method

Using mainly *B. bronchoseptica*, the *Pseudomonas* sp., and other species to a smaller extent as bacterium associates, quantitation of different species or strains of amebas was carried out on BST agar plates by the procedure already described. All plates were incubated at 25° C, although preliminary tests indicated that the incubation time could be shortened by one-half by incubating the plates at 35° C.

Plaques formed by different strains or species of amebas with different bacterium associates were not only enumerated but also carefully examined for size, shape, clarity, color (if any), and other visible features for possible identification criteria. In each plaque count determination, three to four dilutions were employed and each dilution was plaqued in triplicate or quadruplicate. To illustrate the essential points, only representative plates were selected for photographing, and the photographs thus made are presented in Figs. 7–10.

Figure 7A, B, and C demonstrates the relationship between plaque appearance and incubation time. These plaques are typical of those formed by all the pathogenic strains of *N. gruberi* in the growth of *B. bronchoseptica*. Each plate was prepared with a calculated number of 120 organisms of the HB_3 strain. The actual plaque count was 125 after 9 days, 130 after 11 days, and 128 after 15 days. These figures indicate that insignificant errors will be introduced if the plaques of very slow-growing amebas are enumerated within 3 days of the counting period. One interesting point is the appearance of a "center" in each of these plaques, as pointed out earlier when plate growth features were described. Since these centers remained more or less the same size during the 4-day incubation period, they were more likely the "leftovers" of bacterial growth remaining after the amebas moved away from the point of growth rather than "aftergrowth" of bacteria occurring after the amebas had left.

Figure 8 demonstrates the dilution–plaque count relationship in quantitation of the two mostly commonly found small, free-living amebas, namely, *N. gruberi* and *A. rhysodes*, by the plaque count technique employing *B. bronchoseptica* as the associate. It also demonstrates the differences in size increase and appearance of plaques between the pathogenic and wild strains of *N. gruberi*. The plaques formed by the pathogenic strain (HB_2) of *N. gruberi* are typical of those formed by other pathogenic strains, and the plaques formed by the wild strains (NG_2 and NG_7) of *N. gruberi* are typical of those formed by other wild strains.

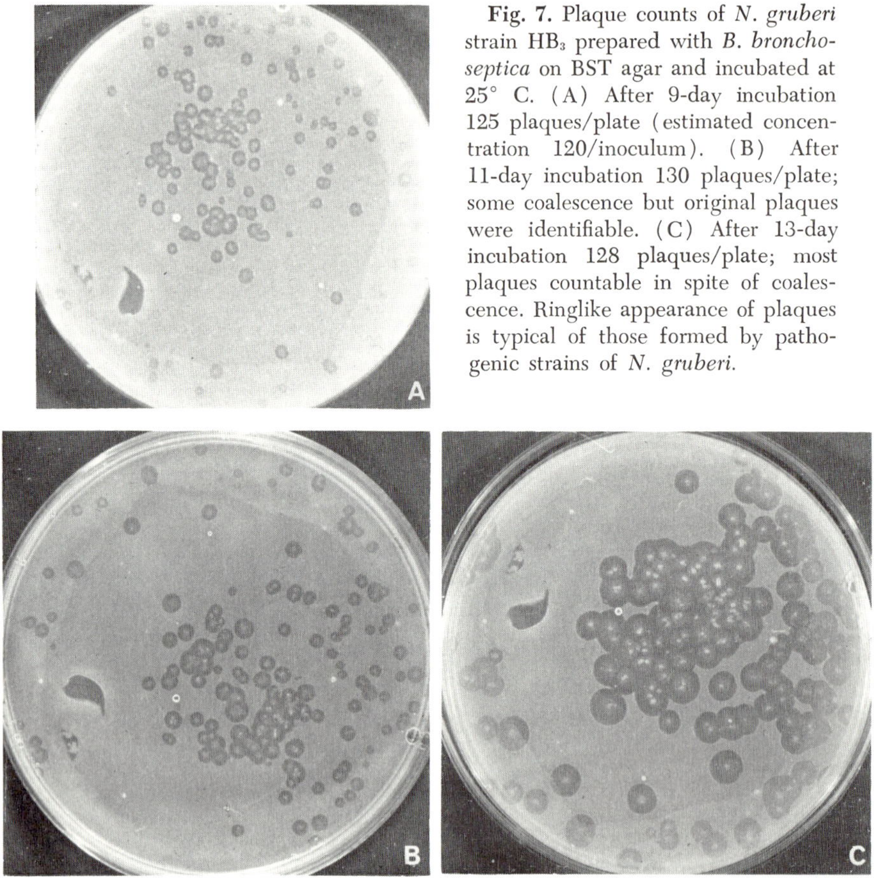

Fig. 7. Plaque counts of *N. gruberi* strain HB_3 prepared with *B. bronchoseptica* on BST agar and incubated at 25° C. (A) After 9-day incubation 125 plaques/plate (estimated concentration 120/inoculum). (B) After 11-day incubation 130 plaques/plate; some coalescence but original plaques were identifiable. (C) After 13-day incubation 128 plaques/plate; most plaques countable in spite of coalescence. Ringlike appearance of plaques is typical of those formed by pathogenic strains of *N. gruberi.*

Figure 8A, C, E, and G shows plaques on plates prepared with four different dilutions of a suspension of strain NG_2 after 4 days of incubation. The actual counts of 11, 24, 48, and 97 were very close to the calculated numbers of 12, 25, 50, and 100 organisms per inoculum. The rapid growth of the wild strains of *N. gruberi* is demonstrated by the considerably larger plaques formed by NG_7 (Dr, s, t) with a 1-day increase in incubation time. The counts of 17, 23, and 32 (Dr, s, t) were not as close to the calculated numbers of 20, 30, and 40 organisms per inoculum. This could have resulted from the coalescence of several plaques, which was not indicated by the plaque appearance.

Figure 8H shows the plaques formed on four plates prepared with a suspension of the pathogenic strain HB_2 after 11 days of incubation. It is worth noting that the plaques on these plates (Hr, s, t, u) are comparable in size to those formed by NG_2 after 4 days. The phenomenon becomes even more striking when one takes into consideration the fact that a large percent of NG_2 trophozoites had already encysted at this stage of incubation, while most of the HB_2 amebas were trophozoites. The actual plate counts of 19, 26, 38, and 51 for the 4 plates (Hr, s, t, u) were quite close to the calculated numbers of 20, 30, 40, and 50 amebas per inoculum, respectively.

The presence of centers in the plaques formed by HB_2 conforms to the appearance of plaques formed by all pathogenic strains of *N. gruberi.* These strains made the plaques resemble "rings" more than true plaques, which characterize those formed by the wild strains.

Figure 8B shows the three plaque count plates prepared with *A. rhysodes* AR_2 after 6 days of incubation. The actual counts of 28, 52, and 72 plaques per plate (Bx, y, z) were also quite close to the calculated numbers of 25, 50, and 75 amebas per inoculum, respectively. One interesting feature observed in these plates is the presence of plaques of highly varied sizes and irregular outline.

For the purpose of comparison, plaque counts were also made on both pathogenic and wild strains of *N. gruberi,* but using the *Pseudomonas* sp. as their associate. *Hartmannella glebae* and *H. agricola,* two slow-growing amebas, were included. The features of these plaque count plates are illustrated by the photographs shown in Fig. 9.

Figure 9A shows the plaques formed by NG_7 after 5 days of incubation, which were not as outstanding as those formed with *B. bronchoseptica.* The actual counts of 26 and 52 plaques per plate (As, t) were in close agreement with the calculated numbers of 25 and 50 amebas per inoculum.

Figure 9B shows two plates prepared with NG_8 after 11 days of incubation. The plaques were rather faint but countable; the actual counts of 28 and 56 for the two plates (Bs, t) agreed well with the calculated number of 25 and 50 per inoculum.

The two plates shown in Fig. 9C were prepared with HB_3 and a suspension of *Pseudomonas* much thicker than that ordinarily used. The plaques formed after 9 days of incubation were small but distinct. Tiny centers were visible in the larger plaques. The 18 and 38 plaques counted on the two plates (Cs, t) agree well with the 20 and 40 estimated in the inocula. With a lighter *Pseudomonas* suspension, the plaques formed by HB_2 after a 10-day incubation (Fig. 9D) were just as faint as those formed by NG_8. The counts of 52 and 102 on these two plates

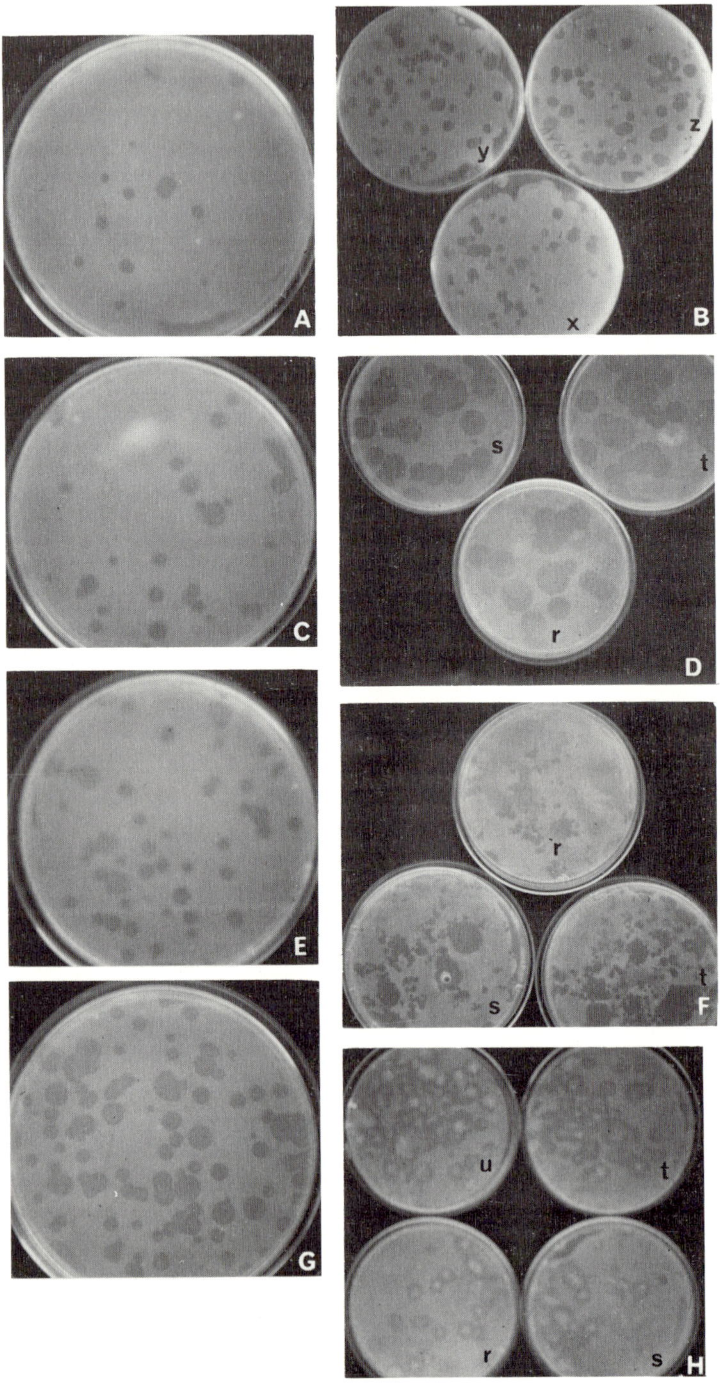
A
y
z
x
B
s
t
r
C
D
E
r
s
t
F
G
u
t
r
s
H

(Ds, t) were, nevertheless, very close to the estimated 50 and 100 in the inocula.

Hartmannella agricola and *H. glebae* behaved quite similar in their plaque formation. Their plaques were small and rather faint even when fairly thick *Pseudomonas* suspensions were used, apparently as a result of their slow growth and encystation on prolonged incubation, which reduced the number of active, growing trophozoites (Fig. 9E and F). The counts of 74 and 24 plaques formed by *H. agricola* (Es, t) after 11 and 9 days of incubation were very close to the 74 and 25 estimated in the inocula, and the counts of 7 and 11 plaques formed by *H. glebae* after 7 days (Fs, t) were much less than the estimated 10 and 20 in the inoculum. These results demonstrate the long incubation time needed to bring out plaques of these slow-growing amebas.

While there is a similarity in size and outline of plaques formed by hartmannellids to those formed by slow-growing pathogenic strains of *N. gruberi*, they can be distinguished from each other by the fact that plaques formed by the former are clear while those formed by the latter show centers.

Another organism found in preliminary experiments capable of showing plaques in amebic association is *A. fecalis*. The formation of plaques by *N. gruberi* strains in the growth of this bacterium was also studied. Plaque count determinations were also made with other species of amebas in association with *A. fecalis*, *B. bronchoseptica*, and *S. lutea*. Photographs of plaquing plates in these determinations are shown in Fig. 10.

Fig. 8. Plaque counts made with different amebas and *B. bronchoseptica* on BST agar plates incubated at 25° C. (A, C, E, and G) *Naegleria gruberi* strain NG_2; 4 days old. (A) 11 Plaques/plate (estimated 12/plate). (C) 24 Plaques/plate (estimated 25/plate). (E) 48 Plaques/plate (estimated 50/plate). (G) 97 Plaques/plate (estimated 100/plate). (B) *A. rhysodes* strain AR_2; 6 days old. x, 28 Plaques/plate (estimated 25/plate); y, 52 plaques/plate (estimated 50/plate); z, 72 plaques/plate (estimated 75/plate). (D) *Naegleria gruberi* strain NG_7; 5 days old. r, 17 Plaques/plate (estimated 20/plate); s, 23 plaques/plate (estimated 30/plate); t, 32 plaques/plate (estimated 40/plate). (F) Mixed suspension of *N. gruberi* strain NG_7, *A. rhysodes* strain AR_2, and *H. agricola;* 7 days old. r, NG_7 1/plate (estimated 2/plate), AR_2 5/plate (estimated 5/plate), and *H. agricola* 27/plate (estimated 30/plate); s, NG_7 4/plate (estimated 4/plate), AR_2 8/plate (estimated 10/plate), and *H. agricola* 51/plate (estimated 60/plate); t, NG_7 6/plate (estimated 8/plate), AR_2 15/plate (estimated 20/plate), and *H. agricola* 82/plate (estimated 90/plate). (H) *Naegleria gruberi* strain HB_2 with *B. bronchoseptica;* 11 days old. r, 19/plate (estimated 20/plate); s, 26/plate (estimated 30/plate); t, 38/plate (estimated 40/plate); u, 51/plate (estimated 50/plate).

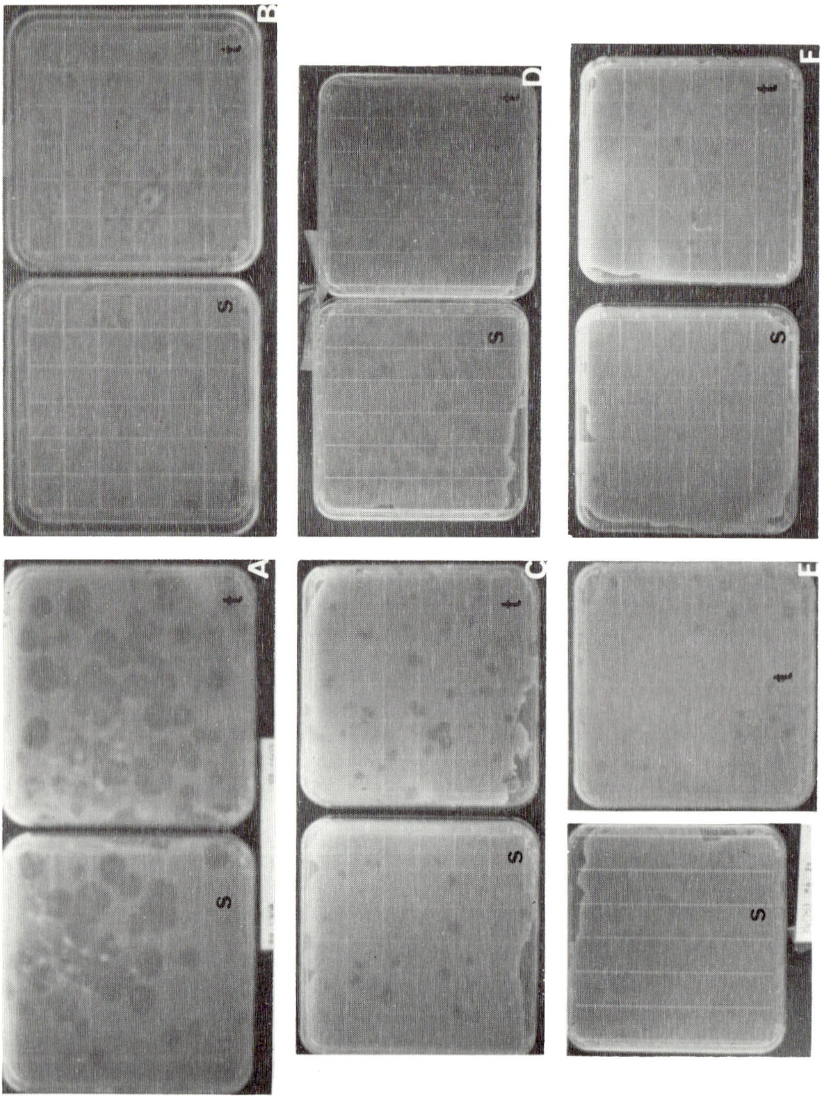

Figure 10A and B demonstrates the lack of sharpness and the marked variation in size of the plaques formed by NG_7 (A) and NG_2 (B). When the plaques became definite, which took 8–9 days, some of them had already coalesced (Ad, e, f; B) and the original plaques were difficult to identify in the coalesced groups. As a result, the actual counts were significantly lower than estimated even at these low ameba concentrations.

Figure 10C shows a plaque plate prepared with strain NG_8 after 13 days of incubation. The plaques were hard to see in daylight but, when illuminated with artificial light from opposite sides, they became visible. The ring appearance of plaques typical of the pathogenic strains of *N. gruberi* was clearly visible in this type of illumination. The count of 55 plaques was quite close to the 60 estimated.

Figure 10D and E shows plaques formed by *S. erythaenusa* in the growth of *B. bronchoseptica.* The red-colored plaques shown in (E) but not in (D) between a period of 6 days of incubation demonstrated the long period of time required for pigment production. The presence of 27 plaques (estimated 30) in (E), which is 4 more than in (D) indicates the slow-growing nature of this ameba.

Figure 10F demonstrates the appearance of plaques formed by *A. rhysodes* AR_1 in the growth of *S. lutea* after 18 days of incubation. It was identical to that of AR_2 observed in association with *B. bronchoseptica.* The long incubation time required was apparently a result of the mild toxic effect of the bacterial pigment; so were the lower plaque counts.

Figure 10G and I shows the plaques formed by *H. glebae* and *H. agricola,* respectively, in the growth of *A. fecalis.* The plaques were more visible than those formed in growth of *Pseudomonas* (Fig. 9E and F), mainly because of the fact that the plates were photographed at a 15° angle. The fact that the plaques formed by *H. glebae* were

---

Fig. 9. Plaque counts of different amebas made with *Pseudomonas.* (A) *Naegleria gruberi* NG_7; 5-day incubation; s, 26 plaques/plate (estimated 25/plate); t, 52 plaques/plate (estimated 50/plate). (B) *Naegleria gruberi* NG_8; 11-day incubation; s, 28 plaques/plate (estimated 30/plate); t, 56 plaques/plate (estimated 60/plate). (C) *Naegleria gruberi* HB_3; 9-day incubation; s, 18 plaques/plate (estimated 20/plate); t, 38 plaques/plate (estimated 40/plate). (D) *Naegleria gruberi* HB_2; 10-day incubation; s, 52 plaques/plate (estimated 50/plate); t, 102 plaques/plate (estimated 100/plate). (E) *Hartmannella agricola;* 9- to 11-day incubation; s, 74 plaques/plate after 9 days (estimated 75/plate); t, 24 plaques/plate after 7 days (estimated 25/plate). (F) *Hartmannella glebae;* 7-day incubation; s, 7 plaques/plate (estimated 10/plate); t, 11 plaques/plate (estimated 20/plate).

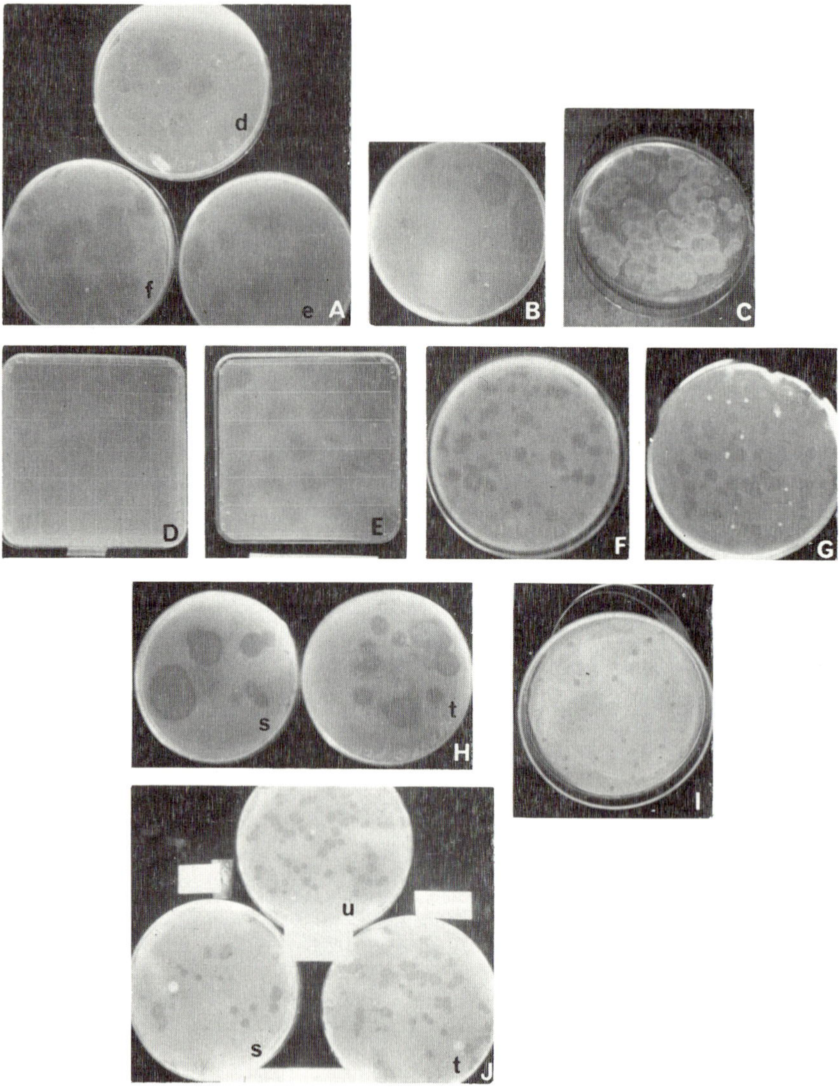

Fig. 10. Plaque counts of *N. gruberi* strains with *A. fecalis* and other species of amebas with *B. bronchoseptica* or *S. lutea.* (A) *Naegleria gruberi* NG_7 with *A. fecalis;* 9-day incubation; d, 6 plaques/plate (estimated 10/plate); e, 11 plaques/plate (estimated 20/plate); f, 24 plaques/plate (estimated 30/plate). (B) *Naegleria gruberi* NG_2 with *A. fecalis;* 9-day incubation; 8 plaques/plate (estimated 10/plate); photographed at 15° angle. (C) *Naegleria gruberi* NG_8 with *A. fecalis;* 13-day incubation; photographed at 15° angle with side illumination. 55 plaques/plate (estimated 60/plate). (D) *Schizopyrenus erythaenusa* with *B. bronchoseptica;* 10-

larger in size than those formed by *H. agricola* was attributable to their longer incubation (*H. glebae,* 15 days; *H. agricola,* 7 days). The counts of 55 (G) and 27 (I) were also close to the estimated numbers of 60 and 30 in the respective inocula.

In Fig. 10H are shown the plaques formed by *S. leptocnemus* in the growth of *A. fecalis.* They were made much more visible by illuminattion from sides. The relatively dark, large area in the large plaques was not attributable to leftover bacterial growth similar to that of the pathogenic strains of *N. gruberi,* but resulted from the side illumination. The plaque counts of 8 (s) and 15 (t) were lower than the 10 and 20 estimated, likely attributable to coalescence of a few of the plaques.

Plaque count plates prepared with strains of *S. russelli* isolated from Lake Chester are shown in photographs of plates prepared with strain SR_6 (P) grown with *B. bronchoseptica* after a 5-day incubation (Fig. 10J). The plaques of this ameba were countable, and round, as are those of the wild strains of *N. gruberi,* but they were very small and not as visible. Top illumination was used to make the plaques more easily visible. Presence of the centerlike spots in some of the plaques was accentuated by the way in which the plates were illuminated. These spots disappeared as the plaques enlarged on further incubation. The counts of 21, 48, and 64 on plates Js, t, and u were not too far from the estimated numbers of 25, 50, and 75 in the inocula, respectively, when coalescence of plaques in plate Ju was taken into consideration.

The plaque count results obtained in this part of the study demonstrate clearly that all small, free-living amebas can be quantitated by the plaquing technique developed in our laboratory, and that *B. bronchoseptica* appears to be the most suitable bacterium-associate for plaquing. The plaque formation time, appearance, color, and other features are

---

day incubation; 23 plaques/plate (estimated 30/plate); (E) Same plate as shown in (D) after 16-day incubation; note that the red pigment developed in plaques. 27 plaques/plate, an increase of 4 plaques in 6 days. (F) *Acanthameba rhysodes* AR_1 with *S. lutea;* 18-day incubation; note the irregularity in size and shape of the plaques. 66 plaques/plate (estimated 100/plate). (G) *Hartmannella glebae* with *A. fecalis;* 15-day incubation; 56 plaques/plate (estimated 60/plate); photographed at a 15° angle. (H) *Singhella leptocnemus* with *A. fecalis;* 12-day incubation; photographed with side illumination; s, 8 plaques/plate (estimated 10/plate); t, 15 plaques/plate (estimated 20/plate). (I) *Hartmannella agricola* with *A. fecalis;* 9-day incubation; photographed at 15° angle; 27 plaques/plate (estimated 30 plate). (J) *Schizopyrenus russelli* P with *B. bronchoseptica,* 5-day incubation; photographed with artificial light straight from top with camera placed at 15° angle; s, 21 plaques/plate (estimated 25/plate); t, 48 plaques/plate (estimated 50/plate); u, 64 plaques/plate (estimated 75/plate).

distinct for different groups of amebas and can be used for isolation and identification. The slow formation of well-outlined plaques with a center appears to be characteristic of the pathogenic strains of *N. gruberi.* The presence of a red color in plaques formed after a long period of incubation appears to be typical of *S. erythaenusa.*

C. Identification and Classification

The morphology of trophozoites and cysts of all species and strains employed has been studied in the fresh cover slip-slide preparations under both light and phase-contrast microscopes. Nuclear changes during mitosis have been studied in both hematoxylin- and Feulgen-stained smears. Findings from these examinations, together with those obtained in both plate and MK cell cultures, are used as a basis for the statements that follow.

The morphological and cytological findings are in complete agreement with those carefully and thoroughly described by Singh (1952) in his study of nine species of small, free-living amebas. It would be superfluous to describe them again. We would, however, like to correct a statement we made early (Chang, 1958a) to the effect that interzonal bodies were not found in our examination of *N. gruberi* during anaphase. That statement was based on observations made on Feulgen-stained smears. Since these bodies are Feulgen-negative, their absence in smears so stained is to be expected. In all examinations made in the study described here, these bodies were found in hematoxylin-stained smears prepared with all strains of *N. gruberi.* Interzonal bodies are illustrated in the photomicrograph of NG_8 shown in Fig. 5E. The location of chromatin granules under the nuclear membrane and the presence of thread-like structures radiating from the nucleolus are illustrated in two photomicrographs of NG_8 in the same figure (Fig. 5D and F).

By the procedure already described, attempts were made to induce flagellate transformation in all species and strains of amebas studied. While 50–75% of amebas of wild strains of *N. gruberi* formed flagellates, few were observed when the procedure was applied to the pathogenic strains. HB strains formed flagellates only when induced (Fig. 4E and F); the NG_8 strain occasionally formed a few flagellates in MK cell cultures (Fig. 5F) during the early period of growth. Flagellate transformation is a mass phenomenon among the wild strains of *N. gruberi,* but it is an occasional phenomenon occurring over a period of about 3 weeks among the pathogenic strains.

The cultural results indicate that schizopyrenids differ from hartmannellids not only in mitotic changes but also in growth rates, the former being a faster-growing group than the latter.

Acanthamoeba rhysodes, which Singh (1952) placed in the *Hartmannella* genus, differs from *Hartmannella* spp. in that it forms filamentous processes from either ectoplasm or endoplasm, assumes the typical mosaic appearance, and grows readily in ordinary bacteriological fluid media.

Singhella leptocnemus was also placed by Singh in the *Hartmannella* genus on the basis of nuclear changes during mitosis. This ameba has some morphological features that are quite different from other *Hartmannella* spp. First, its ectoplasm and endoplasm are entirely indistinguishable. Second, there are many vacuoles in the endoplasm. Third, its cyst has a double wall. On the basis of these features, it is separated from the *Hartmannella* genus. It is named *S. leptocnemus* because it was Singh who first found it in an examination of soil. The elongated forms of trophozoites, on the basis of which the species was named, were also found on BST agar in association with most of the gram-negative bacilli used, not just the non-nutrient agar supplied with *A. aerogenes* observed by Singh.

After taking all the features into consideration, it is felt that Singh's phylogenic classification should be used as a basis in the taxonomic treatment of small, free-living amebas, but the classification should be slightly modified to include morphological and physiological criteria. Hence a modified classification is suggested for use in working on this group of free-living amebas. This classification is as follows.

SUBPHYLUM: Sarcodina Hertwig and Lesser
- CLASS: Rhizopoda von Siebold
  - SUBCLASS: Amoebaea Butschli
    - ORDER: Amoebida Calkins and Ehrenberg
      - SUPERFAMILY: Amoebaceae. Free living
        (Endamoebaceae. Parasitic in animals)
        - FAMILY: Schizopyrenidae. Active limax form common; transient flagellates present or absent; nucleolus origin of polar masses; polar caps and interzonal bodies present or absent
          - GENUS: *Schizopyrenus.* No transient flagellates; single-walled cysts; no polar caps or interzonal bodies in mitosis
            - SPECIES: *S. erythaenusa.* Reddish orange pigment formed in agar cultures with gram-negative bacillary bacteria
              S. russelli. No pigment produced in agar cultures
          - GENUS: *Didascalus.* Morphology and cytology similar to *Schizopyrenus* but small numbers of transient flagellates formed at times
            - SPECIES: *D. thorntoni.* Only species described by Singh (1952)
          - GENUS: *Naegleria* Alexeieff—double-walled cysts; transient flagellates

formed readily; polar caps and interzonal bodies present in mitosis

SPECIES: *N. gruberi* (Schardinger)—Only species established; Singh (1952) disclaimed the *N. soli* he described in 1951

FAMILY: Hartmannellidae. No transient flagellate formed; motility sluggish; no limax form; nucleolus disappearing, probably forming spindle in mitosis; no polar caps or masses, aster and centrosome not known

GENUS: *Hartmannella.* Ectoplasm clear or less granular than endoplasm; single-walled cysts; single vacuole

SPECIES: *H. glebae.* Clear ectoplasm

H. agricola. Ectoplasm less granular than endoplasm

GENUS: *Acanthamoeba.* Filamentous processes from ecto- or endoplasm; growing axenically in fluid bacteriological media

SPECIES: *A. rhysodes*

GENUS: *Singhella.* Double-walled cysts; ecto- and endoplasm indistinguishable; many vacuoles

SPECIES: *Singhella leptocnemus*

The question whether or not these pathogenic strains of *N. gruberi* are those of *Didascalus* was raised in view of their scanty flagellate formation. The formation of polar caps by the nucleolus in prophase and the appearance of interzonal bodies in anaphase during mitosis, together with the double-walled cysts, unquestionably establish them in the *Naegleria* genus. However, the distinct differences between the pathogenic and nonpathogenic forms in growth rate, CPE on MK cells, and flagellate formation cast great doubt as to the justification in treating them as strains of the same species.

It is believed that these pathogenic *Naegleria* amebas should be separated from *N. gruberi,* and we propose that they be named *Naegleria invades* on the basis of their cytolytic property and ability to invade tissues. Confirmation of this proposal will have to wait until FA staining and other serological studies are carried out. To avoid confusion, the establishment of a new species appears justified.

D. Pathogenicity in Animals

The pathogenic nature of HB_2 in mice has been established (Culbertson *et al.*, 1968); NG_8 has just been found to be equally pathogenic to mice (Culbertson and Ensminger, Lilly Research Laboratories, personal communication). In the same communication it was learned that the *S. russelli* strains caused no symptoms in mice after nasal instillation. The pathogenicity of the wild strains of *N. gruberi* is being ascertained at the Lilly Research Laboratories.

In 1963, shortly after the NG_2 strain of *N. gruberi* was isolated, a limited number of experiments were carried out on mice. A suspension containing mostly trophzoites at a concentration of about 1000 amebas per drop was instilled intranasally into eight mice at a dosage of 4 drops per mouse. A similar experiment was performed with a suspension containing mostly cysts. No animal became sick with in a 2-week period. All mice were sacrificed and autopsied; no cerebral pathology was found in any of the sacrificed mice.

A strain of *A. rhysodes*, isolated together with the *S. russelli* from Lake Chester and maintained in MK cell cultures, has been sent to Dr. C. G. Culbertson for pathogenicity tests.

It appears that the pathogenic species of *Naegleria* are virulent in mice by nasal instillation and intracerebral inoculation, while the non-pathogenic strains of *N. gruberi* are not by these routes of inoculation. The pathogenicity of *A. rhysodes* remains to be confirmed.

Until more pathological findings are accumulated, it may be safe to consider *N. invades* the only ameba pathogenic in man.

E. FA Staining

Only the AR_1 and AR_2 strains of *A. rhysodes* have been studied by the FA-staining method. The amebas were grown in HeLa cell cultures in Leighton tubes; the thin slides were removed at scheduled times and fixed in warm acetone. The fixed slides were stained with fluorescein-conjugated γ globulins and examined under a fluorescent microscope. Photomicrographs taken of amebas in these two sets of FA-stained slides are shown in Fig. 11.

As described in the legend for this figure, AR_2 stained more intensely by the homologous antibody than AR_1. Of interest is the fact that the trophozoites were stained uniformly while the cysts showed fluorescence only in the peripheral part, giving a "halo" appearance (Fig. 11B). These results indicate that there exists some strain difference within a species of ameba. This is in agreement with the immobilization results obtained by Adam (1963) in serological experiments made on several strains of *Acanthamoeba.*

F. Resistance of Amebas to Amphotericin B, Chloroquine Sulfate, and Emetine–Hydrogen Chloride

In a screening test employing a large number of antibiotics and anti-amebic agents, only amphotericin B, chloroquine sulfate, and emetine–hydrogen chloride were found to have antiamebic activity at reason-

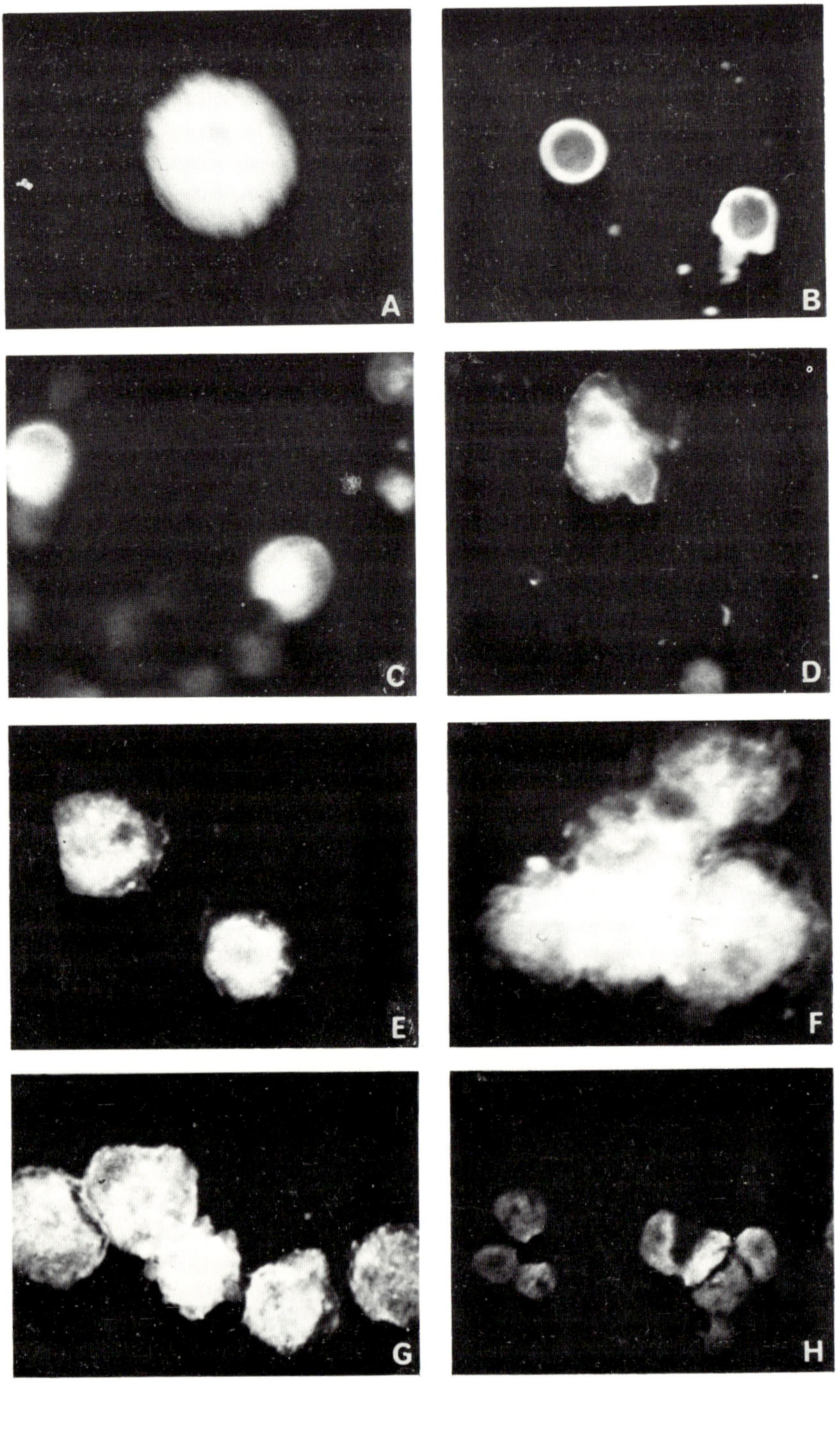
A
B
C
D
E
F
G
H

ably low concentrations. Experiments were then made on all species and strains of amebas employed in the study by (1) incorporating each agent into the maintenance medium, and (2) adding the agent to each of a number of MK cell culture tubes at peak growth. Untreated cell cultures were used as controls. Both test and control tubes were examined daily for antiamebic and cytotoxic effect (CTE). Subcultures were made in case of negative results. Results obtained in the experiments are shown in Table IV, and photomicrographs of some typical cultural findings are shown in Fig. 12.

Table IV shows that all three agents exhibited definite antiamebic activity on the pathogenic *N. invades* amebas when they were incorporated into the maintenance medium at a concentration of 1 μg/ml, but the antiamebic effects required subculturing of the amebas once or twice in the presence of the same agents. At a concentration of 2 μg/ml, an antiamebic effects was observed in the first cultures. There was no, or very little, CTE observed at a concentration of 1 μg/ml of each agent; a noticeable CPE was observed at a 2 μg/ml concentration of amphotericin B in a few transfers. Both chloroquine sulfate and emetine–hydrogen chloride were toxic to MK cells at a 2 μg/ml concentration.

When these agents were added separately to cultures at the peak of amebic growth, no definite antiamebic effect on the pathogenic amebas was observed at a dosage of 1 μg/ml. Effects became definite when a dosage of 2 μg/ml was used.

All other species of amebas, including the wild strains of *N. gruberi*, were not affected by these agents at a 1 μg/ml dosage, and no definite effect was observed at a 2 μg/ml dosage.

Fig. 11. Photomicrographs of FA-stained *A. rhysodes*. (A, C, E, and G) *Acanthamoeba rhysodes* AR_2 grown in Leighton tube cultures of HeLa cells and AFMK cells and stained with fluorescein-conjugated homologous globulin. 125×. (B, D, F, and H) *Acanthamoeba* AR_1 grown in similar cultures and stained with fluorescein-conjugated heterologous globulin. 125×. (A) HeLa cell culture 4 hours after inoculation. Note the heavily stained cyst clump lying on the cell sheet. (B) HeLa cell culture 4 hours after inoculation. Note the peripherally stained cysts, one lying on cell sheet and one phagocytized. (C) HeLa cell culture 144 hours after inoculation. Note the heavily stained trophozoites, the endoplasm being more heavily stained than the ectoplasm. (D) HeLa cell culture 144 hours after inoculation. Note the slightly less fluorescence in this figure in comparison to (C). (E) AGMK cell culture 96 hours after inoculation. Cysts phagocytized in MK cells. (F) AGMK cell culture 144 hours after inoculation. A large clump of cysts are phagocytized in MK cells. (G) AGMK cell culture 16 days after inoculation. Trophozoites are mingled with degenerating MK cells. (H) AGMK cell culture 16 day after inoculation. Note that the trophozoites are less deeply stained in this figure than in (G).

TABLE IV

EFFECTS OF AMPHOTERICIN B, CHLOROQUINE PHOSPHATE, AND EMETINE–HYDROGEN CHLORIDE ON THE GROWTH OF *N. gruberi*, *S. russelli*, AND *A. rhysodes* IN MK CELL CULTURES

Species of ameba	Effects of agents at concentrations stated in micrograms per milliliter of culture fluid					
	Amphotericin B		Chloroquine phosphate		Emetine–hydrogen chloride	
	1	2	1	2	1	2
With agent incorporated in maintenance medium:						
Naegleria gruberi (HB_1, HB_2, HB_3, and NG_8)	No antiamebic effect after first transfer; amebas disappeared after three to four transfers; no CTE on MK cells	Reduced ameba growth after first transfer; no amebas after second transfer; slight CTE on MK cells	Reduced ameba growth after first transfer; amebas disappeared after second transfer; slight CTE on MK cells	Amebas disappeared after first transfer; profound CTE on MK cells	Few amebas after first transfer; no amebas after second transfer; moderate CTE on MK cells	No amebas after 4–5 days after first transfer; marked CTE on MK cells
Naegleria gruberi (wild strains)	No antiamebic effect after seven to eight transfers	Reduced ameba growth after three to four transfers; no amebes after eight transfers	No antiamebic effect after seven to eight transfers	Gradual disappearance of amebes after six transfers	No antiamebic effect after seven to eight transfers	Gradual disappearance of amebas after six transfers

Schizopyrenus russelli (six strains)	[a]	[a]	[a]	[a]	[a]	[a]
Acanthamoeba rhysodes (two strains)	[a]	[a]	[a]	[a]	[a]	[a]
With agent added to cultures at peak of amebic growth:						
Naegleria gruberi (HB_2 and NG_8)	No significant effect; fewer elongated trophozoites	Amebas rounded, reduced in size and activity (Fig. 11A and D)	More rounded amebas after 24 hours; no significant reduced amebas growth	Amebas with large amount of clear ectoplasm in 2 days (Fig. 11B); disappeared in 5 days	Amebas rounded, reduced in size and motility	Most amebas degenerated after 2 days; no amebas after 4 days (Fig. 11C and E)
Naegleria gruberi (NG_2, NG_4, and NG_7)	No antiamebic effect in 4 days	No antiamebic effect in 4 days	No antiamebic effect in 4 days	No antiamebic effect in 4 days	No antiamebic effect in 4 days	More rounded trophozoites
Schizopyrenus russelli	[b]	[b]	[b]	[b]	[b]	[b]
Acanthamoeba rhysodes	[b]	[b]	[b]	[b]	[b]	[b]

[a] No significant effect observed after four transfers.
[b] No significant effect observed in 4 days.

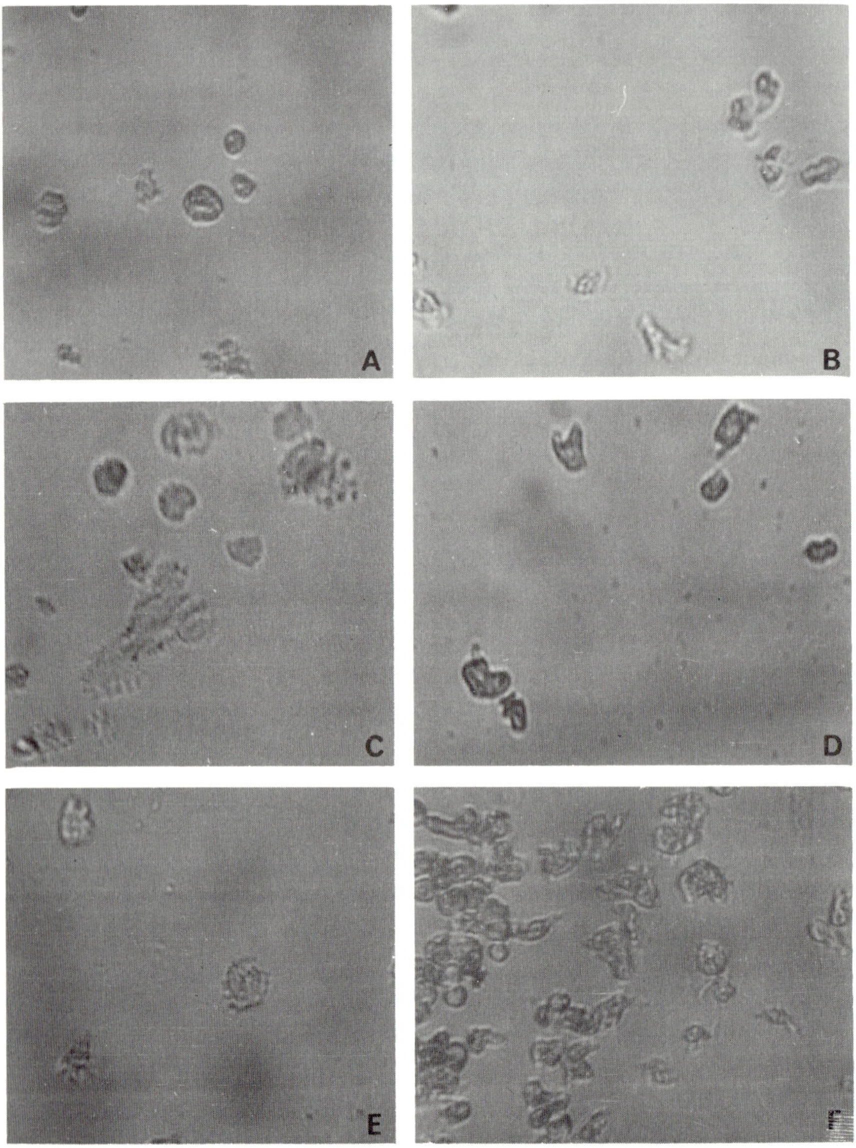

Fig. 12. Antiamebic effects of amphotericin B, emetine–hydrogen chloride and chloroquine on *N. gruberi* HB_2 and NG_s in MK cell cultures; the drug was added at the peak of amebic growth. (A) Photomicrograph of HB_2 in MK cell cultures 3 days after the addition of 2 μg/ml amphotericin B. Note the rounded trophozoites of small size which are in an inactive state. 250×. (B) Photomicrograph of HB_2 in MK cell culture 2 days after the addition of 2 μg/ml chloroquine. Note the appear-

Morphological changes in *N. invades* effected by these agents were: rounding of trophozoites and decrease in motility (Fig. 12A and D) in the early stage of exposure to a 2 μg/ml concentration of amphotericin or emetine–hydrogen chloride, or an appearance of watery ectoplasm in an abnormally large amount (Fig. 12B). These changes were followed by the granular appearance of organisms with loss of motility (Fig. 12C and F). Eventually, the affected amebas disintegrated. Figure 12F shows resistance of NG_7 to a 2 μg/ml concentration of amphotericin B; its rich growth was a result of early degeneration of cells affected by the antibiotic.

This difference in resistance to the three antiamebic agents among the pathogenic amebas and the other species and strains provides one more criterion for separating the pathogenic strains from *N. gruberi* and establishing them as a separate species in the genus *Naegleria.*

From a therapeutic viewpoint these results offer little comfort to clinicians in the treatment of amebic meningoencephalitis. The effective concentration of 2 μg/ml of any of these agents requires a dosage that is above the safety range. Furthermore, it is doubtful that such a concentration could be reached in the affected part of the brain, even if the level of 2 μg/ml were maintained in the blood or cerebrospinal fluid.

IV. Conclusions and Summary

Methods of isolation, cultivation, enumeration, and identification have been developed and studied as to their applicability with four pathogenic and four wild strains of *N. gruberi,* six strains of *S. russelli,* two strains of *A. rhysodes,* and one strain each of *S. erythaenusa, H. glebae, H. agricola,* and *S. leptocnemus.* Results obtained in this study justify the following conclusions.

---

ance of an unusually large amount of ectoplasm. 250×. (C) Photomicrograph of HB_2 in MK cell culture 4 days after the addition of 2 μg/ml emetine–hydrogen chloride. Note the granular appearance of rounded trophozoites and also of MK cells. 250×. (D) Photomicrograph of NG_8 in MK cell culture 3 days after the addition of 2 μg/ml amphotericin B. Note the resemblence between this photomicrograph and (A). 250×. (E) Photomicrograph of NG_8 in MK cell culture 4 days after the addition of 2 μg/ml emetine–hydrogen chloride. Note the similarity in appearance of trophozoites in this photomicrograph to that in (C) 250×. (F) Photomicrograph of *N. gruberi* NG_7 in MK cell culture 4 days after the addition of 2 μg/ml amphotericin. Note the absence of antiamebic effect. 250×.

(1) All small, free-living amebas grow on BST agar in association with most gram-negative bacillary bacteria, including *Pseudomonas pyocyanea* and *S. lutea,* the mildly toxic pigments of which are usually tolerated by the amebas after a period of cultural association.

(2) Certain cultural appearances can be used as an aid in the identification of amebas, for example, the production of reddish pigment is diagnostic for *S. erythaenusa.*

(3) Schizopyronids, excluding the pathogenic strains of *Naegleria,* grow significantly faster on bacteria in plate cultures than hartmannellids, providing another criterion for establishment of these two families. Members of both families exist in the cystic stage in old cultures. The pathogenic strains of *Naegleria* grow very slowly in these cultures and form small numbers of cysts.

(4) All amebas grow in MK cell cultures. The pathogenic strains of *Naegleria* exhibit marked CPE and grow much faster than the other species and strains which exhibit no CPE. No cysts are formed in cell cultures by the pathogenic strains, while cysts are the main forms of other amebas in the terminal stage.

(5) A plaque count method has been developed and found useful and accurate for quantitation of all species of amebas. The most suitable bacterium associate for plaquing is *B. bronchoseptica.* The time for plaque development, and the plaque appearance, size, color, and other features are useful in ameba identification and isolation.

(6) Morphological and cytological observations, together with cultural characteristics in both plate and MK cell cultures, confirmed all the features elaborately described by Singh in his study of nine small amebas. From these observations a modification of Singh's classification is suggested. In this classification *H. rhysodes* and *H. leptocnemus* are established as separate genera with the species names retained—*Acanthaamoeba rhysodes* and *Singhella leptocnemus.* The growth and cultural characteristics of the pathogenic strains of *Naegleria* justify their separation from *N. gruberi* and establishment of a separate species; *N. invades* is suggested.

(7) FA staining of the two strains of *A. rhysodes* indicates that there exist strain differences among amebas in the same species which can be used to identify amebas that are morphologically indistinguishable from one another.

(8) Preliminary results indicate that the wild strains of *N. gruberi* are not pathogenic to mice by nasal instillation.

(9) Amphotericin B, chloroquine sulfate, and emetine–hydrogen chloride exhibit an anti–amebic effect at a concentration of 2 μg/ml on the

pathogenic strains of *Naegleria* in MK cell cultures but apparently not on the wild strains of *N. gruberi* and other genera. This further indicates that these pathogenic strains of *Naegleria* are physiologically different from *N. gruberi* and justifies the establishment of a separate species in the genus *Naegleria.*

V. Recommendations for Research

Findings of this study strongly indicate that the pathogenic strains of *Naegleria* are physiologically quite different from *N. gruberi* commonly encountered in examination of water and sewage effluent and soils, although morphologically they are indistinguishable. It becomes apparent that the wild strains of *N. gruberi* frequently present in these environments should not be linked with the occurrence of human brain infections. An analogy to this relationship is the presence of *Bacillus anthracis* and other nonpathogenic bacilli, such as *B. cereus* and *B. megatherium* in soils. Morphologically they resemble one another, but pathogenetically *B. anthracis* is quite different from the last-mentioned two.

The fact that the growth requirement of the pathogenic *Naegleria* is more suited to a parasitic (CPE) than to a free-living (feeding on bacteria) form of life suggests that some aquatic form or forms of life may serve as their hosts. In this connection the finding of *Hartmannella tahitiensis* as the cause of mass mortalities of the oyster *Crassostrea commercialis* in Tahiti as reported by Cheng (1970) is interesting. In examination of the photomicrographs shown in Cheng's report, we find that the ameba involved looks much more like a *Singhella* sp., since the cytoplasm is entirely homogenous and contains three to eight vacuoles.

Studies in search of possible hosts for the pathogenic *Naegleria* in the lakes and the estuary where cases of human meningoencephalitis have occurred, together with analysis of the water for amebas and other ecological factors, may shed light on the epidemiology of this "mysterious" disease.

The involvement of an indoor swimming pool in this disease is hard to understand. In addition to considering the possibility of the existence of carriers in whom brain invasion is precipitated by the washing of amebas into the upper nasal cavity during swimming or diving, the pool itself should also be studied. The pool walls, the floor, and the filter

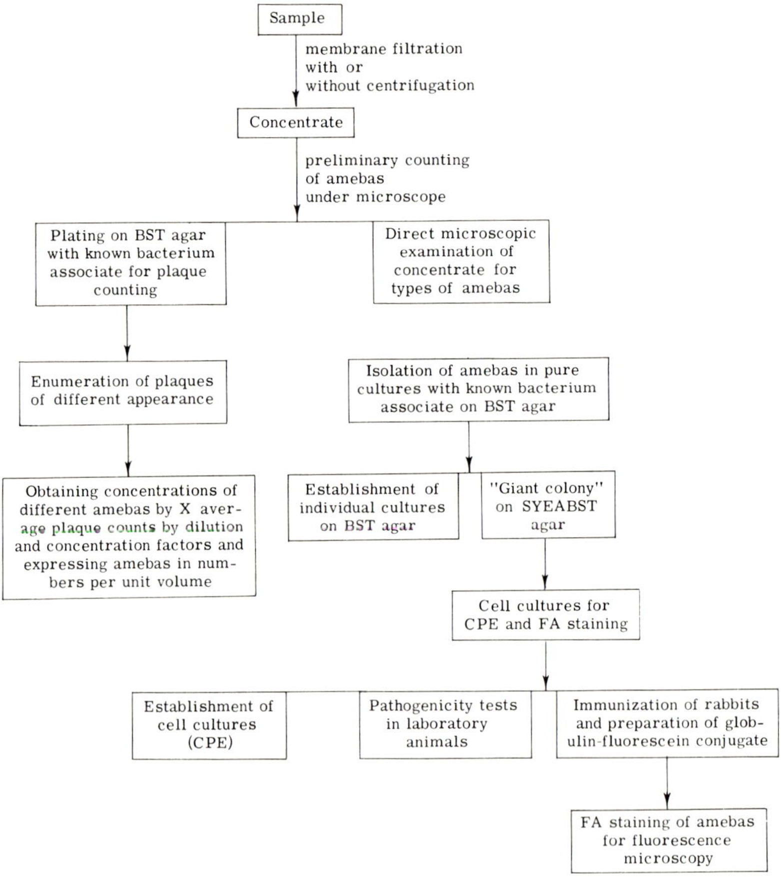

Fig. 13. Procedures for isolation, identification, and determination of pathogenicity of amebas.

should be examined for amebas, and amebic fauna should be analyzed for the presence of pathogenic *Naegleria*.

To facilitate such ecological studies, a scheme of procedure has been prepared in an outline form and is shown in Fig. 13. We hope that this scheme will be useful to those interested in such investigations.

ACKNOWLEDGMENT

The fluorescent antibody–staining work described in this chapter was performed by Dr. Chien Liu of the University of Kansas Medical Center, Lawrence, Kansas.

References

Adam, K. M. G. (1963). *In* "Progress in Protozoology" (J. Ludvik, J. Lom, and J. Vávra, eds.), p. 75. Academic Press, New York.

Appley, J., Clarke, S. K. R., Roome, A. P. C. H., Sandry, S. A., Saygi, G., Silk, B., and Warhurst, D.C. (1970). Primary amoebic meningoencephalitis in Britain. *Brit. Med. J.* **1**, 596–599.

Armstrong, J. A., and Pereira, M. (1967). Identification of "Ryan Virus" as an amoeba of the genus *Hartmannella. Brit. Med. J.* **1**, 212–214.

Berg, G., Harris, E. K., Chang, S. L., and Busch, K. A. (1963). Quantitation of viruses by the plaque technic. *J. Bacteriol.* **85**, 691–700.

Butt, C. G. (1966). Primary amoebic meningoencephalitis. *New Engl. J. Med.* **274**, 1473–1476.

Butt, C. G., Baro, C., and Knorr, R. W. (1968). *Naegleria*(sp) identified in amoebic encephalitis. *Amer. J. Clin. Pathol.* **50**, 568–574.

Callicott, J. H., Jr., Nelson, E. C., Jones, M. M., dos Santos, J. G., Utz, J. P., Duma, R. J., and Morrison, J. V., Jr. (1968). Meningocephalitis due to pathogenic free-living amoeba. *J. Amer. Med. Ass.* **206**, 579–582.

Carter, R. (1968). Primary amoebic meningo-encephalitis: Clinical, pathological and epidemiological features of six fatal cases. *J. Pathol. Bacteriol.* **96**, 1–25.

Černa, L. (1969). Amoebic meningo-encephalitis: A new isolate. *Science* **163**, 575–576.

Černa, L., and Novăk, K. (1968). Amoebic meningoencephalitis: Sixteen fatalities. *Science* **160**, 92.

Černa, L., Zimak, V., and Novăk, K. (1969). Amoebic meningoencephalitis: Axenic culture of Naegleria. *Science* **163**, 575.

Chang, R. S., Pan, I.-H., and Rosenau, B. J. (1966). On the "Lipovirus." *J. Exp. Med.* **124**, 1153–1166.

Chang, S. L. (1958a). Cultural, cytological and ecological observations on the amoeba stage of *Naegleria gruberi. J. Gen. Microbiol.* **18**, 565–578.

Chang, S. L. (1958b). Cytological and ecological observations on the flagellate transformation of *Naegleria gruberi. J. Gen. Microbiol.* **18**, 579–585.

Chang, S. L. (1960). Growth of small free-living amoebae in various bacterial and in bacteria-free cultures. *Can. J. Microbiol.* **6**, 397–405.

Chang, S. L., and Kabler, P. W. (1956). Detection of cysts of *E. histolytica* in tap water by the use of membrane filter. *Amer. J. Hyg.* **64**, 170–180.

Chang, S. L., and Negherbon, W. O. (1947). Studies on Haemoflagellates II. A study of the growth rates of Leishmania donovani, *L. brasiliansis, L. tropica*, and *Trypanosoma cruzi* in culture. *J. Infec. Dis.* **80**, 172–184.

Chang, S. L., Berg, G., Busch, K. A., Stevenson, R. E., Clarke, N. A., and Kabler, P. W. (1958). Application of the "most probable number" method for estimating concentrations of animal viruses by the tissue culture technique. *Virology* **6**, 27–42.

Chang, S. L., Berg, G., Clarke, N. A., and Kabler, P. W. (1960). Survival and protection against chlorination of human enteric pathogens in freeliving nematodes isolated from water supplies. *Amer. J. Trop. Med. Hyg.* **9**, 136–142.

Cheng, T. C. (1970). *Hartmannella tahitiensis* sp.n., an amoeba associated with mass mortalities of the oyster *Crassostrea commercialis* in Tahiti, French Polynesia. *J. Invertebr. Pathol.* **15**, 405–419.

Chi, L., Vogel, J. E., and Shilokov, A. (1959). Selective phagocytosis of nucleated erythrocytes by cytotoxic amoeba in cell cultures. *Science* **130,** 1763.

Culbertson, C. G. (1961). Pathogenic *acanthamoeba* (*Hartmannella*). *Amer. J. Clin. Pathol.* **35,** 195–202.

Culbertson, C. G., Smith, J. W., and Minner, J. R. (1958). *Acanthamoeba:* Observations on animal pathogenicity. *Science* **127,** 1506.

Culbertson, C. G., Smith, J. W., Cohen, H. K., and Minner, J. R. (1959). Experimental infection of mice and monkeys by *Acanthamoeba. Amer. J. Pathol.* **35,** 185–197.

Culbertson, C. G., Ensminger, P. W., and Overton, W. M. (1966). *Hartmennella* (*Acanthamoeba*): Experimental Chronic, granulomatous brain infections produced by new isolates of low virulence. *Amer. J. Clin. Pathol.* **46,** 305–314.

Culbertson, C. G., Ensminger, P. W., and Overton, W. M. (1968). Pathogenic *Naegleria* sp.—Study of a strain isolated from human cerebrospinal fluid. *J. Protozool.* **15,** 353–363.

Duma, R. J., Ferrell, H. W., Nelson, E. C., and Jones, M. M. (1969). Primary amebic meningoencephalitis. *New Engl. J. Med.* **281,** 1315–1323.

Fowler, M. C., and Carter, R. (1965). Acute pyogenic meningitis probably due to *Acanthamoeba* sp: A preliminary report. *Brit. J. Med.* **2,** 740–742.

Gurr, E. (1962). "Staining: Practical and Theoretical," 631 pp. Williams & Wilkins, Baltimore, Maryland.

Jahnes, W. G., Fullmer, H. M., and Li, C. P. (1957). Free-living amoeba as contaminants in monkey kidney tissue culture. *Proc. Soc. Exp. Biol. Med.* **96,** 484–488.

Little, J. B., and Chang, R. S. (1968). Effect of ionizing radiation on all division in an amoeboid cell. *Radiat. Res.* **35,** 132–146.

Liu, C., and Rodina, P. (1966). Immunofluorescent studies of human cell culture and chick embryos inoculated with the ameboid cell—"Lipovirus" Complex. *J. Exp. Med.* **124,** 1167–1178.

McCroan, J. E., and Patterson, J. (1970). Primary amoebic meningo-encephalitis. *Georgia Morbidity and Mortality Weekly Report* **19** (#42) 413–414.

Patras, D., and Andujar, J. J. (1966). Meningoencephalitis due to *Hartmannella* (*Acanthamoeba*). *Amer. J. Clin. Pathol.* **46,** 226–233.

Singh, B. N. (1952). Nuclear division in nine species of small freeliving amoebae and its bearing on the classification of the order amoebeda. *Phil. Trans. Roy. Soc. London, Ser. B* **236,** 405–461.

Symmers, W. St. C. (1969). Primary amoebic meningo-encephalitis in Britain. *Brit. Med. J.* **2,** 449–454.

Wang, S. S., and Feldman, H. A. (1961). Occurrence of acanthamoebae in tissue cultures inoculated with human pharyngeal swabs. *Antimicrob. Ag. Chemother.* **1,** 50–53.

Wang, S. S., and Feldman, H. A. (1967). Isolation of Hartmannella species from human throats. *New Engl. J. Med.* **277,** 1174–1179.

Warhurst, D. C., Roome, A. P. C. H., and Saygi, G. (1970). *Naegleria* sp. from human cerebrospinal fluid. *Trans. Roy. Soc. Trop. Med. Hyg.* **64,** 19–21.

Wenyon, C. M. (1926). "Protozoology," 2 Vols. Bailliere, London.

Author Index

Numbers in italics refer to the pages on which the complete references are listed.

C

N

T

U

Subject Index

G

H

N

T